Carotid Artery Stenosis

Current and Emerging Treatments

Carotid Artery Stenosis

Current and Emerging Treatments

edited by

Seemant Chaturvedi, M.D.
Wayne State University
Detroit, Michigan, U.S.A.

Peter M. Rothwell, M.D., Ph.D.
University of Oxford
Radcliffe Infirmary
Oxford, U.K.

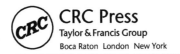

CRC Press
Taylor & Francis Group
Boca Raton   London   New York

CRC Press is an imprint of the
Taylor & Francis Group, an **informa** business
A TAYLOR & FRANCIS BOOK

CRC Press
Taylor & Francis Group
6000 Broken Sound Parkway NW, Suite 300
Boca Raton, FL 33487-2742

First issued in paperback 2019

ISBN-13: 978-0-8247-5417-4 (hbk)
ISBN-13: 978-0-367-39240-6 (pbk)

Library of Congress Cataloging-in-Publication Data

Catalog record is available from the Library of Congress

Visit the Taylor & Francis Web site at
http://www.taylorandfrancis.com

and the CRC Press Web site at
http://www.crcpress.com

We dedicate this book
to our families for their support over the years and
to our clinical teachers, particularly
Henry Barnett, Vladimir Hachinski, Robert Lisak, and Charles Warlow,
who stimulated and nurtured
our interest in carotid disease and stroke.

Preface

Carotid artery stenosis (CAS) is a major cause of ischemic stroke. Each year in the US and Europe alone, there are nearly two million strokes and CAS is estimated to account for up to 20% of these events. Carotid disease is also a leading cause of transient ischemic attacks or "mini-strokes", and is likely to be an increasingly important public health problem in both the developed and developing worlds as populations age.

For the last three decades, treatment of patients with CAS has involved medical therapy with antithrombotics, lipid-lowering and blood pressure-lowering drugs in most patients and surgical treatment with carotid endarterectomy (CEA) in some. However, in recent years medical treatments have improved and there has been increasing interest in carotid artery stenting as a possible alternative to conventional surgery. Several randomized trials of stenting are ongoing or have recently been completed and there have been advances in catheter design and distal protection devices. Surgical treatment is also changing with increased use of local anesthesia and new data on the risks and benefits of ancillary techniques, such as routine patching and synthetic grafts. Of equal importance, our understanding of which patients are most at risk of stroke without treatment and therefore have the most to gain from timely intervention is also advancing.

A multidisciplinary book, summarizing the latest evidence on optimal medical, surgical, and intravascular interventional treatment of CAS, as well as recent advances in our understanding of its epidemiology, pathology, and imaging, is therefore required. The goal of this book is to provide a "state-of-the-art" review of all of these areas, with particular emphasis on the latest evidence about treatment. We are therefore indebted to all of our co-authors and colleagues who have helped us to achieve this goal by providing comprehensive reviews of the "state of the art" in their particular clinical and research specialties.

We hope that this book will be of interest to all healthcare professionals who are involved in the management of patients with CAS, including neurologists, vascular surgeons, neurosurgeons, neuroradiologists, general interventional radiologists, and internists. Ultimately, we hope that patients will benefit from the application in routine clinical practice of the advances outlined in this book and that it will stimulate further research into the many questions that still remain unanswered.

Seemant Chaturvedi MD
Wayne State University,
Detroit, MI
Peter M. Rothwell MD PhD
Oxford University,
Oxford, UK

Contents

Contributors

Pierre Amarenco   Department of Neurology and Stroke Centre, Bichat, Claude Bernard University Hospital and Medical School, Denis Diderot University, Paris VII and Formation de Recherche en Neurologie Vasculaire (Association Claude Bernard), Paris, France

Brian H. Annex   Division of Cardiology, Department of Medicine, Duke University School of Medicine, Durham, North Carolina, U.S.A.

Mark K. Borsody   Stroke Program and Department of Neurology, Wayne State University, Detroit, Michigan, U.S.A.

Martin M. Brown   Institute of Neurology, University College London, London, U.K.

Seemant Chaturvedi   Department of Neurology, Detroit Medical Center, Wayne State University, Detroit, Michigan, U.S.A.

Robert Côté   Department of Neurology and Neurosurgery, McGill University, Montreal General Hospital, Montreal, Canada

Lucy Coward   Institute of Neurology, University College London, London, U.K.

Michael Daffertshofer   Department of Neurology, University of Heidelberg, Universitätsklinikum Mannheim, Germany

Graeme J. Hankey   Stroke Unit, Department of Neurology, Royal Perth Hospital and School of Medicine and Pharmacology, University of Western Australia, Perth, Australia

Michael G. Hennerici   Department of Neurology, University of Heidelberg, Universitätsklinikum Mannheim, Germany

Catalina C. Ionita   Cerebrovascular Program, Department of Neurology and Neurosciences, University of Medicine and Dentistry of New Jersey, Newark, New Jersey, U.S.A.

L. Jaap Kappelle   University Department of Neurology, University Medical Center Utrecht and Rudolf Magnus Institute of Neuroscience, Utrecht, The Netherlands

Jawad F. Kirmani   Cerebrovascular Program, Department of Neurology and Neurosciences, University of Medicine and Dentistry of New Jersey, Newark, New Jersey, U.S.A.

Catharina J. M. Klijn   University Department of Neurology, University Medical Center Utrecht and Rudolf Magnus Institute of Neuroscience, Utrecht, The Netherlands

Christopher D. Kontos   Division of Cardiology, Department of Medicine, Duke University School of Medicine, Durham, North Carolina, U.S.A.

Philippa Lavallée   Department of Neurology and Stroke Centre, Bichat, Claude Bernard University Hospital and Medical School, Denis Diderot University, Paris VII and Formation de Recherche en Neurologie Vasculaire (Association Claude Bernard), Paris, France

Hugh Markus   Clinical Neuroscience, St. George's Hospital Medical School, London, U.K.

Jeffrey Minuk   Department of Neurology and Neurosurgery, McGill University, Sir M.B. Davis-Jewish General Hospital, Montreal, Canada

A. Ross Naylor   The Department of Vascular Surgery, Leicester Royal Infirmary, Leicester, U.K.

David Pelz   Department of Diagnostic Radiology and Clinical Neurological Sciences, London Health Sciences Centre, University Campus, London, Ontario, Canada

L. Creed Pettigrew Stroke Program of the Sanders-Brown Center on Aging and the Department of Neurology, University of Kentucky College of Medicine, Lexington, Kentucky, U.S.A.

Adnan I. Qureshi Cerebrovascular Program, Department of Neurology and Neurosciences, University of Medicine and Dentistry of New Jersey, Newark, New Jersey, U.S.A.

Kumar Rajamani Department of Neurology, Wayne State University, Detroit, Michigan, U.S.A.

Peter M. Rothwell Stroke Prevention Research Unit, University Department of Neurology, University of Oxford, Radcliffe Infirmary, Oxford, U.K.

Houta S. Sabet Stroke Program of the Sanders-Brown Center on Aging and the Department of Neurology, University of Kentucky College of Medicine, Lexington, Kentucky, U.S.A.

J. David Spence Stroke Prevention and Atherosclerosis Research Centre, Robarts Research Institute, London, Ontario, Canada

Pierre-Jean Touboul Department of Neurology and Stroke Centre, Bichat, Claude Bernard University Hospital and Medical School, Denis Diderot University, Paris VII and Formation de Recherche en Neurologie Vasculaire (Association Claude Bernard), Paris, France

Andrew R. Xavier Cerebrovascular Program, Department of Neurology and Neurosciences, University of Medicine and Dentistry of New Jersey, Newark, New Jersey, U.S.A.

1

Introduction

Peter M. Rothwell

Stroke Prevention Research Unit, University Department of Neurology, University of Oxford, Radcliffe Infirmary, Oxford, U.K.

Seemant Chaturvedi

Department of Neurology, Detroit Medical Center, Wayne State University, Detroit, Michigan, U.S.A.

Somewhere between 15 and 20% of patients presenting with transient ischemic attack (TIA) or non-disabling ischemic stroke have a significant stenosis at or around the bifurcation of the ipsilateral carotid artery and about 5–10% of asymptomatic elderly individuals have significant stenosis of at least one carotid artery. The purpose of this book is to summarize current knowledge about the natural history and optimal treatment of patients with carotid disease and to consider future directions for research and therapy. However, it is appropriate to first briefly review how our current understanding and practice have developed. The recent history of the development of medical treatments for vascular disease is well known and so we have confined ourselves to a brief review of the history of our understanding of the role of carotid stenosis in causing TIA and stroke, and of the development of surgical and endovascular treatment.

1. PATHOPHYSIOLOGY

The knowledge of the relationship between atheromatous disease of the extracranial carotid and vertebral arteries and the occurrence of ischemic stroke goes back to the nineteenth century. In 1856, Virchow described carotid thrombosis in a patient with sudden onset ipsilateral visual loss in whom the ophthalmic and retinal arteries were patent (1). In 1888, Penzoldt reported a patient who had developed sudden permanent loss of vision in the right eye and later sustained a left hemiplegia (2). At post-mortem she was found to have had thrombotic occlusion of the right distal common carotid artery and a large area of cerebral softening in the right cerebral hemisphere. In 1905, Chiari performed a number of pathological studies which led him to suggest that emboli could break away from ulcerated carotid plaques in the neck and cause cerebral infarction(3,4). Clinical research on carotid disease was given a major boost by the development of cerebral arteriography by Egas Moniz in 1927 (5), and the subsequent demonstration of stenosis and occlusion of the carotid arteries in life (6,7).

The hypothesis that carotid disease was an important cause of ischemic stroke and that thromboembolism was the predominant mechanism was re-emphasized in the 1950s and 1960s by Miller Fisher (8,9). The work of Fisher and others prompted the development in the 1950s and 1960s of several operative techniques, the aim of which was to restore the flow of blood to the brain in patients with stenosis or occlusion of the extracranial carotid or vertebral circulations (10). The development of extracranial/intracranial (EC/IC) bypass surgery and carotid endarterectomy are described below. Several other surgical techniques have been tried, although unlike endarterectomy and EC/IC bypass, they have not been tested in randomized controlled trials. These include various bypass procedures for occlusion of the proximal neck and aortic arch vessels (11), vertebral artery endarterectomy, reconstruction or bypass (12), and various arterial transpositions involving anastomosis of the subclavian and vertebral arteries into the common carotid artery (13).

Patients with complete occlusion of the internal carotid artery are not suitable for carotid endarterectomy or angioplasty. Patients with symptomatic carotid occlusion have an annual risk of ipsilateral ischemic stroke of around 5% (14,15). Many of these strokes are likely to be caused by embolism from the occluded carotid artery, but there is evidence that cerebral hypoperfusion is also important (16,17). With developments in microsurgical techniques in the 1960s, it became possible to perform EC/IC bypass surgery in such patients in order to increase cerebral perfusion (18). The most commonly performed procedure involved anastomosis of branches of the superficial temporal artery to the middle cerebral artery. This operation became very popular for symptomatic carotid occlusion in the 1970s and early 1980s. As a consequence of this, a large randomized controlled trial was performed (19). Although EC/IC bypass does appear to be effective in increasing cerebral perfusion in some patients (20), the trial reported no reduction in the risk of stroke. Since the trial was reported in 1985, the use of EC/IC bypass surgery has declined dramatically. However, recent studies have suggested that it is possible to identify a subgroup of patients with carotid occlusion who have severe cerebral hypoperfusion and a particularly high risk of ipsilateral ischemic stroke (21,22). Further randomized trials are ongoing in this subgroup (23).

2. EARLY CAROTID SURGERY

Carotid endarterectomy was introduced in the 1950s and became popular in the 1970s and early 1980s, but it was not until 1991 that it was shown to be of value in patients with a recently symptomatic 70–99% carotid stenosis (24,25). However, the history of carotid artery surgery goes back much further. The first operations on the carotid artery were ligation procedures for trauma or hemorrhage. The first report was in Benjamin Bell's surgery in 1793 (26). However, most early ligations resulted in the death of the patient. The first successful ligation was performed by a British naval surgeon, David Fleming, in 1803 (27). This operation was performed for late carotid rupture following neck trauma in an attempted suicide. The first successful ligation for carotid aneurysm was performed five years later in London by Astley Cooper (28). By 1868, Pilz was able to collect 600 recorded cases of carotid ligation for cervical aneurysm or hemorrhage with an overall mortality of 43% (29). In 1878, an American surgeon named John Wyeth reported a 41% mortality in a collected study of 898 common carotid ligations, and contrasted this with a 4.5% mortality for ligation of the external carotid artery (30).

There were relatively few developments for the next 70 years. However, in 1946, a Portuguese surgeon, Cid Dos Santos, introduced thromboendarterectomy for the restoration of flow in peripheral vessels (31). The first successful reconstruction of the carotid artery was performed by Carrea et al., in Buenos Aires in 1951 (32). However, this was not an endarterectomy. Rather they performed an end-to-end anastomosis of the left external carotid artery and the distal internal carotid artery in a man of 41 with a recently symptomatic severe carotid stenosis.

3. CAROTID ENDARTERECTOMY

There is a debate about who performed the first true carotid endarterectomy. In 1954, Eastcott et al., published a case report detailing a carotid resection performed in May 1954 on a 66-year-old woman with recurrent left carotid TIAs and a severe stenosis on angiography (33). The patient made an uneventful recovery and was relieved of her TIAs. However, in 1975, DeBakey reported that he had performed a carotid endarterectomy on a 53-year-old man in August 1953 (34). However, it was the report by Eastcott et al., which provided the impetus for the further development of carotid surgery. Over the next five years there were numerous other reports of the operation being performed and several technical improvements were suggested. The operation became extremely popular in the 1960s and 1970s.

By the early 1980s there were over 100,000 procedures per year in the USA alone (35). However, at this point in time, there was no evidence from randomized controlled trials that the operation was of any value. This prompted several eminent clinicians to question the widespread use of the operation in the early 1980s (36–39) which led to a fall in the number of operations being done and set the scene for a number of large, randomized controlled trials.

There have been five randomized controlled trials of carotid endarterectomy for symptomatic carotid stenosis (24,25,40–42). The first two studies were relatively small and did not produce reliable results (40,41). The larger VA Cooperative Symptomatic Carotid Stenosis Trial (VA #309) reported a non-significant trend in favor of surgery (42), but was stopped in 1991 when the European Carotid Surgery Trial (ECST) and the North American Symptomatic Carotid Endarterectomy Trial (NASCET) demonstrated a clear reduction in the overall risk of stroke in operated patients with recently symptomatic severe (70–99%) carotid stenosis (24,25). The final report from the NASCET and a subsequent pooled analysis of individual patient data from all trials showed that endarterectomy was also of benefit in patients with recently symptomatic 50–69% stenosis (43,44). However, other research done in parallel has shown that the benefit also depends to a significant extent on other clinical characteristics (45–47).

4. CAROTID ANGIOPLASTY

Transluminal angioplasty was first used in the limbs in the 1960s (48), and then subsequently in the renal and coronary arteries. Angioplasty was introduced cautiously in the cerebral circulation because of fears of plaque rupture and embolism causing stroke. Angioplasty of stenoses of the proximal vertebral artery (49), the basilar artery (50), the distal internal carotid artery and proximal middle cerebral artery stenosis (51,52), were performed in the 1980s. During the past 10 years angioplasty and stenting at the carotid bifurcation has increased in popularity and is now under investigation as a potential alternative to endarterectomy. Thus far, there have been five small randomized controlled trials of angioplasty +/− stenting vs. endarterectomy (53–57). Taken together they suggest that angioplasty +/− stenting is associated with a similar procedural risk to endarterectomy but a possibly increased rate of restenosis. However, improvements in cerebral protection devices may reduce the procedural risks (58), and several further trials of angioplasty and stenting with cerebral protection vs. endarterectomy are ongoing.

5. INTERVENTION FOR ASYMPTOMATIC CAROTID STENOSIS

About 5–10% of the general population aged over 60 years have at least one asymptomatic carotid stenosis (59). However, the natural history of asymptomatic carotid stenosis was only reliably defined in large studies in the 1980s when carotid ultrasound became available. Several large studies showed that the prognosis was much more benign than that of recently symptomatic stenosis, with a risk of ipsilateral ischemic stroke of less than 2% per year in patients with severe asymptomatic stenosis (60,61). Despite inconclusive results from some small early randomized trials of endarterectomy for asymptomatic carotid stenosis vs. medical treatment alone (62–65), the number of operations done for asymptomatic stenosis in North America increased dramatically in the 1980s (35). In 1993, the VA trial demonstrated a significant reduction in the risk of the combined outcome of stroke and TIA in the endarterectomy group, but did not have the power to demonstrate a reduction in the risk of stroke alone (66). In 1995, the Asymptomatic Carotid Artery Study (ACAS) (67) demonstrated a clearly significant reduction in the risk of ipsilateral ischemic stroke in patients with 60–99% asymptomatic stenosis: a reduction in the five-year actuarial risk of ipsilateral ischemic stroke or operative death from 11 to 5.1% ($p < 0.001$). Unlike the ECST and NASCET trials, the ACAS trial included the risks of stroke and death due to carotid angiography in the overall outcome. However, the operative risk of stroke and death due to endarterectomy was much lower than in the randomized controlled trials of endarterectomy for symptomatic stenosis, an observation that was confirmed by analyses of case series from routine clinical practice (68). More recently, the much larger Asymptomatic Carotid Surgery Trial (ACST) showed a very similar absolute benefit to that in ACAS, despite a higher operative risk (69). Several questions remain, particularly about the benefit of surgery in specific subgroups, the potential for selection of patients on the basis of an increased risk of stroke without surgery, and the long-term benefits of surgery (70), but there is no doubt that endarterectomy for asymptomatic stenosis is of modest overall benefit. Whether it is a cost effective intervention and whether screening will do more good than harm are less certain (71).

6. CONCLUSIONS

Considerable progress was made during the last century in our understanding of the role of carotid stenosis in the etiology of stroke, and in the development of surgical and endovascular techniques to remove stenoses. The last two decades have seen the demonstration of the benefit of carotid endarterectomy over medical treatment alone for patients with symptomatic carotid stenosis and to a lesser extent in patients with asymptomatic stenosis. We will soon have reliable data on the relative effectiveness of carotid angioplasty and stenting, and progress is now being made in using risk models to determine which individual patients have the most to gain from these interventions. Future challenges include the determination of the role of new technologies, such as the detection of cerebral microemboli (72), in routine clinical practice and the determination of the effect of improvements in medical treatments on the need for surgical and endovascular interventions (73). The only certainty as we look to the future is the continuing need for high-quality clinical research.

REFERENCES

1. Gurdjian ES. History of occlusive cerebrovascular disease, I: from Wepfer to Moniz. Arch Neurol 1979; 36:340–343.
2. Penzoldt F. Uber thrombose (autochtone oder embolische) der carotis. Dtsch Arch f Klin Med 1891; 28:80–93.
3. Fields WS, Lemak NA. A History of Stroke. New York: Oxford University Press, 1989.
4. Chiari H. Uber des verhalten des teilungswinkels der carotis communis bei der endarteritis chronica deformans. Verh Dtsch Ges Pathol 1905; 9:326–330.
5. Moniz E. L'encephalographic arterielle: son importance dans la localisation des tumeurs cerebrales. Rev Neurol (Paris) 1927; 2:72–90.
6. Moniz E, Lima A, de Lacerda R. Hemiplegies par thrombose de la carotide interne. Presse Med 1937; 45:977–980.
7. Johnson HC, Walker AE. The angiographic diagnosis of spontaneous thrombosis of the internal and common carotid arteries. J Neurosurg 1951; 8:631–659.
8. Fisher M. Occlusion of the internal carotid artery. Arch Neurol Psychiatry 1951; 65:346–377.
9. Fisher M. Occlusion of the carotid arteries. Arch Neurol Psychiatry 1954; 72:187–204.
10. Thompson JE. The evolution of surgery for the treatment and prevention of stroke: the Willis Lecture. Stroke 1996; 27:1427–1434.
11. Thompson JE. Surgery for Cerebrovascular Insufficiency (Stroke). Springfield, Illinois: Charles C Thomas Publishing, 1968.
12. Berguer R. Advances in vertebral artery surgery. In: Veith FJ, ed. Current Critical Problems in Vascular Surgery. St Louis, MO: Quality Medical Publishing Inc., 1991:404–408.
13. Edwards WH Jr, Tapper SS, Edwards WH Sr, Mulherin JL Jr, Martin RS, Jenkins JM. Subclavian revascularisation: a quarter century experience. Ann Surg 1994; 219:673–678.
14. Hankey GJ, Warlow CP. Prognosis of symptomatic carotid artery occlusion. Cerebrovasc Dis 1991; 1:245–256.
15. Cote R, Barnett HJM, Taylor DW. Internal carotid occlusion: a prospective study. Stroke 1983; 14:898–901.
16. Bullock R, Mendelow AD, Bone I, Patterson J, MacLeod WN, Allardice G. Cerebral blood flow and CO_2 responsiveness as an indicator of collateral reserve capacity in patients with carotid artery disease. Br J Surg 1985; 72:348–351.

17. Norrving B, Nilsson B, Risberg J. rCBF in patients with carotid occlusion. Resting and hypercapnic flow related to collateral pattern. Stroke 1982; 13: 155–162.
18. Yasargil MG, Krayenbuhl HA, Jacobson JH. Microneurosurgical arterial reconstruction. Surgery 1970; 67:222–223.
19. EC/IC Bypass Study Group. Failure of extracranial-intracranial arterial bypass to reduce the risk of ischaemic stroke. N Engl J Med 1985; 313:1191–1200.
20. Powers WJ, Grubb RL, Raichle ME. Clinical results of extracranial-intracranial bypass surgery in patients with hemodynamic cerebrovascular disease. J Neurosurg 1989; 70:61–67.
21. Klijn CJM, Kappelle LJ, Tulleken CJF, van Gijn J. Symptomatic carotid artery occlusion: a reappraisal of haemodynamic factors. Stroke 1997; 28:2084–2093.
22. Grubb RL, Derdeyn CP, Fritsch SM, Carpenter DA, Yundt KD, Videen TO, Spitznagel EL, Powers WJ. Importance of haemodynamic factors in the prognosis of symptomatic carotid occlusion. JAMA 1998; 280:1055–1060.
23. Adams HP. Occlusion of the internal carotid artery: Reopening a closed door? JAMA 1998; 280:1093–1094.
24. European Carotid Surgery Trialists' Collaborative Group. MRC European Carotid Surgery Trial: interim results for symptomatic patients with severe (70–99%) or with mild (0–29%) carotid stenosis. Lancet 1991; 337:1235–1243.
25. North American Symptomatic Carotid Endarterectomy Trial Collaborators. Beneficial effect of carotid endarterectomy in symptomatic patients with high-grade carotid stenosis. N Engl J Med 1991; 325:445–453.
26. Wood JR. Early history of the operation of ligature of the primitive carotid artery. N Y J Med July 1857:1–59.
27. Keevil JJ. David Fleming and the operation for ligation of the carotid artery. Br J Surg 1949; 37:92–95.
28. Cooper A. Account of the first successful operation performed on the common carotid artery for aneurysm in the year 1808 with the post-mortem examination in the year 1821. Guy's Hosp Rep 1836; 1:53–59.
29. Hamby WB. Intracranial Aneurysms. Springfield, Illinois: Charles C, Thomas Publishing, 1952.
30. Wyeth JA. Prize essay: essays upon the surgical anatomy and history of the common, external and internal carotid arteries and the surgical anatomy of the innominate and subclavian arteries. Trans AMA (Appendix) [Philadelphia, Pa] 1878; 29:1–245.
31. Dos Santos JC. From embolectomy to endarterectomy or the fall of a myth. J Cardiovasc Surg 1976; 17:113–128.
32. Carrea R, Mollins M, Murphy G. Surgical treatment of spontaneous thrombosis of the internal carotid artery in the neck: carotid-carotideal anastomosis. Report of a case. Acta Neurol Latin Am 1955; 1:71–78.
33. Eastcott HHG, Pickering GW, Rob CG. Reconstruction of internal carotid artery in a patient with intermittent attacks of hemiplegia. Lancet 1954; 2: 994–996.
34. DeBakey ME. Successful carotid endarterectomy for cerebrovascular insufficiency. JAMA 1975; 233:1083–1085.

35. Gillum RF. Epidemiology of carotid endarterectomy and cerebral arteriography in the United States. Stroke 1995; 26:1724–1728.
36. Warlow CP. Carotid endarterectomy: Does it work? Stroke 1994; 15:964–967.
37. Chambers BR, Norris J. The case against surgery for asymptomatic carotid stenosis. Stroke 1984; 15:964–967.
38. Barnett HJM, Plum F, Walton JN. Carotid endarterectomy – an expression of concern. Stroke 1984; 15:941–943.
39. Jonas S. Can carotid endarterectomy be justified? No. Arch Neurol 1987; 44: 652–654.
40. Fields WS, Maslenikov V, Meyer JS, Hass WK, Remington RD, MacDonald M. Joint study of extracranial arterial occlusion. V Progress report on prognosis following surgery or non-surgical treatment for transient cerebral ischaemic attacks and cervical carotid artery lesions. JAMA 1970; 211:1993–2003.
41. Shaw DA, Venables GS, Cartilidge NEF, Bates D, Dickinson PH. Carotid endarterectomy in patients with transient cerebral ischaemia. J Neurol Sci 1984; 64:45–53.
42. Mayberg MR, Wilson SE, Yatsu F, Weiss DG, Messina L, Hershey LA, Colling C, Eskridge J, Deykin D, Winn HR. Carotid endarterectomy and prevention of cerebral ischaemia in symptomatic carotid stenosis. JAMA 1991; 266:3289–3294.
43. North American Symptomatic Carotid Endarterectomy Trialists' Collaborative Group. The final results of the NASCET trial. N Engl J Med 1998; 339: 1415–1425.
44. Rothwell PM, Gutnikov SA, Eliasziw M, Fox AJ, Taylor W, Mayberg MR, Warlow CP, Barnett HJM. (for the Carotid Endarterectomy Trialists' Collaboration). Pooled analysis of individual patient data from randomised controlled trials of endarterectomy for symptomatic carotid stenosis. Lancet 2003; 361:107–116.
45. Rothwell PM, Warlow CP. (on behalf of the European Carotid Surgery Trialists' Collaborative Group) Prediction of benefit from carotid endarterectomy in individual patients: a risk modeling study. Lancet 1999; 353:2105–2110.
46. Rothwell PM, Eliasziw M, Gutnikov SA, Warlow CP, Barnett HJM (for the Carotid Endarterectomy Trialists' Collaboration). Effect of endarterectomy for symptomatic carotid stenosis in relation to clinical subgroups and to the timing of surgery. Lancet 2004; 363:915–924.
47. Rothwell PM, Mehta Z, Howard SC, Gutnikov SA, Warlow CP. From subgroups to individuals: general principles and the example of carotid endartectomy. Lancet 2005; 365:256–265.
48. Dotter CT, Judkins MP. Transluminal treatment of arteriosclerotic obstruction. Description of a new technique and a preliminary report of its application. Circulation 1964; 30:654–670.
49. Schutz H, Yeung HP, Chiu MC, Terbrugge K, Ginsberg R. Dilatation of vertebral-artery stenosis. N Engl J Med 1981; 304:732.
50. Sundt TM Jr, Smith HC, Campbell JK, Vlietstra RE, Cucchiara RF, Stanson AW. Transluminal angioplasty for basilar artery stenosis. Mayo Clin Proc 1980; 55:673–680.

51. Clark WM, Barnwell SL, Nesbit G, O'Neill OR, Wynn ML, Coull BM. Safety and efficacy of percutaneous transluminal angioplasty for intracranial atherosclerotic stenosis. Stroke 1995; 26:1200–1204.
52. Marks MP, Marcellus M, Norbash AM, Steinberg GK, Tong D, Albers GW. Outcome of angioplasty for atherosclerotic intracranial stenosis. Stroke 1999; 30:1065–1069.
53. Endovascular versus surgical treatment in patients with carotid stenosis in the Carotid and Vertebral Artery Transluminal Angioplasty Study (CAVATAS investigators): a randomised trial. Lancet 2001; 357:1729–1737.
54. Naylor AR, Bolia A, Abbott RJ, Pye IF, Smith J, Lennard N, Lloyd AJ, London NJ, Bell PR. Randomised study of carotid angioplasty and stenting versus carotid endarterectomy: a stopped trial. J Vasc Surg 1998; 28:326–334.
55. Alberts MJ (for the Publications Committee of the WALLSTENT). Results of a multicantre prospective randomised trial of carotid artery stenting vs. carotid endarterectomy. Stroke 2001; 32:325.
56. Brooks WH, McClure RR, Jones MR, Coleman TL, Breathitt L. Carotid angioplasty and stenting versus carotid endarterectomy: randomized trial in a community hospital. J Am Coll Cardiol 2001; 38:1589–1595.
57. Yadav JS, Wholey MH, Kuntz RE, Fayad P, Katzen BT, Mishkel GJ, Bajwa TK, Whitlow P, Strickman NE, Jaff MR, Popma JJ, Snead DB, Cutlip DE, Firth BG, Ouriel K. Protected carotid-artery stenting versus endarterectomy in high-risk patients. N Engl J Med 2004; 351:1493–1501.
58. Reimers B, Corvaja N, Moshiri S, Sacca S, Albiero R, Di Mario C, Pascatto P, Colombo A. Cerebral protection with filter devices during carotid artery stenting. Circulation 2001; 104:12–15.
59. Jose MO, Touboul PJ, Mas JL, Laplane D, Bousser MG. Prevalence of asymptomatic internal carotid artery stenosis. Neuroepidemiology 1987; 6:150–152.
60. Hennerici M, Hulsbomer H-B, Hefter H, Lammerts D, Rautenberg W. Natural history of asymptomatic extracranial arterial disease. Results of a long-term prospective study. Brain 1987; 110:777–791.
61. Chambers BR, Norris JW. Outcome in patients with asymptomatic neck bruits. N Engl J Med 1986; 315:860–865.
62. Clagget GP, Youkey JR, Brigham RA, Orecchia PM, Salander JM, Collins GJ Jr, Rich NM. Asymptomatic cervical bruit and abnormal ocular pneumoplesmography: a prospective study comparing two approaches to management. Surgery 1984; 96:823–830.
63. Mayo Asymptomatic Carotid Endarterectomy Study Group. Effectiveness of carotid endarterectomy for asymptomatic carotid stenosis. Stroke 1989; 20;844–849.
64. The Casanova Study Group. Carotid surgery versus medical therapy in asymptomatic carotid stenosis. Stroke 1991; 22:1229–1235.
65. Lagneau P. Stenoses carotidiennes asymptomatiques. J Mal Vasc 1993; 18: 209–212.
66. Hobson RW 2nd, Weiss DG, Fields WS, Goldstone J, Moore WS, Towne JB, Wright CB. Efficacy of carotid endarterectomy for asymptomatic carotid stenosis. N Engl J Med 1993; 328:221–227.

67. Asymptomatic Carotid Atherosclerosis Study Group. Carotid endarterectomy for patients with asymptomatic internal carotid artery stenosis. JAMA 1995; 273:1421–1428.
68. Rothwell PM, Slattery J, Warlow CP. A systematic comparison of the risks of stroke and death due to carotid endarterectomy for symptomatic and asymptomatic stenosis. Stroke 1996; 27:266–269.
69. Halliday A, Mansfield A, Marro J, Peto C, Peto R, Potter J, Thomas D. Prevention of disabling and fatal strokes by successful carotid endarterectomy in patients without recent neurological symptoms: randomised controlled trial. Lancet 2004; 363:1491–1502.
70. Rothwell PM, Goldstein LB. Carotid endarterectomy for asymptomatic stenosis: Asymptomatic Carotid Surgery Trial. Stroke 2004; 35:2425–2427.
71. Whitty CJ, Sudlow CL, Warlow CP. Investigating individual subjects and screening populations for asymptomatic carotid stenosis can be harmful. J Neurol Neurosurg Psychiatry 1998; 64:619–623.
72. Malloy JE, Markus HS. Asymptomatic embolism predicts stroke and TIA risk in carotid artery stenosis. Stroke 1999; 30:1440–1443.
73. Chaturvedi S. Should the multicenter carotid endarterectomy trials be repeated? Arch Neurol 2003; 60:774–775.

2

Epidemiology of Carotid Artery Stenosis

Robert Côté

*Department of Neurology and Neurosurgery, McGill University,
Montreal General Hospital, Montreal, Canada*

Jeffrey Minuk

*Department of Neurology and Neurosurgery, McGill University,
Sir M.B. Davis-Jewish General Hospital, Montreal, Canada*

1. INTRODUCTION

Carotid artery stenosis (CAS) is most often the consequence of atherosclerosis which has a predilection for large and medium-sized systemic arteries and can lead to infarction of different organs including the heart and the brain. Through its diverse clinical manifestations, atherosclerosis is a leading cause of disability and mortality (1,2) despite lifestyle modifications and new pharmacological interventions (3). Atherosclerotic disease of the extracranial and intracranial carotid arteries is responsible for a substantial proportion of all strokes (4,5), and stenotic lesions in particular account for approximately 15–20% of all ischemic strokes (4–8), which remain a major cause of morbidity and mortality. Furthermore, in population studies (9), the presence of carotid stenosis detected by ultrasound is a strong predictor of mortality in itself.

The atherostenotic process occurs at preferential sites in the carotid circulation which includes the extracranial carotid bifurcation, most often within the first 2 cm from the origin of the internal carotid and less often the intracranial portion in the siphon and at the origin of the middle and anterior cerebral arteries (10). This distribution however has been shown to vary according to race, with an increased prevalence of intracranial arterial disease in Oriental and Black populations (11–13). This phenomenon is reflected in the higher incidence rate of small vessel ischemic strokes reported among Blacks compared with that in the White population (14). The detection of carotid stenosis by clinical examination is possible through the identification of a cervical bruit; however, this physical finding lacks adequate accuracy and reliability (15,16). Methods of imaging the carotid arteries vary and include noninvasive measures such as high resolution Doppler ultrasonography, magnetic resonance angiography, and spiral CT technology, all of which have been shown to possess reasonable sensitivity and specificity as well as concordance when compared to conventional cerebral angiography (17–20). However, despite advances in the technology of carotid artery imaging, there remain several methodological issues to be addressed especially with regard to the optimal method to visualize and measure carotid stenosis (21).

2. RISK FACTORS

Several risk factors have been associated with carotid atherosclerotic disease and in particular with stenotic lesions (see Table 1). In population studies, age and male sex are among the strongest and most consistent risk factors for carotid stenosis (22–27) with the risk of higher grade stenosis being twice as frequent in men compared to women (23) although in older age, the sex difference appears to attenuate (26,27). Among the modifiable risk factors, systolic hypertension in particular has been found to be closely associated with the severity of carotid atherosclerosis in several population studies

Table 1   Conditions Associated with Carotid Artery Stenosis

Risk factors
Age (22–27)
Male sex (22–27)
Hypertension (22–24,28)
Cigarette smoking (29–31)
Diabetes mellitus (32)
Hypercholesterolemia (33)
Lifestyle patterns (physical inactivity, diet...) (34)
Genetic influences (31,35–37)
Biological markers
Homocysteine (44,45)
Fibrinogen (41,42)
Prothrombin fragments 1.2 (46)
C-reactive protein (38)
Adhesion molecules (38)

from Europe, North America, and Asia (22–24,28). In the recent study by Su et al. (28), hypertensive patients when compared to normotensives had an odds ratio of 4.8 for the development of a carotid stenosis ($\geq 50\%$). Cigarette smoking has also been associated with an increased risk of vascular disease and more specifically carotid stenosis (29–31). The Cardiovascular Health Study (29), a community-based study of older adults, reported prevalences of clinically significant carotid stenosis ($\geq 50\%$) of 4.4% in never-smokers, 7.3% in former smokers, and 9.5% in current smokers ($p < 0.0001$). In a previous report, Whisnant et al. (30) reported in a hospital-based study that the duration of cigarette smoking was the strongest independent predictor of severe carotid atherosclerosis when compared to other risk factors such as age, hypertension, and male sex. Recent evidence also suggests a potential gene–environment interaction in smokers for the development of early carotid atherosclerosis through the promotion of endotoxin receptors (31). The presence of diabetes mellitus, particularly type 2, increases the risk of atherosclerosis and its complications including carotid occlusive disease (32). Some studies (26,33) have also found cholesterol to be closely associated with severity of carotid stenosis. In particular, the Framingham Study (33) reported on the increased risk of moderate carotid stenosis ($\geq 25\%$) according to the presence of certain risk factors such as hypertension, cigarette smoking, and cholesterol. They utilized a different approach for risk analysis, which included time-integrated measurements of risk factors using mean levels of these factors collected from examinations over the previous 34 years. This long-term approach was found to better reflect the individuals' past exposure to these risk factors rather than a single contemporaneous measurement. Specifically, the authors reported that the association between these risk factors and the degree of carotid stenosis was more consistent if the time-integrated approach was used rather than a single measurement; this was especially true for total cholesterol and hypertension. For example, in men, the odds ratio for carotid stenosis associated with an increase of 20 mmHg in systolic blood pressure was 2.11 (95% CI, 1.51–2.97) with the time-integrated analysis but only 1.12 and non-significant with the single current measurement approach. Also, the odds ratio for carotid stenosis for an increase of 0.26 mmol in total cholesterol was 1.10, significant for the time-integrated analysis but non-significant if current cholesterol levels only were used. Unfavorable lifestyle patterns have been previously related to cardiovascular disease and premature death. In a recent report, Luedemann et al. (34) have shown an increased risk of severe asymptomatic carotid atherosclerosis in individuals with an unfavorable lifestyle pattern which included physical inactivity and less than optimal dietary patterns. The interaction in this study between smoking status and lifestyle factors was interesting in that any beneficial effects of a favorable lifestyle were outweighed by the smoking status for both current and ex-smokers. In addition to the association of traditional risk factors with carotid artery stenosis, recent evidence suggests a substantial genetic influence at least for the expression of subclinical atherosclerosis as reflected by studies evaluating the carotid intima-media thickness (IMT) or the presence of carotid plaques (35–37). In particular, the San Antonio Family Heart Study (35) reported a substantive genetic influence on the formation of focal carotid artery plaque which is believed to represent a more advanced stage of atherosclerosis compared to the intima-media thickness.

Recently there has also been a growing interest in the diagnostic and prognostic potential of biological markers of inflammation and thrombosis such as homocysteine, fibrinogen, prothrombin fragments, C-reactive protein, and adhesion molecules and their positive association with the presence and severity of atherosclerotic carotid disease (38–46). In this regard the Framingham Study (44) reported an odds ratio for carotid stenosis ($\geq 25\%$) of 2.0 for individuals with the highest plasma homocysteine levels when compared to those with lower levels. Similar odds ratios for the presence of moderate-to-severe carotid plaques have also been reported with higher levels of C-reactive protein and soluble intercellular adhesion molecule-1 (ICAM-1) in the Rotterdam Study (38), although others could not confirm a clear association between soluble levels of adhesion molecules such as ICAM-1 and vascular cell adhesion molecule-1 (VCAM-1), and symptomatic carotid disease (47). In addition, prothrombin fragment 1.2, a marker of thrombin upregulation, has been associated (OR, 2.04; 95% CI, 1.10–3.78) with the presence of carotid stenosis ($\geq 50\%$) in selected groups of patients including asymptomatic individuals (46).

Finally, the presence of carotid atherosclerotic disease including plaques and stenosis is strongly correlated to incident ischemic heart disease and coronary disease as well as to peripheral vascular disease in selected groups and in population studies (48–50). The prevalence of clinically significant carotid stenosis ($\geq 50\%$) has been recently reported to vary between 14 and 33% in different high risk groups investigated for either coronary insufficiency or peripheral vascular disease (51,52). These observations reflect the systemic nature of the atherosclerotic involvement which accompanies carotid stenosis.

3. ASYMPTOMATIC CAROTID ARTERY STENOSIS

In general population studies, the prevalence of carotid artery plaque has been reported to vary from 13 to above 30% and to increase with age, reaching more than 80% in the elderly population (23,25,26,53). On the other hand, clinically significant asymptomatic extracranial carotid stenosis most often defined as 50% or greater is less prevalent, ranging from 1.5 to 9% (22–24,54–57) but with a higher reported prevalence of 28% in elderly men in their late seventies, as recently documented in a Swedish study (53). In North America, both the Cardiovascular Health Study and the

Framingham cohort reported prevalence rates for ≥50% carotid stenosis in the population above 65 years old of between 5 and 7% in women and between 7 and 9% in men (24,57).

Although the presence of carotid stenosis increases threefold the risk of stroke in population studies (58), the level of risk remains relatively low in absolute terms with a range between < 1 and 1.5% annually (54,59–61). In particular, the Cardiovascular Health Study reported in more than 5000 elderly individuals an ipsilateral stroke rate of 5% at 5 years distal to a > 70% asymptomatic carotid stenosis documented by cervical ultrasound (59). In comparison, higher risk groups with prevalent cardiovascular disease present a higher risk of stroke with associated asymptomatic carotid stenosis which varies between 2.5 and 3.4% per annum (62–66); this is comparable to the reported prognosis of medically treated patients enrolled in carotid endarterectomy trials for asymptomatic carotid disease (67,68) or long-term observation of stroke risk in the territory of an asymptomatic carotid stenosis in symptomatic carotid endarterectomy trials (69,70). Clearly, however, the degree of stenosis in addition to the type of population studied will have a major influence on stroke risk with an increase in annual risk which can reach between 4.2 and 8.8% in patients with a higher degree of stenosis in the range of 80% or more (62,66,71). In some studies, an increase in the mortality rate mostly due to co-existing cardiovascular disease could explain lower stroke rates in individuals with a similar degree of carotid stenosis (72,73). Of some importance as well is the presumed cause of the ischemic stroke which occurs distally to an asymptomatic carotid stenosis; recent data from the North American Symptomatic Carotid Endarterectomy Trial (NASCET) suggest that more than 45% of ischemic strokes which occur in patients with substantial asymptomatic carotid stenosis (60–99%) are attributable to either lacunes or a cardioembolic source (69,74). In addition, recent data also suggest a low stroke risk distally to a nearly occluded (95–99%) or occluded but never symptomatic carotid artery; this is probably due at least in part to a compensatory cerebral hemodynamic state in these individuals, which possibly reflects an adequate intracerebral collateral circulation (69,75).

Several natural history studies (62,66,73,76,77) have reported that disease progression is closely associated with cerebral ischemic events including stroke. In the prospective study by Mackey et al. (66), 639 patients followed for an average of 3.6 years had at least two separate ultrasound evaluations and thus were available for assessment of carotid disease progression. In particular, those patients who progressed to a degree of stenosis of ≥ 80% had a sixfold risk ($p < 0.0001$) of a vascular event compared to patients who did not progress to that level. In addition, the presence of certain risk factors (including degree of stenosis (≥ 50%), age, presence of coronary disease, hypertension, and peripheral vascular disease) was associated with an increased risk of ischemic vascular events including stroke and transient ischemic attacks (TIAs).

The presence of asymptomatic carotid stenosis in patients considered for elective surgery and in particular coronary artery bypass grafting (CABG) represents a problematic and high-risk clinical situation. Even though the overall risk of perioperative stroke in CABG surgery is low (2%), it clearly is higher for individuals with severe extracranial carotid stenosis or occlusion (78–80) with rates close to 8% in the case of a completely occluded carotid artery (79). Conversely, other reports could not confirm this level of risk with a comparable degree of asymptomatic carotid disease in the context of elective vascular surgery (81,82).

Some controversy still persists with regard to the screening and monitoring of occlusive carotid disease (83–87). Some have advocated screening of selected groups with a potentially higher prevalence for carotid stenosis, such as individuals with cervical bruits or elderly hypertensives, or in patients evaluated for cardiac or peripheral arterial surgery (84,87). However, the benefit of this approach has never been documented, and furthermore, others believe that based on the available evidence with regard to the prevalence of severe asymptomatic carotid stenosis and the limited impact of carotid endarterectomy in this context, it would be difficult to justify such recommendations which would probably not only be non-cost-effective (85) but also be potentially harmful in certain cases (86). Furthermore, although some authorities have suggested repeating carotid ultrasound evaluations at regular intervals (6–12 months) in patients with known asymptomatic occlusive carotid disease of a moderate or severe degree, others were unable to document a strong predictive potential for repeat ultrasonography in the prediction of clinical events of interest essentially because of both low clinical event rates and slow progression of arterial disease (83).

4. SYMPTOMATIC CAROTID ARTERY STENOSIS

Although much is known about the incidence and prevalence of transient ischemic attacks, ischemic stroke, and asymptomatic carotid artery disease, relatively little is known about the actual incidence and prevalence of symptomatic carotid artery disease. This is primarily due to the difficulty in ascribing with certainty causation between both the presence and the degree of carotid stenosis and clinical symptoms. Epidemiological studies on ischemic stroke subtypes do offer some information regarding the incidence of stroke associated with carotid artery stenosis. In one population of primarily white Americans (6), the overall incidence of ischemic stroke associated with a carotid artery stenosis of > 50% was 27 per 100,000. Incidence rates were 3–4-fold higher in white men than in white women. Although the overall age- and sex-adjusted ischemic stroke incidence is higher in black Americans compared with non-blacks, the incidence of stroke in the association with a carotid artery stenosis of >50% is lower amongst black Americans compared with non-blacks (17/100,000 vs. 27/ 100,000) (14).

Some stroke databases have examined the frequency of either moderate-to-high grade carotid stenosis or carotid occlusion in subjects with various stroke subtypes. In the Oxford Community Stroke Project (88), approximately 40% of those presenting with either total or partial anterior circulation infarctions had an appropriate carotid stenosis >50% or a carotid occlusion. Conversely, in the Lausanne Stroke Registry (4), approximately 13% of patients with a hemispheric stroke had an ipsilateral carotid stenosis of >50%. In a recent pooled analysis of randomized controlled trials of endarterectomy for symptomatic carotid stenosis ($n = 6092$), 25% of those with either a TIA or an ischemic stroke had a carotid stenosis between 50 and 69%, while 21% had a stenosis >70% (89).

In the Northern Manhattan Stroke Study (8), approximately 10% of patients had strokes attributed to extracranial atherosclerotic disease. This matches results seen in the National Institute of Neurological Disorders and Stroke–Stroke Data Bank (90) in which 9% of patients had a stroke occurring in the setting of severe carotid stenosis (>80%). The Yonsei Stroke Registry (91) found that 16.5% of strokes were attributable to large artery atherothrombosis in an Asian population.

4.1. Modes of Clinical Presentation

The mechanisms by which carotid artery stenosis produces clinical symptoms include distal embolization (atheroembolism), hypoperfusion, or distal propagation of carotid artery thrombus. Regardless of the precise mechanism, TIAs and acute ischemic stroke (AIS) are the typical clinical manifestations of symptomatic carotid artery disease.

4.1.1. Transient Ischemic Attacks

Transient ischemic attacks are defined as a temporary focal neurological deficit of presumed ischemic origin lasting < 24 h (92). Most TIAs, however, last <15 minutes (92). The branch of the internal carotid artery affected determines the specific symptoms of TIA.

Transient monocular blindness (TMB), also known as amaurosis fugax, accounts for approximately 24% of TIAs occurring in the carotid artery territory (93). Patients may describe the classical descending curtain-like effect though most simply describe the visual obscuration as a fog or darkening (92). Symptoms typically last <5 minutes (92). Hollenhorst described the presence of cholesterol crystals ("Hollenhorst plaques") in the retinal circulation of patients with cerebrovascular disease, but most subjects with TMB do not have such crystals (94). Other authors have documented with ophthalmoscopy, a variety of materials in the retinal circulation during episodes of TMB (95,96).

Hemispheric TIAs or transient hemispheric attacks (THAs) account for approximately 75% of carotid territory TIAs and 60% of all TIAs (93). Like TMB, THAs typically have durations of <15 minutes (92). The usual symptoms include aphasia or dysphasia, hemiparesis, or hemisensory impairment either in isolation or in combination, restricted to one side of the body. Very rarely, limb shaking can occur as a manifestation of a THA (97). Such THAs typically occur in the setting of very high-grade carotid stenosis (98).

The correlation with severe carotid artery stenosis appears greatest in those patients who have experienced separate episodes of both TMB and THA in the same vascular territory compared to those who have experienced one type of TIA only (92).

4.1.2. Crescendo TIAs

This term refers to the occurrence of multiple TIAs over the period of several days or hours that may be increasing in their duration and severity. Many consider such TIAs to be a sign of impending cerebral infarction (99,100). Crescendo TIAs are very often associated with ipsilateral high-grade carotid stenosis (99,100).

4.1.3. Ischemic Stroke

A variety of stroke subtypes both in the ocular and in the hemispheric circulations can occur as manifestations of symptomatic carotid artery stenosis. Ocular infarctions include branch retinal artery occlusions, central retinal artery occlusions, and ischemic optic neuropathy.

Hemispheric infarctions in the setting of carotid artery stenosis can occur within major large vessel territories (anterior and middle cerebral arteries), within branches of the major large vessels, within the deep perforating vessel branches, or within "watershed" or "border-zone" territories (vascular territories at the borders of the anterior and middle cerebral arteries, the middle and posterior cerebral arteries, or at the level of the lenticulostriate perforating arteries).

In the medically treated arm of the North American Symptomatic Carotid Endarterectomy Trial (NASCET), about 78% of recurrent strokes in those with carotid stenosis between 70 and 99% involved major large vessels of the circle of Willis during a 5-year follow-up while only 15% of recurrent strokes occurred in the territory of perforating vessels (74). The risk of recurrent stroke in a large vessel territory increased as the degree of symptomatic carotid stenosis increased (101). Border-zone type infarctions appear to be more common in those with stenosis > 90% rather than lesser degrees of stenosis (102). Some authors consider subcortical or lacunar infarctions to be related directly to high-grade internal carotid artery stenosis (103), while others consider the association coincidental (104).

Clinical manifestations of AIS include, either in isolation or in various combinations, aphasia or dysphasia, hemiparesis, hemisensory impairment, and hemianopsia. Certain clinical characteristics may be useful in differentiating ischemic stroke due to carotid artery stenosis from that due to cardioembolism. The presence of fractional arm weakness (proximal arm weakness different from hand weakness) may suggest stroke due to carotid artery disease whereas an impaired level of consciousness and dysphasic syndromes suggest cardioembolism (90).

4.2. Overall Natural History of Symptomatic Carotid Artery Stenosis

Considerable information regarding the natural history of symptomatic carotid artery stenosis has been gathered from the medically treated (control) arms from several large randomized controlled trials of carotid endarterectomy in symptomatic individuals (101,105,106). In general, the risk of recurrent ischemic events correlates positively with the degree of carotid stenosis as measured at the time of initial presentation (101).

According to the NASCET study (105), the 2-year rate of any ipsilateral stroke in medically treated patients with 70–99% carotid artery stenosis was 26%, and the 2-year and 5-year rates of ipsilateral stroke for more moderate symptomatic stenosis (50–69%) were 14.6 and 22%, respectively. For carotid stenosis of < 50%, the 5-year risk of ipsilateral stroke was close to 19%. Approximately 2.4% of patients with carotid stenosis between 70 and 99% died of cardiac related disease at 2 years and approximately 9% of patients with stenosis between 50 and 69% died of cardiac related disease at 5 years. In the European Carotid Surgery Trial (ECST) (101), the 3-year risk of ipsilateral major stroke in medically treated patients with carotid stenosis between 80 and 99% was approximately 21%. In the smaller Veterans Affairs Cooperative Trial for Symptomatic Carotid Stenosis (106), 20% of medically treated patients with symptomatic high-grade carotid stenosis (50–99%) experienced recurrent stroke or TIA over an approximate 12 month follow-up period.

4.3. Factors Influencing the Natural History of Symptomatic Carotid Stenosis

4.3.1. Near Occlusion of the Carotid Artery

Near occlusion refers to a very severe degree of stenosis, usually in the range of 95–99%. The near occluded artery usually demonstrates a "string sign" on conventional angiography (107). Although the annual risk of ipsilateral stroke increased with the degree of symptomatic stenosis, this annual risk drops in those with near occlusion and approaches the annual risk seen in those with 50–59% stenosis (89,108). Expanded collateral circulation and reduced intraluminal diameter with reduced perfusion pressure (which may reduce the risk of atheroembolism) are postulated to explain this somewhat more benign prognosis with near occlusion.

4.3.2. Hemispheric vs. Retinal Ischemic Events

In general, retinal ischemic events or TMB carry a more favorable prognosis with respect to recurrent stroke than do THAs (109,110). The 3-year risk of ipsilateral stroke for patients presenting with TMB is approximately half that for patients who have experienced a THA. This improved outlook for TMB is not enjoyed, however, by patients who have three or more of the risk factors among the following: age >75 years, male sex, a previous THA or stroke, carotid stenosis between 80 and 94%, a history of intermittent claudication, or absent collateral circulation on angiography (111).

4.3.3. Symptomatic Carotid Occlusion

The annual rate of recurrent stroke in patients with symptomatic carotid artery occlusion has been reported to vary between 0 and 20% (112). The combined annual incidence of stroke and TIA from 20 studies is 5.5% while the annual incidence of stroke ipsilateral to the carotid occlusion is 2.1% (112). The annual risk of stroke may be higher in those who continue to experience ongoing symptoms after symptomatic carotid occlusion (113).

Hemodynamic failure as defined by an increased oxygen extraction fraction on positron emission tomography (PET) scanning appears to identify a subgroup of patients with carotid occlusion at an even higher risk of recurrent stroke (114). In a cohort of 81 patients with an average follow-up of 31 months, those demonstrating hemodynamic failure on PET had ipsilateral stroke rates 5–6-fold higher than those without hemodynamic failure (115).

4.3.4. Miscellaneous Factors

Factors known to influence the natural history of symptomatic internal carotid artery stenosis are listed in Table 2.

Because of its poor long-term outcome, symptomatic bilateral carotid occlusion, although relatively uncommon, deserves mention. Wade et al. (122) reported the outcome of 34 conservatively treated subjects with symptomatic bilateral carotid occlusions after a mean follow-up of 42 months. Of these, 53% had suffered a recurrent cerebrovascular event (TIA or AIS) during follow-up with an annual stroke rate of 13% per patient year. In another cohort of 21 patients with symptomatic bilateral carotid occlusion (123), medically treated patients ($n = 8$) had a mortality rate of 75% during a mean follow up period of 6 years. However, one study, a meta-analysis of the outcome of patients with symptomatic occlusion of either the internal carotid artery or an intracranial artery (117), commented on the

Table 2 Factors Associated with the Risk of Stroke in the Setting of Symptomatic Carotid Stenosis

Factors Associated with Increased Risk of Stroke	Factors Associated with a Lower Risk of Stroke
Hemispheric transient ischemic attacks (109,110)	Retinal transient ischemic attacks (109,110)
Presence of leukoaraiosis on neuroimaging (116)	Near occlusion of the symptomatic artery (108)
Presence of intracranial artery stenosis on angiography (117,118)	Presence of collateral circulation on angiography (121)
Contralateral carotid occlusion (119)	
Presence of plaque ulceration (120)	

"protective effect" of bilateral carotid occlusion relative to unilateral carotid occlusion or intracranial arterial occlusion.

5. CONCLUSIONS

The importance of carotid artery stenosis stems not only from its role as a cause of ischemic stroke but also from its being a vascular condition which is amenable to several therapeutic interventions from either a medical or an interventional perspective. One of the greatest challenges has been to more precisely define higher risk profiles for individuals with different degrees of carotid occlusive disease beyond the presence of traditional vascular risk factors. Some answers, however, might be forthcoming through the application of newer approaches which might identify unstable atherosclerotic plaques, such as computer-assisted image analysis (124) and specific magnetic resonance imaging techniques (125), ultrasonographic measurement of carotid plaque area (126), and assessment of cerebrovascular reactivity and detection of microembolisms based on transcranial Doppler ultrasonography in individuals with high-grade carotid stenosis or occlusion (127–129). In addition, recent studies have reported an association between high levels of certain markers of inflammation such as C-reactive protein and progression of arterial disease including the carotid arteries (130). These different approaches provide opportunities to better identify potentially higher risk individuals with carotid occlusive disease and permit to better justify and apply diverse therapeutic interventions.

REFERENCES

1. Braunwald E. Shattuck lecture – Cardiovascular medicine at the turn of the millennium: triumphs, concerns, and opportunities. N Engl J Med 1997; 337: 1360–1369.

2. Beaglehole R. Global cardiovascular disease prevention: time to get serious. Lancet 2001; 358:661–663.
3. Yusuf S. Two decades of progress in preventing vascular disease. Lancet 2002; 360:2–3.
4. Bogousslavsky J, Van Melle G, Regli F. (for the Lausanne Stroke Registry Group). The Lausanne Stroke Registry: Analysis of 1,000 Consecutive Patients With First Stroke 1988; 19:1083–1092.
5. Wolf PA, D'Agostino RB. Epidemiology of stroke. In: Barnett HJM, Mohr JP, Stein BM, Yatsu FM, eds. Stroke Pathophysiology, Diagnosis, and Management. Philadelphia: Churchill Livingstone, 1986:3–28.
6. Petty GW, Brown RD, Whisnant JP, Sicks JD, O'Fallon WM, Wiebers DO. Ischemic stroke subtypes. A population-based study of incidence and risk factors. Stroke 1999; 30:2513–2516.
7. Sacco RL. Extracranial carotid stenosis. N Engl J Med 2001; 345:1113–1118.
8. Sacco RL. Ischemic stroke. In: Gorelick PB, Alter M, eds. Handbook of Neuroepidemiology. New York: Marcel Dekker Inc, 1994:77–121.
9. Joakimsen O, Bonna KH, Mathiesen EB, Stensland-Bugge E, Arnesen E. Prediction of mortality by ultrasound screening of a general population for carotid stenosis. The Tromso Study. Stroke 2000; 31:1871–1876.
10. Mohr JP, Gautier JC, Pessin MS. Internal carotid artery disease. In: Barnett HJM, Mohr JP, Stein BM, Yatsu FM, eds. Stroke Pathophysiology, Diagnosis, and Management. Philadelphia: Churchill Livingstone, 1998:355–400.
11. Fisher M. Atherosclerosis. In: Caplan LR, ed. Brain Ischemia: Basic Concepts and Clinical Relevance. New York: Springer-Verlag, 1995:135–149.
12. Inzitari D, Hachinski VC, Taylor W, Barnett HJM. Racial differences in the anterior circulation in cerebrovascular disease. How much can be explained by risk factors? Arch Neurol 1990; 47:1080–1084.
13. Wityk RJ, Lehman D, Klag M, Coresh J, Ahn H, Litt B. Race and sex differences in the distribution of cerebral atherosclerosis. Stroke 1996; 27: 1974–1980.
14. Woo D, Gebel J, Miller R, Kothari R, Brott T, Khoury J, Salisbury S, Skukla R, Pancioli A, Jauch E, Broderick J. Incidence rates of first-ever ischemic stroke subtypes among blacks. A population-based study. Stroke 1999; 30:2517–2522.
15. Sauve JS, Laupacis A, Ostbye T, Feagan B, Sackett DL. Does this patient have a clinical important carotid bruit? JAMA 1993; 270:2843–2845.
16. Ingall TJ, Homer D, Whisnant JP, Baker HL, O'Fallon WM. Predictive value of carotid bruit for carotid atherosclerosis. Arch Neurol 1989; 46:418–422.
17. Wityk RJ, Beauchamp NJ. Diagnostic evaluation of stroke. In: Morgenstern LG, ed. Neurologic Clinics. Philadelphia: W.B. Saunders Company, 2000: 357–378.
18. Johnston DCC, Goldstein LB. Clinical carotid endarterectomy decision making. Noninvasive vascular imaging versus angiography. Neurology 2001; 56:1009–1015.
19. Nederkoorn PJ, van der Graff Y, Hunink M. Duplex ultrasound and magnetic resonance angiography compared with digital subtraction angiography in carotid artery stenosis. Stroke 2003; 34:1324–1332.

20. Schwartz SW, Chambless LE, Baker WH, Broderick JP. (for the Asymptomatic Carotid Atherosclerosis Study Investigators). Consistency of doppler parameters in predicting arteriographically confirmed carotid stenosis. Stroke 1997; 28:343–347.

21. Rothwell PM, Pendlebury ST, Wardlaw J, Warlow CP. Critical appraisal of the design and reporting of studies of imaging and measurement of carotid stenosis. Stroke 2000; 31:1444–1450.

22. Willeit J, Kiechl S. Prevalence of risk factors of asymptomatic extracranial carotid artery atherosclerosis. A population-based study. Arteriosclero Thromb 1993; 13:661–668.

23. Prati P, Vanuzzo D, Casaroli M, Di Chiara A, De Biasi F, Feruglio GA, Touboul PJ. Prevalence and determinants of carotid atherosclerosis in a general population. Stroke 1992; 23:1705–1711.

24. O'Leary DH, Polak JF, Kronmal RA, Kittner SJ, Bond G, Wolfson SK, Bommer W, Price TR, Gardin JM, Savage PJ. (on behalf of the CHS Collaborative Research Group). Distribution and correlates of sonographically detected carotid artery disease in the cardiovascular health study. Stroke 1992; 23:1752–1760.

25. Li R, Duncan BB, Metcalf PA, Crouse JR, Sharrett ARE, Barnes R. [for the Atherosclerosis Risk in Communities (ARIC) Study Investigators]. B-mode-detected carotid artery plaque in a general population. Stroke 1994; 25: 2377–2383.

26. Fabris F, Zanocchi M, Bo M, Fonte G, Poli L, Bergoglio I, Ferrario E, Pernigotti L. Carotid plaque, aging, and risk factors. A study of 457 subjects. Stroke 1994; 25:1133–1140.

27. Joakimsen O, Bonaa KH, Stensland-Bugge E, Jacobsen BK. Age and sex differences in the distribution and ultrasound morphology of carotid atherosclerosis. The Tromso Study. Arteriosclero Thromb Vasc Biol 1999; 19: 3007–3013.

28. Su TC, Jeng JS, Chien KL, Sung FC, Hsu HC, Lee YT. Hypertension status is the major determinant of carotid atherosclerosis. A community-based study in Taiwan. Stroke 2001; 32:2265–2271.

29. Tell GS, Polak JF, Ward BJ, Kittner SJ, Savage PJ, Robbins J. Relation of smoking with carotid artery wall thickness and stenosis in older adults. The Cardiovascular Health Study. The Cardiovascular Health Study (CHS) collaborative Research Group. Circulation 1994; 90:2905–2908.

30. Whisnant JP, Homer D, Ingall TJ, Baker HL, O'Fallon WM, Wiebers DO. Duration of cigarette smoking is the strongest predictor of severe extracranial carotid artery atherosclerosis. Stroke 1990; 21:707–714.

31. Risley P, Jerrard-Dunne P, Sitzer M, Buehler A, von Kegler S, Markus HS. Promoter polymorphism in the endotoxin receptor (CD14) is associated with increased carotid atherosclerosis only in smokers. The Carotid Atherosclerosis Progression Study (CAPS). Stroke 2003; 34:600–604.

32. Beckman JA, Creager MA, Libby P. Diabetes and atherosclerosis. Epidemiology, pathophysiology, and management. JAMA 2002; 287:2570–2581.

33. Wilson PWF, Hoeg JM, D'Agostino RB, Silbershatz H, Belanger AM, Poehlmann H, O'Leary D, Wolf PA. Cumulative effects of high cholesterol levels,

high blood pressure, and cigarette smoking on carotid stenosis. N Engl J Med 1997; 337:516–522.

34. Luedemann J, Schminke U, Berger K, Piek M, Willich SN, Doring A, John U, Kessler C. Association between behavior-dependent cardiovascular risk factors and asymptomatic carotid atherosclerosis in a general population. Stroke 2002; 33:2929–2935.

35. Hunt KJ, Duggirala R, Goring HHH, Williams JT, Almasy L, Blangero J, O'Leary DH, Stern MP. Genetic basis of variation in carotid artery plaque in the San Antonio Family Heart Study. Stroke 2002; 33:2775–2780.

36. Fox CS, Polak JF, Chazaro I, Cupples A, Wolf PA, D'Agostino RA, O'Donnell CJ. Genetic and environmental contributions to atherosclerosis phenotypes in men and women. Heritability of Carotid Intima-Medial Thickness in the Framingham Heart Study. Stroke 2003; 34:397–401.

37. Duggirala R, Villalpando CG, O'Leary DH, Stern MP, Blangero J. Genetic basis of variation in carotid artery wall thickness. Stroke 1996; 27:833–837.

38. van der Meer HIM, de Maat MPM, Bots ML, Breteler MMB, Meijer J, Kiliaan AJ, Hofman A, Witteman JCM. Inflammatory mediators and cell adhesions molecules as indicators of severity of atherosclerosis. The Rotterdam Study. Arteriosclero Thromb Vasc Biol 2002; 22:838–842.

39. Rohde LE, Lee RT, Rivero J, Jamacochian M, Arroyo LH, Briggs W, Rifai N, Libby P, Creager MA, Ridker PM. Circulating cell adhesion molecules are correlated with ultrasound-based assessment of carotid atherosclerosis. Arteriosclero Thromb Vasc Biol 1998; 18:1765–1770.

40. De Caterina R, Basta G, Lazzerini G, Dell'Omo G, Petrucci R, Morale M, Carmassi F, Pedrinelli R. Soluble vascular cell adhesion molecule-1 as a biohumoral correlate of atherosclerosis. Arteriosclero Thromb Vasc Biol 1997; 17:2646–2654.

41. Qizilbash N. Fibrinogen and cerebrovascular disease. Eur Heart J 1995; 16: 42–46.

42. Schmidt H, Schmidt R, Niederkorn K, Horner S, Becsagh P, Reinhart B, Schumacher M, Weinrauch V, Kostner GM. β-fibrinogen gene polymorphism ($C_{148} \rightarrow T$) is associated with carotid atherosclerosis. Results of the Austrian Stroke Prevention Study. Arteriosclero Thromb Vasc Biol 1998; 18:487–492.

43. Grotta JC, Yatsu FM, Pettigrew LC, Rhoades H, Bratina P, Vital D, Alam R, Earls R, Picone C. Prediction of carotid stenosis progression by lipid and hematologic measurements. Neurology 1989; 39:1325–1331.

44. Selhub J, Jacques PF, Bostom AG, D'Agostino RB, Wilson PWF, Belanger AJ, O'Leary DH, Wolf PA, Schaefer EJ, Rosenberg IH. Association between plasma homocysteine concentrations and extracranial carotid-artery stenosis. N Engl J Med 1995; 332:286–291.

45. Welch GN, Loscalzo J. Homocysteine and atherothrombosis. N Engl J Med 1998; 338:1042–1050.

46. Côté R, Wolfson C, Solymoss S, Mackey A, Leclerc JR, Simard D, Rouah F, Bourque F. Hemostatic markers in patients at risk of cerebral ischemia. Stroke 2000; 31:1856–1862.

47. Nuotio K, Lindsberg PJ, Carpen O, Soinne L, Lehtonen-Smeds EMP, Saimanen E, Lassila R, Sairanen T, Sarna S, Salonen O, Kovanen PT,

Kaste M. Adhesion molecule expression in symptomatic and asymptomatic carotid stenosis. Neurology 2003; 60:1890–1899.

48. Craven TE, Ryu JE, Espeland MA, Kahl FR, McKinney WM, Toole JF, McMahan MR, Thompson CJ, Heiss G, Crouse JR. Evaluation of the associations between carotid artery atherosclerosis and coronary artery stenosis. A case-control study. Circulation 1990; 82:1230–1242.

49. Khoury Z, Schwartz R, Gottlieb S, Chenzbraun A, Stern S, Keren A. Relation of coronary artery disease to atherosclerotic disease in the aorta, carotid, and femoral arteries evaluated by ultrasound. Am J Cardiol 1997; 80:1429–1433.

50. Ebrahim S, Papacosta O, Whincup P, Wannamethee G, Walker M, Nicolaides AN, Dhanjil S, Griffin M, Belcaro G, Rumley A, Lowe GDO. Carotid plaque, intima media thickness, cardiovascular risk factors, and prevalent cardiovascular disease in men and women. The British Regional Heart Study. Stroke 1999; 30:841–850.

51. Zimarino M, Cappelletti L, Venarucci V, Gallina S, Scarpignato M, Acciai N, Calafiore AM, Barsotti A, De Caterina R. Age-dependence of risk factors for carotid stenosis: an observational study among candidates for coronary arteriography. Atherosclerosis 2001; 159:165–183.

52. Cina CS, It SC, Safar HA, Maggisano R, Bailey R, Clase CM. Prevalence and progression of internal carotid artery stenosis in patients with peripheral arterial occlusive disease. J Vasc Surg 2002; 36:75–82.

53. Lernfelt B, Forsberg M, Blomstrand C, Mellstrom D, Volkmann R. Cerebral atherosclerosis as predictor of stroke and mortality in representative elderly population. Stroke 2002; 33:224–229.

54. Mineva PP, Manchev IC, Hadjiev DI. Prevalence and outcome of asymptomatic carotid stenosis: a population-based ultrasonographic study. Eur J Neurol 2002; 9:383–388.

55. Manchev IC, Mineva PP, Hadjiev DI. Prevalence of stroke risk factors and their outcomes. A population-based longitudinal epidemiological study. Cerebrovasc Dis 2001; 12:303–307.

56. Pujia A, Rubba P, Spencer MP. Prevalence of extracranial carotid artery disease detectable by echo-Doppler in an elderly population. Stroke 1992; 23:818–822.

57. Fine-Edelstein JS, Wolf PA, O'Leary DH, Poehlman H, Belanger AJ, Kase CS, D'Agostino RB. Precursors of extracranial carotid atherosclerosis in the Framingham Study. Neurology 1994; 44:1046–1050.

58. Manolio TA, Kronmal RA, Burke GL, O'Leary DH, Price TR. (for the CHS Collaborative Research Group). Short-term predictors of incident stroke in older adults. The Cardiovascular Health Study. Stroke 1996; 27:1479–1486.

59. Longstreth WT, Shemanski L, Lefkowitz D, O'Leary DH, Polak JF, Wolfson SK. (for the Cardiovascular Health Study Collaborative Research Group). Asymptomatic internal carotid artery stenosis defined by ultrasound and the risk of subsequent stroke in the elderly. The Cardiovascular Health Study. Stroke 1998; 29:2371–2376.

60. Belcaro G, Nicolaides AN, Laurora G, Cesarone MR, De Sanctis M, Incandela L, Barsotti A. Ultrasound morphology classification of the arterial

wall and cardiovascular events in a 6-year follow-up study. Arteriosclero Thromb Vasc Biol 1996; 16:851–856.

61. Ogren M, Hedblad B, Isacsson S-O, Janzon L, Jungquist G, Lindell S-E. Ten year cerebrovascular morbidity and mortality in 68 year old men with asymptomatic carotid stenosis. Brit Med J 1995; 310:1294–1298.

62. Bock RW, Gray-Weale AC, Mock PA, Robinson DA, Irwig L, Lusby RJ. The natural history of asymptomatic carotid artery disease. J Vasc Surg 1993; 17:160–171.

63. Norris JW, Zhu CZ, Bornstein NM, Chambers BR. Vascular risks of asymptomatic carotid stenosis. Stroke 1991; 22:1485–1490.

64. Bogousslavsky J, Despland PA, Regli F. Asymptomatic tight stenosis of the internal carotid artery: long-term prognosis. Neurology 1986; 36:861–863.

65. Meissner I, Wiebers DO, Whisnant JP, O'Fallon M. The natural history of asymptomatic carotid artery occlusive lesions. JAMA 1987; 258:2704–2707.

66. Mackey AE, Abrahamowicz M, Langlais Y, Battista R, Simard D, Bourque F, Leclerc J, Côté R. (and the Asymptomatic Cervical Bruit Study Group). Neurology 1997; 48:896–903.

67. Executive Committee for the Asymptomatic Atherosclerosis Study. Endarterectomy for asymptomatic carotid artery stenosis. JAMA 1995; 273:1421–1428.

68. Hobson RW, Weiss DG, Fields WAS, Goldstone J, Moore WAS, Towne JB, Wright CB, and the Veterans Affairs Cooperative Study Group. Efficacy of carotid endarterectomy for asymptomatic carotid stenosis. N Engl J Med 1993; 328:221–227.

69. Inzitari D, Eliasziw M, Gates P, Sharpe BL, Chan RKT, Meldrum HE, Barnett HJM. (for the North American Symptomatic Carotid Endarterectomy Trial Collaborators). The causes and risk of stroke in patients with asymptomatic internal carotid artery stenosis. N Engl J Med 2000; 342:1693–1700.

70. The European Carotid Surgery Trialists Collaborative Group. Risk of stroke in the distribution of an asymptomatic carotid artery. Lancet 1995; 345: 209–212.

71. Erzurum VZ, Littooy FN, Steffen G, Chmura C, Mansour MA. Outcome of nonoperative management of asymptomatic high-grade carotid stenosis. J Vasc Surg 2002; 36:663–667.

72. Autret A, Saudeau D, Bertrand PH, Pourcelot L, Marchal C, De Boisvilliers S. Stroke risk in patients with carotid stenosis. Lancet 1987; 1:888–890.

73. Hennerici M, Hulsbomer HB, Hefter H, Lammerts D, Rautenberg W. Natural history of asymptomatic extracranial arterial disease. Results of a long-term prospective study. Brain 1987; 110:777–791.

74. Barnett HJM, Gunton RW, Eliasziw M, Fleming L, Sharpe B, Gates P, Meldrum H. Causes and severity of ischemic stroke in patients with internal carotid artery stenosis. JAMA 2000; 283:1429–1436.

75. Powers WJ, Derdeyn CP, Fritsch SM, Carpenter DA, Yundt KD, Videen TO, Grubb RL. Benign prognosis of never-symptomatic carotid occlusion. Neurology 2000; 54:878–882.

76. Rockman CB, Riles TS, Lamparello PJ, Giangola G, Adelman MA, Stone D, Guareschi C, Goldstein J, Landis R. Natural history and management of the

asymptomatic, moderately stenotic internal carotid artery. J Vasc Surg 1997; 25:423–431.

77. Roederer GO, Langlois YE, Jager KA, Primozich JF, Beach KW, Phillips DJ, Strandness DE. The natural history of carotid arterial disease in asymptomatic patients with cervical bruits. Stroke 1984; 15:605–613.

78. Stamou SC, Hill PC, Dangas G, Pfister AJ, Boyce SW, Dullum MKC, Bafi AS, Corso PJ. Stroke after coronary artery bypass. Incidence, predictors, and clinical outcome. Stroke 2001; 32:1508–1513.

79. Dashe JF, Pessin MS, Murphy RE, Payne DD. Carotid occlusive disease and stroke risk in coronary artery bypass graft surgery. Neurology 1997; 49: 678–686.

80. Hogue CW, Murphy SF, Schechtman KB, Davila-Roman VG. Risk factors for early or delayed stroke after cardiac surgery. Circulation 1999; 100: 642–647.

81. Gerraty RP, Gates PC, Doyle JC. Carotid stenosis and perioperative stroke risk in symptomatic and asymptomatic patients undergoing vascular or coronary surgery. Stroke 1993; 24:1115–1118.

82. Furlan AJ, Craciun ARE. Risk of stroke during coronary artery bypass graft surgery in patients with internal carotid artery disease documented by angiography. Stroke 1985; 16:797–799.

83. Lewis RF, Abrahamowicz M, Côté R, Battista RN. Predictive power of duplex ultrasonography in asymptomatic carotid disease. Ann Intern Med 1997; 127:13–20.

84. Strandness DE. Screening for carotid disease and surveillance for carotid restenosis. Vasc Surg 2001; 14:200–205.

85. Lee TT, Solomon NA, Heidenreich PA, Oehlert J, Garber AM. Cost-effectiveness of screening for carotid stenosis in asymptomatic persons. Ann Intern Med 1997; 126:337–346.

86. Whitty CJM, Sudlow CLM, Warlow CP. Investigating individual subjects and screening populations for asymptomatic carotid stenosis can be harmful. J Neurol Neurosurg Psychiatry 1998; 64:619–623.

87. Obuchowski NA, Modic MT, Magdinec M, Masaryk TJ. Assessment of the efficacy of noninvasive screening for patients with asymptomatic neck bruits. Stroke 1997; 28:1330–1339.

88. Bamford J, Sandercock P, Dennis M, Burn J, Warlow C. Classification and natural history of clinically identifiable subtypes of cerebral infarction. Lancet 1991; 337:1521–1526.

89. Rothwell PM, Gutnikov SA, Eliasziw M, Fox AJ, Taylor W, Mayberg MR, Warlow CP, Barnett HJM. (for the Carotid Endarterectomy Trialists' Collaboration). Pooled analysis of individual patient data from randomised controlled trials of endarterectomy for symptomatic carotid stenosis. Lancet 2003; 361:107–116.

90. Timsit SG, Sacco RL, Mohr JP, Foulkes MA, Tatemichi TK, Wolf PA, Price TR, Hier DB. Early clinical differentiation of cerebral infarction from severe atherosclerotic stenosis and cardioembolism. Stroke 1992; 23:486–491.

91. Lee BI, Nam HS, Heo JH, Kim DI. Yonsei Stroke Registry. Cerebrovasc Dis 2001; 12:145–151.

92. Pessin MS, Duncan GW, Mohr JP, Poskanzer DC. Clinical and angiographic features of carotid transient ischemic attacks. N Engl J Med 1977; 296: 358–362.

93. Brown RD, Petty GW, O'Fallon WM, Wiebers DO, Whisnant JP. Incidence of transient ischemic attacks in Rochester Minnesota, 1985–1989. Stroke 1998; 29:2109–2113.

94. Hollenhorst RW. Significance of bright plaques in the retinal arterioles. JAMA 1961; 178:23–29.

95. Fisher CM. Observations of the fundus oculi in transient monocular blindness. Neurology 1959; 9:337–347.

96. McBrien DJ, Bradley RD, Ashton N. The nature of retinal emboli in stenosis of the internal carotid artery. Lancet 1963; 1:697–699.

97. Baquis GD, Pessin MS, Scott RM. Limb shaking—a carotid TIA. Stroke 1985; 16:444–448.

98. Tatemichi TK, Young WL, Prohovnik I, Gitelman DR, Correll JW, Mohr JP. Perfusion insufficiency in limb shaking transient ischemic attacks. Stroke 1990; 21:341–347.

99. Wilson SE, Mayberg MR, Yatsu F, Weiss DG. Crescendo transient ischemic attacks: a surgical imperative. J Vasc Surg 1993; 17:249–256.

100. Bruno A, Jeffries L, Lakind E, Qualls C. Predictors of cerebral infarction following transient ischemic attacks. J Stroke Cerebrovasc Dis 1993; 3:23–28.

101. European Carotid Surgery Trialists' Collaborative Group. Randomised trial of endarterectomy for recently symptomatic carotid stenosis: final results of the MRC European Carotid Surgery Trial (ECST). Lancet 1998; 351: 1379–1387.

102. Del Sette M, Eliasziw M, Streifler JY, Hachinski VC, Fox AJ, Barnett HJM. [for the North American Symptomatic Carotid Endarterectomy Trial (NAS-CET) Group]. Internal borderzone infarction; a marker of severe stenosis in patients with symptomatic internal carotid artery disease. Stroke 2000; 31:631–636.

103. Tejada J, Diez-Tejedor E, Hernandez-Echebarria L, Balboa O. Does a relationship exist between carotid stenosis and lacunar infarction? Stroke 2003; 34:1404–1411.

104. Boiten J. Ischemic lacunar stroke in the European Carotid Surgery Trial: risk factors, distribution of carotid stenosis, effect of surgery and type of recurrent stroke. Cerebrovasc Dis 1996; 6:281–287.

105. North American Symptomatic Carotid Endarterectomy Trialists' Collaborative Group. The final results of the NASCET trial. N Engl J Med 1998; 339:1415–1425.

106. Mayberg MR, Wilson SE, Yatsu F, Weiss DG, Messina L, Hershey LA, Colling C, Eskridge J, Deykin D, Winn HR. (for the Veteran Affairs Cooperative Study Program 309 Trialist Group). Carotid endarterectomy and prevention of cerebral ischemia in symptomatic carotid stenosis. JAMA 1991; 226:3289–3294.

107. Mehigan JT, Olcott C IV. The carotid "string" sign: differential diagnosis and management. Am J Surg 1980; 140:137–142.

108. Morgenstern LB, Fox AJ, Sharpe BL, Eliasziw M, Barnett HJM, Grotta J. [for the North American Symptomatic Carotid Endarterectomy Trial (NAS-

CET) Group]. The risks and benefits of carotid endarterectomy in patients with near occlusion of the carotid artery. Neurology 1997; 48:911–915.

109. Streifler JY, Eliasziw M, Benavente OR, Harbison JW, Hachinski VC, Barnett HJM, Simard D. [for the North American Symptomatic Carotid Endarterectomy Trial (NASCET) Group]. The risk of stroke in patients with first-ever retinal vs. hemispheric transient ischemic attacks and high-grade carotid stenosis. Arch Neurol 1995; 52:246–249.

110. Benavente OR, Eliasziw M, Streifler JY, Fox AJ, Barnett HJM. [for the North American Symptomatic Carotid Endarterectomy Trial (NASCET) Group]. Prognosis after transient monocular blindness associated with carotid-artery stenosis. N Engl J Med 2001; 345:1084–1090.

111. Barnett HJM, Meldrum HE, Eliasziw M. [for the North American Symptomatic Carotid Endarterectomy Trial (NASCET) Group]. The appropriate use of carotid endarterectomy. CMAJ 2002; 166:1169–1179.

112. Klijn CJM, Kappelle LJ, Tulleken CAF, van Gijn J. Symptomatic carotid artery occlusion: a reappraisal of hemodynamic factors. Stroke 1997; 28: 2084–2093.

113. The EC/IC bypass Study Group. Failure of extracranial-intracranial arterial bypass to reduce risk of ischemic stroke: results of an international randomized trial. N Engl J Med 1985; 313:1191–1200.

114. Kappelle LJ, Klijn CJ, Tulleken CA. The management of patients with symptomatic carotid artery occlusion. Clin Exp Hypertension 2002; 24:631–637.

115. Grubb RL, Derdeyn CP, Fritsch SM, Carpenter DA, Yundt KD, Videen TO, Spitznagel EL, Powers WJ. Importance of hemodynamic factors in the prognosis of symptomatic carotid occlusion. JAMA 1998; 280:1055–1060.

116. Streifler JY, Eliasziw M, Benavente OR, Alamowitch S, Fox AJ, Hachinski VC, Barnett HJM. [for the North American Symptomatic Carotid Endarterectomy Trial (NASCET) Group]. Prognostic importance of leukoaraiosis in patients with symptomatic internal carotid artery stenosis. Stroke 2002; 33:1651–1655.

117. Klijn CJ, Kappelle LJ, Algra A, van Gijn J. Outcome in patients with symptomatic occlusion of the internal carotid artery or intracranial arterial lesions: a meta-analysis of the role of baseline characteristics and type of antithrombotic treatment. Cerebrovasc Dis 2001; 12:228–234.

118. Kappelle LJ, Eliasziw M, Fox AJ, Sharpe BL, Barnett HJM. Importance of intracranial atherosclerotic disease in patients with symptomatic stenosis of the internal carotid artery. The North American Symptomatic Carotid Endarterectomy Trial. Stroke 1999; 30:282–286.

119. Gasecki AP, Eliasziw M, Ferguson GG, Hachinski VC, Barnett HJM. [for the North American Symptomatic Carotid Endarterectomy Trial (NASCET) Group]. Long-term prognosis and effect of endarterectomy in patients with symptomatic severe stenosis and contralateral carotid stenosis or occlusion: results from NASCET. J Neurosurg 1995; 83:778–782.

120. Eliasziw M, Streifler JY, Fox AJ, Hachinski VC, Ferguson GG, Barnett HJM. Significance of plaque ulceration in symptomatic patients with high-grade stenosis. North American Symptomatic Carotid Endarterectomy Trial. Stroke 1994; 25:304–308.

121. Henderson RD, Eliasziw M, Fox AJ, Rothwell PM, Barnett HJM. Angiographically defined collateral circulation and risk of stroke in patients with severe carotid artery stenosis. The North American Symptomatic Carotid Endarterectomy (NASCET) Group. Stroke 2000; 31:128–132.

122. Wade JPH, Wong W, Barnett HJM, Vandervoot P. Bilateral carotid occlusion of internal carotid arteries. Brain 1987; 110:667–682.

123. AbuRahama AF, Copeland SE. Bilateral internal carotid artery occlusion: natural history and surgical alternatives. Cardiovasc Surg 1998; 6:579–583.

124. Aly S, Bishop CC. An objective characterization of atherosclerotic lesion. An alternative method to identify unstable plaque. Stroke 2000; 31:1921–1924.

125. Murphy RE, Moddy ARE, Morgan PS, Martel AL, Delay GS, Allder S, MacSweeney ST, Tennant WG, Gladman J, Lowe J, Hunt BJ. Prevalence of complicated carotid atheroma as detected by magnetic resonance direct thrombus imaging in patients with suspected carotid artery stenosis and previous acute cerebral ischemia. Stroke 2003; 107:3053–3058.

126. Spence JD, Eliasziw M, DiCicco M, Hackam DG, Galil R, Lohmann T. Carotid plaque area; a tool for targeting and evaluating vascular preventive therapy. Stroke 2002; 33:2916–2922.

127. Markus H, Cullinane M. Severely impaired cerebrovascular reactivity predicts stroke and TIA risk in patients with carotid artery stenosis and occlusion. Brain 2001; 124:457–467.

128. Silvestrini M, Vernieri F, Pasqualetti P, Matteis M, Passarelli F, Troisi E, Caltagirone C. Impaired cerebral vasoreactivity and risk of stroke in patients with asymptomatic carotid artery stenosis. JAMA 2000; 283:2122–2127.

129. Molloy J, Markus HS. Asymptomatic embolisation predicts stroke and TIA risk in patients with carotid artery stenosis. Stroke 1999; 30:1440–1443.

130. van der Meer HIM, de Maat MPM, Hak AE, Kiliaan AJ, Iglesias del Sol A, van der Kuip DAM, Nijhuis RLG, Hofman A, Witteman JCM. C-reactive protein predicts progression of atherosclerosis measured at various sites in the arterial tree. The Rotterdam Study. Stroke 2002; 33:2750–2755.

3

Pathophysiology

Hugh Markus

Clinical Neuroscience, St. George's Hospital Medical School, London, U.K.

The great majority of cases of carotid artery stenosis result from atherosclerotic disease, with only a small minority being due to other causes including carotid dissection, radiation induced damage, and post-carotid endarterectomy restenosis. Most atherosclerotic carotid stenoses remain asymptomatic. A complex interaction of factors, still incompletely understood, determines whether a particular stenosis becomes symptomatic. The pathophysiology of symptomatic carotid stenosis can be considered as a number of stages, each of which may have differing risk factors and differing opportunities for intervention. These are listed below:

1. early atherosclerotic lesion;
2. progression to plaque and stenosis formation;
3. plaque instability;
4. thrombosis on the "activated" plaque and distal embolization; and
5. intracerebral vessel flow disruption and cerebral infarction.

Carotid stenosis could theoretically cause focal ischemia either through a reduction in flow or through embolization, or through a combination of the two. A number of lines of evidence, presented later in this chapter, support embolism being the predominant disease process, although in a minority of patients, hemodynamic stroke can occur.

In this chapter the processes leading to the initial atherosclerotic stenotic lesion will first be discussed, followed by the possible cellular and molecular processes that result in plaque instability. The clinical evidence that plaques become "active" and unstable will then be reviewed. The role of hemodynamic factors both in determining whether an embolus results in ischemic symptoms and as a primary process in stroke in patients with carotid stenosis will be discussed.

1. ATHEROSCLEROSIS

Atherosclerosis is a progressive disease characterized by the accumulation of lipids and fibrous elements in the large arteries (1,2). Early sub-clinical lesions consist of sub-endothelial accumulations of cholesterol-engorged macrophages, called "foam cells". Autopsy studies have shown that these "fatty streaks" can be found in the aorta in the first decade of life, the coronary arteries in the second decade, and the cerebral arteries in the third or fourth decade (1). Although not clinically significant, these fatty streaks are the precursors of more advanced lesions characterized by the accumulation of smooth muscle cells (SMCs) and lipid-rich necrotic debris. Typically a fibrous cap consisting of SMCs and an extracellular matrix encloses a lipid-rich necrotic core. This "fibrous plaque" can become increasingly complex with ulceration at the luminal surface, hemorrhage from new vessels growing into the lesion from the media of the blood vessel wall, and calcification. Advanced lesions can progressively stenose the vessel to result in a reduction in blood flow, but the most important clinical complication occurs with thrombus formation, often associated with the rupture or erosion of the luminal surface of the plaque. This can lead to in-situ thrombosis, believed to be most important in the pathogenesis of myocardial infarction, or distal embolization, which is more important in the pathogenesis of stroke.

Atherosclerosis is a complex process with multiple disease pathways interacting at each stage. For almost a century lipid deposition was felt to be central to the disease process. Although aspects of this lipid oxidation hypothesis appear to play a role, more recently the importance of other interacting disease processes has been appreciated. Increasing evidence suggests inflammation plays a crucial role at all stages of the process from plaque initiation to plaque activation, while endothelial dysfunction has also been implicated particularly in the earlier stages (3). The molecular mechanisms underlying atherosclerosis have been greatly clarified by studies in a range of animal models. Mice deficient in apolipoproteinE (apoE) or the low-density lipoprotein (LDL) receptor develop atherosclerosis when fed high-cholesterol diets, and are the models most used in such studies. The crossing of these animals with mice that have been engineered to over-express or lack genes of interest has led to a growing list of proteins that accelerate or retard the rate of lesion growth and/or lesion composition (2). These provide a unique insight into mechanisms, but may not always be directly representative of the much more slowly developing and progressive lesion occurring in humans. Furthermore there are no good animal models of plaque rupture.

In experimental animals fed a high-fat cholesterol diet, the first morphological changes in the arterial wall are accumulation of lipoprotein particles and their aggregates in the intima at sites of lesion predilection (1). Within days or weeks, monocytes can be seen adhering to the surface of the endothelium and these then transmigrate across the endothelial layer into the intima. Here they proliferate and differentiate into macrophages which ingest lipoproteins, forming foam cells. As time passes, these foam cells die, contributing their lipid-filled contents to the necrotic core of the lesion. Accumulation of SMCs occurs via migration from the medial layer, and these secrete fibrous elements leading to the production of fibrous plaques which gradually increase in size. Initially these lesions grow outwards towards the adventitia but after a certain point, they begin to expand into the lumen. Continued lesion growth occurs by migration of further mononuclear cells from the blood. This is accompanied by cell proliferation, extracellular matrix production, and the accumulation of extracellular lipids.

1.1. Initiation of Atherosclerosis

The endothelium is thought to play a crucial role in the early stages of atherogenesis. With its tight intercellular junction complex, it functions as a selectively permeable barrier between blood and the vessel wall. It produces a number of effector molecules that regulate thrombosis, inflammation, vascular tone, and vascular remodeling. Impaired endothelial function has been associated with a number of risk factors in humans including hypertension (4). This may relate to reduced release or bio-availability of nitric oxide, synthesized by endothelial nitric oxide synthase. The normal endothelium does not in general support binding of white blood cells or platelets. However, early after the initiation of an atherogenic diet in animal models, patches of arterial endothelial cells begin to express surface selective adhesion molecules that bind to various classes of leukocytes, including vascular cell adhesion molecule-1 (VCAM-1). Interestingly these foci of increased adhesion molecule expression overlap with sites in the arterial tree that are particularly prone to developing atheroma (3). Considerable evidence suggests that impaired endogenous protective mechanisms occur at branch points in arteries, where the endothelial cells may experience disturbed flow (5). Cells in the tubular regions of arteries where the blood flow is uniform and laminar are ellipsoid in shape and aligned in the direction of flow. In contrast, cells in regions of arterial branching, where the flow is disturbed, have polygonal shapes and no particular orientation (1). These latter areas show increased permeability to macromolecules such as LDL and are preferential sites for lesion formation (6). Shear stress may mediate part of these differences. For example reduced laminar shear stress may reduce the local production of endothelium-derived nitric oxide.

A primary initiating event is the accumulation of LDL in the sub-endothelium (Fig. 1). This is accentuated by higher circulating LDL levels and reduced by high-density lipoprotein (HDL) levels which carry cholesterol from tissue to liver to form bile in the process of reversed cholesterol transport. In addition to LDL, other ApoB-containing lipoproteins including lipoprotein(a) can accumulate. Low-density lipoprotein is retained in the vessel wall through interactions with proteoglycans and other molecules. In a mouse model, LDL with defective binding to proteoglycans is not retained by the vessel wall and such mice, fed an atherogenic diet, have markedly reduced aortic atherosclerosis (7). A number of different hypotheses have been developed to explain the initial initiating step of atherosclero-

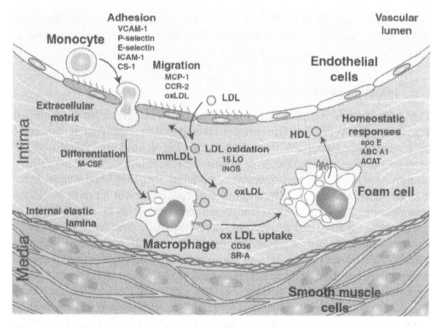

Figure 1 Initiating events in the development of early atherosclerosis. Low-density lipoprotein is subject to oxidative modifications in the sub-endothelial space, progressing from minimally modified LDL (mmLDL) to extensively oxidized LDL (ox LDL). Monocytes attach to endothelial cells that have been induced to express cell adhesion molecules by mmLDL and inflammatory cytokines. Adherent monocytes migrate into the sub-endothelial space and differentiate into macrophages. Uptake of oxLDL via scavenger receptors leads to foam cell formation. OxLDL cholesterol taken up by scavenger receptors is subject to esterification and storage in lipid droplets, is converted to more soluble forms, or is exported to extracellular HDL acceptors via cholesterol transporters, such as ABC-A1. *Source*: From Ref. 2.

sis. The response to injury hypothesis suggests that endothelial injury causes increased permeability to atherogenic lipoproteins. The response to retention hypothesis suggests that the primary step is the entry of LDL into the vessel wall. Therefore whether atherosclerosis is initiated depends on the difference between the arterial wall influx and efflux of atherogenic lipoproteins.

Whatever the initial mechanism, this trapped LDL then undergoes modification including oxidation, lipolysis, and proteolysis. A particularly important process is lipid oxidation as a result of exposure to the oxidative waste of vascular cells. Such modifications initially give rise to "minimally oxidized" LDL species that have pro-inflammatory activity but can still be recognized by LDL receptors. In contrast, extensively modified or highly oxidized LDL is not bound by LDL receptors, but rather by several so-called scavenger receptors expressed on macrophages (2) and SMCs, and two such receptors, SR-A and CV36, appear to play an important role (1). The rapid uptake of highly oxidized LDL particles by macrophages then leads to foam cell formation before it can be taken up sufficiently rapidly by macrophages to form foam cells. This oxidative modification presumably involves reactive oxygen species produced by endothelial cells and macrophages, but several enzymes have been implicated including myeloperoxidase, sphingomyelinase, secretory phospholipase A2, and inducible nitric oxide synthase.

Inflammation appears to play an important part in these early stages (Fig. 2). Leukocytes adherent to the endothelium secondary to endothelial dysfunction penetrate into the intima. Monocyte chemotactic protein-1 (MCP-1) is responsible for the direct migration of monocytes into the intima at sites of lesion formation (8). Once resident in the arterial wall, these inflammatory cells participate and perpetuate a local inflammatory response. The macrophages express scavenger receptors for modified lipoproteins, permitting them to ingest lipid and become foam cells. In addition to MCP-1, macrophage colony-stimulating factor (M-CSF) contributes to the differentiation of blood monocytes into macrophage foam cells (9). Mice carrying a naturally occurring mutation in M-CSF exhibit an almost complete absence of macrophages, and are very resistant to atherosclerosis (9). T cells are also activated causing them to release inflammatory cytokines such as γ-interferon and tumor necrosis factor-β that can in turn stimulate macrophages (2).

1.2. Fibrous Plaque Formation

Fibrous plaques are characterized by a central core of extracellular lipid, mostly cholesterol and its ester, and the accumulation of SMCs and SMC-derived extracellular matrix. The transition from the fatty streak to the more complex lesion is characterized by the migration of SMCs from the medial layer of the artery, past the internal elastic lamina, and into the intimal or sub-endothelial space (Fig. 2). Intimal SMCs may proliferate and take up

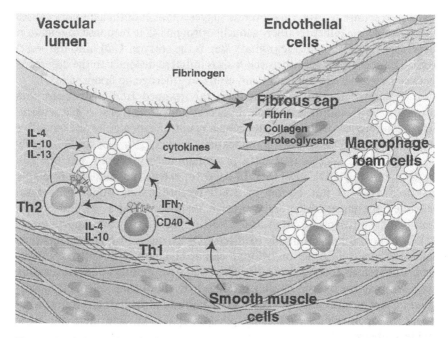

Figure 2 Atherosclerotic lesion progression. Interactions between macrophage foam cells, Th1 and Th2 T cells establish a chronic inflammatory process. Cytokines secreted by lymphocytes and macrophages exert both pro- and anti-atherogenic effects on each of the cellular elements of the vessel wall. Smooth muscle cells migrate from the medial portion of the arterial wall, proliferate, and secrete extracellular matrix proteins that from a fibrous plaque. *Source*: From Ref. 2.

modified lipoproteins, contributing to foam cell formation, and synthesize the extracellular matrix that leads to development of the fibrous cap (2). Activated macrophages and T cells release fibrogenic mediators, including a variety of peptide growth factors that promote the replication of SMCs and contribute to the production by these cells of a dense extracellular matrix. This phase is influenced by interactions between macrophages and T cells which result in a broad range of cellular and humoral responses and the acquisition of many features of a chronic inflammatory state (2).

Considerable evidence indicates that immune activation is ongoing in atherosclerotic lesions, although it is uncertain as to which are the most significant antigens responsible for this activation (2). Bacterial and viral antigens, heat shock proteins, and neoepitopes (antigenic epitopes resulting from the formation of adducts between oxidized lipids in oxidized LDL and apoB or arterial wall components) have all been implicated (2).

On this theme there has been considerable interest in the role of infective agents, particularly *Chlamydia pneumoniae*, in the pathogenesis of atherosclerosis. Epidemiological studies reported the increased prevalence of antibodies directed against *C. pneumoniae, Helicobacter pylori*, herpes simplex virus, and cytomegalovirus in patients with coronary artery disease compared with normal controls. However the results of prospective studies have been less consistent. A number of studies have reported evidence of infection with *C. pneumoniae* in the arterial plaque. This could release lipopolysaccharide (endotoxin) and heat shock proteins which themselves could stimulate the production of pro-inflammatory mediators by vascular endothelial cells, SMCs, and infiltrating leukocytes (3). Whether such an infection represents a primary part of the pathogenic process or is a secondary infection in an already disrupted plaque remains controversial. Chronic infection could also predispose to atherosclerosis by non-specifically increasing systemic inflammation which has been implicated in atherosclerosis (10). If infection did play a causal role, its treatment might reduce vascular event rates. An initial study suggested antibiotic therapy could reduce recurrent myocardial infarction rate, but subsequent larger studies have failed to consistently confirm this finding (11).

1.3. Advanced Lesions and Lesion Stability

Although atherosclerotic lesions can produce symptoms by progressive narrowing of the vessel lumen, acute events resulting in myocardial infarction or stroke are generally thought to arise from plaque rupture (Fig. 3) and thrombosis (2). Most of the human data on mechanisms have been derived from pathological studies of acute coronary events rather than cerebral vasculature. Thrombus in-situ mediated acute coronary events depend primarily on the composition and vulnerability of the plaque rather than the severity of stenosis. Post-mortem and atherectomy studies have demonstrated that plaques removed from patients with unstable coronary syndromes have larger lipid-filled cores and thinner fibrous caps. These fibrous caps contain larger numbers of activated macrophages and T lymphocytes, but smaller numbers of SMCs and less collagen content than plaques from patients with stable angina (12). The likelihood of plaque rupture is a balance between the tensile strength of the plaque and the stresses exerted on it. Interestingly, in a model system, a decrease in fibrous cap thickness markedly increased the circumferential stress on the plaque, whereas an increase in stenosis severity actually decreased circumferential stress (13). The progression of advanced coronary plaques in humans may involve repetitive cycles of microhemorrhage and thrombosis (2).

Maintenance of the fibrous cap reflects matrix production and degradation. Breakdown of collagen, the principal connective tissue component of the fibrous cap, is dependent on the balance between the proteolytic enzymes, the metalloproteinases (MMPs), and their inhibitors, tissue inhibitors of metalloproteinase (TIMPs) (12). Again inflammation appears to play

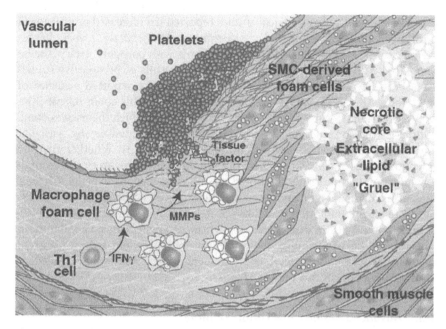

Figure 3 Plaque rupture and thrombosis. Necrosis of macrophage and smooth muscle cell-derived foam cells leads to the formation of a necrotic core and the accumulation of extracellular cholesterol. Macrophage secretion of matrix metalloproteinases and neovascularization contribute to weakening of the fibrous plaque. Plaque rupture exposes blood components to tissue factor, initiating coagulation, the recruitment of platelets, and the formation of a thrombus. *Source*: From Ref. 2.

a crucial role, with high levels of MMPs being demonstrated at the site of the inflammatory infiltrate in the fibrous cap. T cells produce interferon-γ, which inhibits the production of matrix by SMCs, and macrophages produce various proteinases in addition to the MMPs, which degrade the extracellular matrix. Rupture frequently occurs at lesion edges, which are rich in foam cells. Smooth muscle cell apoptosis or programmed cell death has been demonstrated in unstable plaques. T cells can induce macrophages to secrete MMPs by stimulation of CD40, and in addition, through the production of interleukin-1, can promote SMC apoptosis (12).

1.4. Plaque Thrombogenicity

Following plaque rupture, the necrotic core containing tissue factor and plaque lipids is exposed to the circulating blood components initiating the coagulation cascade, platelet adherence, and thrombosis. In addition to causing vessel occlusion by thrombosis and distal embolization, this thrombosis appears to be an important mechanism in plaque progression. This is largely based on data from the coronary circulation suggesting that progression of advanced coronary plaques in humans may involve repetitive cycles of micro-hemorrhage and thrombosis (2). The thrombogenicity of the necrotic core is likely to depend on the presence of tissue factor, a key protein in the initiation of the coagulation cascade. Tissue factor production by endothelial cells and macrophages is enhanced by oxidized LDL and infection (1).

1.5. Molecular Mechanism of Plaque Instability in the Carotid Plaque

Most of the data on plaque changes leading to symptomatic status in humans have been obtained from the coronary circulation. There may be important differences in the carotid circulation. In the coronary circulation, plaque rupture leading to thrombosis and occlusion of the vessel at the site of the plaque appears to play an important role. Frequently rupture occurs in non-stenotic plaques. In the carotid circulation, the risk of symptomatic status increases with increasing degrees of stenosis, and plaque thrombosis primarily produces symptoms by distal embolization. Vessel occlusion at the site of an activated plaque may occur but is much less common. This may reflect the larger diameter of the carotid compared with that of the coronary artery.

A number of studies have compared carotid plaques removed at endarterectomy from symptomatic and asymptomatic patients. There are difficulties in interpreting some of these data. Carotid endarterectomy is sometimes performed some weeks after the onset of symptoms, by which time repair processes may have altered findings. Patients suffering any form of symptoms including amaurosis fugax, hemispheric transient ischemic attack, and stroke have been grouped together (12). Importantly, any changes could reflect secondary changes following rupture and thrombosis, rather than primary initiating changes.

A recent review (12) identified 21 studies, but excluded 10 due to methodological flaws. Plaque rupture or ulceration were more common in symptomatic patients (48% vs. 31%, $p < 0.001$), but lumen thrombus (40% vs. 35%) and intra-plaque hemorrhage (48% vs. 50%) were equally common in symptomatic and asymptomatic plaques. The other markers of increased risk were difficult to pool between studies due to different methods of assessment. However, most studies showed that the fibrous cap of symptomatic carotid plaques was thinner and inflammation more common, with greater numbers of macrophages and T cells detected in the cap. In one study the quantity of extractable lipid was found to be greater in symptomatic plaques (14); this would be consistent with ultrasound studies which demonstrate that echolucent lipid-rich plaques are more often associated with symptoms. Detailed histological studies have demonstrated some subtle differences between plaques removed from symptomatic and asymptomatic patients

(12). In symptomatic patients the necrotic core is placed nearer to the fibrous cap and the minimum cap thickness is less. This may predispose to rupture. It is striking that only 50% of symptomatic patients have evidence of ulceration or plaque rupture (12). This could reflect healing due to the delay between symptom onset and removal of plaque at endarterectomy. Alternatively other processes could play a role. Endothelial erosions with secondary platelet adhesion and embolization, without frank plaque rupture, might be important.

2. CAROTID LOCALIZATION OF ATHEROSCLEROSIS

The carotid bulb and proximal artery is a site of predilection for plaque and subsequent stenosis. The vast majority of carotid stenoses occur at this site. This localization is likely to reflect anatomical factors resulting in secondary hemodynamic alterations. Plaque tends to form at sites of arterial bifurcation which result in distortion of laminar flow.

The importance of anatomical factors is highlighted by a recent study in 1300 community normal volunteers using carotid ultrasound. The angle of origin of the internal carotid artery in relation to the common carotid artery was associated with both increased carotid bulb intima-media thickness (IMT), a marker of early atherosclerosis, and the presence of plaque. These relationships persisted after controlling for other cardiovascular risk factors (15). The more dorsal the angle, the greater the risk. The relationship was site-specific, not being present for common carotid IMT. This suggests that a more dorsal angle of origin results in local hemodynamic changes which themselves increase the risk of atherosclerosis. This is consistent with previous experimental work. It has been shown that adaptive intimal thickening is caused by a reduced longitudinal wall shear stress, and that this results in reduced local endothelial production of nitric oxide (16,17). This view is also supported by results from flow models studying the influence of the insertion angle of an end-to-side anastomosis on wall shear stress distribution around this artificial bifurcation. With increasing insertion angles, longitudinal wall shear stress was reduced near the top of the inserted vessel opposite the flow divider (18). This is mainly due to the fact that at this position, the blood flow features a stagnation point, which oscillates in strength and position leading to an alteration and reduction of the longitudinal wall shear (19). These interactions could also influence adaptive intimal thickening in arterial wall segments near the carotid bifurcation. Ultrasound studies in humans have found an association between reduced near wall shear stress at the carotid bifurcation and increased IMT (20).

Genetic factors may influence why some atheroslerotic individuals suffer carotid stenosis, while others do not. In a community carotid ultrasound study, a parental history of young stroke was strongly associated with an increased internal carotid bulb IMT, but the association with common carotid artery IMT was much weaker (21). In contrast there was no relation-ship between a parental history of myocardial infarction and carotid bulb IMT, but a highly significant association with common carotid IMT. This genetic influence could be mediated through anatomical differences resulting in altered flow and shear stresses as described above. This is consistent with twin studies which have suggested that ultrasonically determined carotid atherosclerosis has a significant genetic component of risk (22).

Non-invasive ultrasound imaging studies have shown that an early change in atherosclerotic disease of the carotid bifurcation is an adaptive vasodilation. Carotid arterial diameter positively correlates with carotid IMT (23). Data from the Bruneck Study, a large prospective community-based ultrasound study, has provided information on the progression of established carotid atherosclerosis (24,25). Two distinct types of progression were identified; a slow continuous type named "diffuse dilative atherosclero-sis" and a non-linear rapid and unpredictable type named "focal stenotic atherosclerosis" (26). Early lesions tend to develop slowly and lumen obstruction is counterbalanced, or overcompensated for, by the compensa-tory arterial dilatation. Significant lumen obstruction does not occur even when plaques grow to 3 or 4 mm in diameter. This slow progression was found to be associated with both conventional factors such as hypertension and hyperlipidemia, and less well-established risk factors such as high body iron stores, heavy drinking, and infections. In contrast more advanced pla-ques were found to frequently progress by episodic marked increases in size followed by stable periods. This could be exacerbated by inadequate vascular remodeling and adaptive vasodilation. No association was found between this process and conventional risk factors. It was suggested this occurred due to plaque disruption and subsequent healing (26). This is analogous with the role of repetitive rupture and microhemorrhage suggested as a mechanism of coronary plaque progression.

The main variables determining whether a stenosis is hemodynami-cally significant are cross-sectional area, stenosis length, and blood viscosity. Of these, cross-sectional area is most important. Studies in humans, during cross-clamping of the common carotid artery for intracerebral aneurysms, have shown that a sudden fall in pressure distal to the stenosis occurs when the luminal diameter reaches < 2 mm; little detectable change in flow or pressure occurred until this point (27). This is consistent with in vitro studies in excised human internal carotid arteries when hemodynamic disturbance only occurred when the cross-sectional area was reduced to 4–5 mm^2. The length of stenosis is a less important factor, and lesions in tandem only produced cumulative effects if the stenoses were separated by more than 3 cm (27).

3. IMPORTANCE OF EMBOLISM IN CAROTID STROKE: EVIDENCE FROM CLINICAL STUDIES

The term "embolism" was coined by Virchow in the context of gangrene of the lower limbs caused by clots from the heart. He suggested this process could also cause cerebral damage (28). However the role of embolism from carotid plaque in the pathogenesis of stroke was largely overlooked until the 1960s, despite the fact that as long ago as 1905, Chiari had drawn attention to the frequency of atherosclerosis in the region of the carotid bifurcation, and had suggested that embolization of atheromatous material might cause stroke (29). For some time the more popular theory was that thrombosis at the site of the carotid plaque resulted in local vessel occlusion. However, considerable evidence from the 1950s onwards has led to the widespread acceptance of the predominant role of embolism in stroke pathogenesis in patients with carotid stenosis. This of course does not exclude the primary role of hemodynamic compromise or in-situ thrombosis in a minority of patients.

A number of lines of evidence support the importance of embolization. Angiographic studies within a few hours after stroke showed the combination of carotid stenosis without occlusion, and distal intracerebral vessel occlusion at the site of impaction of emboli (30). Transcranial Doppler monitoring studies similarly showed middle cerebral artery occlusion, often transient, which is consistent with embolization to distal vessels (31). Studies in the late 1950s and 1960s directly visualized embolization in the retinal vessels. Miller Fischer performed careful ophthalmoscopic examinations and saw white bodies passing slowly through the retinal arteries during an attack of transient monocular blindness (32). The appearance and friability suggested they were emboli largely composed of platelets. These findings were confirmed by Ross Russell (33) whilst other investigators noticed cholesterol emboli in the retinal vessels which became impacted and did not move (34). Plaque thrombus, the substrate for embolization, is more common as the degree of stenosis increases, and this explains the association between the degree of stenosis and stroke risk (35). Further support for the role of embolization was provided following the introduction of CT imaging. Infarction was frequently in the territory of distal branches of the intracerebral vessels rather than in the border-zone or watershed areas, which might be expected to be preferentially affected if hemodynamic factors were most important. Further indirect evidence was provided by the observation that retinal and cerebral transient ischemic attacks (TIAs) usually occurred separately rather than coincidentally. This would favor multiple emboli rather than a single episode of hemodynamic compromise. More recently, direct evidence for the role of embolization has been provided by transcranial Doppler ultrasound (TCD) detection of circulating emboli (Fig. 4).

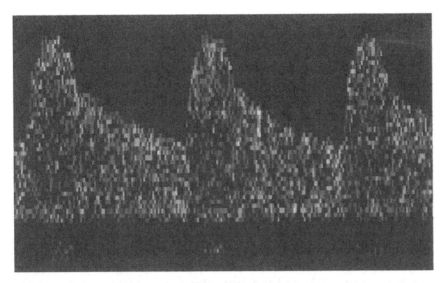

Figure 4 A Doppler embolic signal recorded in the ipsilateral middle cerebral artery in a patient with a symptomatic carotid stenosis. It can seen as a short duration high-intensity signal within the Doppler flow waveform. (Copyright with author.)

This technique allows us, for the first time, to visualize circulating emboli (36). They appear as short-duration high-intensity signals within the Doppler spectrum. In patients with carotid stenosis, recording is usually performed from the ipsilateral middle cerebral artery. Emboli are detected as high-intensity signals, because they reflect and backscatter more ultrasound than the surrounding smaller red blood cells. In vitro and animal studies have demonstrated that the technique has very high sensitivity and specificity, and can detect a wide variety of materials including platelet aggregates, thrombus, and atheromatous debris (37). The smallest size of embolus that can be detected remains uncertain because platelet, thrombus, or atheroma emboli smaller than 200 μm could not be individually introduced into experimental systems (37).

Doppler embolus detection has shown that asymptomatic embolization is surprisingly frequent. During recordings of 1 h, most studies have detected ipsilateral middle cerebral artery embolic signals in about 40% of patients with recently symptomatic carotid stenosis (38–41). A recent study using a prototype ambulatory system, in which recordings were performed continuously for 5 h, detected embolic signals in 11 of 12 patients (42). Although at first surprising, this high embolic load is consistent with previous studies showing multiple asymptomatic retinal emboli, and a pathological study in patients with carotid artery stroke who had multiple additional small areas of infarction (43). It emphasizes the dynamic nature of the embolic process. Therefore the clinical consequence of a single embolus is likely to depend on multiple factors, including embolus size, emboli frequency or "total embolic load", collateral supply, and the state of the vascular bed into which embolization occurs (44). The relevance of Doppler emboli signals as a marker of disease activity is supported by studies demonstrating that embolic signals are more frequent in categories of carotid stenosis patients known to be at a higher risk of recurrent stroke: in symptomatic vs. asymptomatic stenosis (39), with higher degrees of stenosis, with plaque ulceration (40,45–47), and with more recent symptoms (48). Furthermore, small studies have shown that embolic signals are an independent predictor of future stroke and TIA risk in both symptomatic and asymptomatic carotid stenosis (40–51) although no studies have yet been sufficiently powered to demonstrate association with stroke risk alone (Fig. 5).

Current technology does not allow reliable differentiation between platelet, thrombus, and cholesterol emboli. However in patients with symptomatic carotid stenosis, the number of embolic signals is reduced by antiplatelet agents (52), and they were almost completely abolished by the

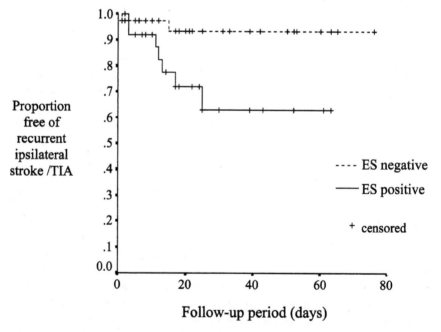

Figure 5 Prediction of stroke and TIA risk by Doppler embolic signals. The presence of embolic signals during a 1 h recording from the ipsilateral middle cerebral artery in patients with recently symptomatic carotid stenosis, predicted recurrent ipsilateral stroke, and TIA rate. *Source*: Modified From Ref. 39.

nitric oxide inhibitor, *S*-nitrosoglutathione (GSNO), which is a powerful inhibitor of platelet adhesion and aggregation (53). In contrast heparin has less effect on their frequency (54). This finding is consistent with recent trials which have shown that antiplatelet agents are, if anything, more effective than anticoagulants in preventing stroke recurrence (55), although these trials included patients with all types of ischemic stroke rather than being focused on carotid artery stroke.

4. HEMODYNAMIC FACTORS IN CAROTID STENOSIS STROKE

In the mid-20th century, hemodynamic insufficiency was a popular explanation for cerebral ischemic symptoms, particularly TIA, in patients with carotid artery stenosis (34). By analogy with peripheral arterial disease, the concept of "cerebral intermittent claudication" was proposed, although it is now accepted this does not apply to the majority of patients with TIA. In addition to the evidence highlighting the importance of embolization presented above, a number of other studies have suggested hemodynamic factors are not of primary importance in the majority of cases of carotid artery stroke. When blood pressure was artificially lowered, by means of hexamethonium and postural tilting, in 35 patients who had either experienced TIAs or known carotid artery disease, only one developed symptoms of focal cerebral ischemia before non-focal syncopal symptoms occurred. These non-focal symptoms signified global rather than focal ischemia of the brain (56). This is supported by the finding that hypotension, caused by cardiac dysrhythmias or other cardiac dysfunctions, usually results in syncope rather than focal ischemic symptoms. The striking difference in stroke risk between asymptomatic carotid stenosis and symptomatic carotid stenosis also argues against a hemodynamic cause, as does the clustering of increased recurrent stroke risk in the months following a symptomatic event. Furthermore, very tight carotid stenosis with distal collapse has been associated with a lower stroke rate than tight stenosis without collapse (57). Interestingly the frequency of asymptomatic emboli was lower in patients with very tight stenosis (40).

Cerebral hemodynamics can be measured distal to a carotid stenosis. Due to cerebral autoregulation, resting cerebral blood flow is usually preserved despite tight stenosis. However more detailed investigations can demonstrate hemodynamic compromise. As perfusion pressure distal to the stenosis falls, the resistance arterioles dilate to maintain cerebral blood flow. This results in an increase in cerebral blood volume. By measuring the cerebral blood volume to blood flow ratio, one can estimate the hemodynamic stress that the circulation is being placed under. Occasionally, if this is particularly severe and results in a drop in cerebral blood flow, a compensatory rise in oxygen extraction fraction (the amount of oxygen that is extracted from a unit volume of blood) can be shown. This measurement requires positron emission tomography (PET). A simpler way of estimating hemodynamic reserve is to measure cerebral blood flow before and after the administration of a vasodilator (58). In a compromised circulation, the vessels are already partially or fully vasodilated to maintain blood flow, and therefore the cerebral blood flow rise in response to the vasodilator is reduced. The vasodilators most commonly used are carbon dioxide (given in a concentration of 5–8% in air) or the carbonic anhydrase inhibitor acetazolamide. Many studies have used TCD measurement of cerebral blood flow velocity as a surrogate marker of cerebral blood flow. This appears valid as the middle cerebral artery diameter does not change during carbon dioxide inhalation (59). These studies have shown that in a subgroup of patients with carotid occlusion and tight carotid stenosis (>70%), there is impaired vasodilatory reserve or reactivity. Reactivity was found to be reduced in symptomatic compared with asymptomatic patients, and the presence of an impaired reactivity correlated with the extent of collateral supply, particularly the integrity of the Circle of Willis. In patients with carotid occlusion an impaired reactivity has been found to predict future TIA and stroke risk, but the evidence in asymptomatic carotid stenosis is less convincing (60–62) (Fig. 6).

It appears that hemodynamic factors may be more important in patients with carotid occlusion. The risk of stroke in this group is lower than that in patients with tight symptomatic carotid stenosis, again supporting the predominant role of embolization in stroke due to carotid stenosis. The role of extracranial–intracranial (ECIC) bypass and hemodynamic assessment of patients with carotid occlusion is discussed elsewhere in this volume.

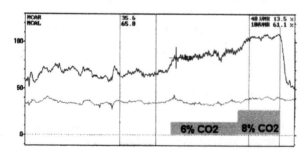

Figure 6 Impaired cerebral hemodynamics in a patient with carotid artery stenosis, measured using transcranial Doppler ultrasound. Increased inspired carbon dioxide (first 6% in air and then 8% in air) is given, which results in a marked increase in middle cerebral artery flow in normal individuals. In a patient with a hemodynamically significant carotid stenosis, this reactivity may be reduced or absent. In this patient with a right carotid occlusion, reactivity is normal in the left middle cerebral artery (top) but absent in the right middle cerebral artery (bottom). Severely impaired reactivity has been associated with an increased future stroke risk, particularly in patients with carotid artery occlusion. (Copyright with author.)

Although hemodynamic factors may not play a primary role in the pathogenesis of ischemic symptoms in most patients with carotid stenosis, they should not be entirely overlooked. There are a minority of patients in whom the distribution of infarction is consistent with hemodyamic factors being important. This includes infarcts both in the cortical border-zone areas between the middle cerebral artery and the anterior cerebral artery anteriorly, and the posterior cerebral artery posteriorly. It also includes patients with internal border-zone infarcts in the deep white matter, in the border-zone between the anterior, middle, and posterior artery main branch supply, and the deep arterial supply. There are also occasional patients with tight hemodynamically significant carotid stenosis who do develop stroke during an episode of systemic hypoperfusion. This may, for example, occur during cardiopulmonary bypass.

Hemodynamic factors are also likely to interact with embolization in determining whether emboli become symptomatic. Collateral supply, particularly by the Circle of Willis, plays a crucial role. For example, carotid occlusion can be accompanied by massive hemispheric infarction in the absence of a functioning Circle of Willis or be completely asymptomatic in the presence of adequate collateral supply. Hemodynamic factors, both perfusion pressure and intracerebral vessel responses, may determine whether an embolus results in permanent vessel occlusion or fragments with reperfusion.

It has been suggested that hemodynamic compromise secondary to internal carotid artery occlusion or stenosis can result in subtle cerebral damage without frank infarction, which can cause cognitive impairment. Some studies have shown an improvement in cognitive functioning following carotid endarterectomy, but this finding has not been consistent and could be influenced by biases such as natural recovery in function following symptomatic events (63). Improvement could also result from removal of an actively embolizing site. Changes in cerebral metabolism, which have improved following endarterectomy, have been reported with magnetic resonance spectroscopy. In particular a reduction in the neuronal marker *N*-acetyl aspartate (NAA) and an increase in the marker of anaerobic metabolism lactate have been found (64). However a recent study has failed to replicate these findings and has shown no relationship between NAA concentration and impairment of cerebral hemodynamics (65).

5. THE ACTIVE "CAROTID PLAQUE" IN HUMANS: CLINICAL STUDIES

Carotid stenosis is not a static process, but the plaque may become intermittently "active". This is emphasized by the marked difference in stroke risk between recently symptomatic tight carotid stenosis (10–20% in the first year) compared with asymptomatic carotid stenosis (2% per year). Multiple other lines of clinical evidence support the transient nature of this plaque activation. The risk of ischemic stroke ipsilateral to a severe carotid stenosis is higher soon after symptomatic presentation and then declines rapidly, even though the stenosis itself rarely regresses (66). Transient ischemic attacks also tend to cluster in time. The early recurrence rate following TIA or stroke is particularly high for carotid stenosis. Asymptomatic emboli detected with transcranial Doppler are much more frequent in patients with symptomatic carotid stenosis compared with asymptomatic stenosis (40), and rapidly reduce in frequency following a symptomatic event (38,48).

Natural history data, predominantly from the medical arms of the North American Symptomatic Carotid Endarterectomy Trial (NASCET) and the European Carotid Surgery Trial (ECST) (66,67), have shown that the risk of recurrent ipsilateral stroke after TIA or stroke remains elevated for about 2 years and then falls towards the risk seen in patients with asymptomatic stenosis (Fig. 7). The risk is particularly elevated within the first 6 months. If anything, the very early risk has been underestimated and two recent studies suggest it may be even higher (68,69). Possible cellular mechanisms of plaque instability, and information derived from the comparison of symptomatic and asymptomatic plaques on histological examination, were discussed earlier. Angiographic studies have demonstrated that plaque ulceration is associated with a higher recurrent stroke risk, initially for higher degrees of stenosis (70), and more recently across

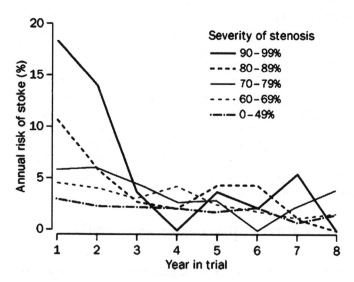

Figure 7 Data from the medical arm of the ECST study showing the risk of any major stroke in control patients by severity of stenosis and in each of the 8 years after randomization. *Source*: From Ref. 66.

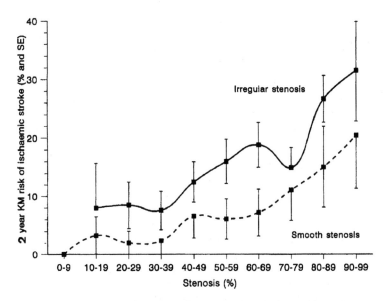

Figure 8 European Carotid Surgery Trial risk associated with ulceration two-year Kaplan-Meier (KM) risk of ischemic stroke in the territory of the symptomatic carotid artery according to the degree of carotid stenosis and angiographic appearance of the plaque surface in patients randomized to medical treatment only.

the full range from 10 to 99% stenosis (Fig. 8) (71). Patients presenting with hemispheric stroke and TIA have been found to have a higher risk of recurrent stroke than patients presenting with retinal ischemia (72). Some evidence suggests that systemic factors may be important. Active plaques in one vascular bed appear to be associated with active plaques in a remote location. This is supported by studies looking at multiple plaques in the coronary circulation using intravascular angioscopy and thermography (73), and also from angiographic data from the ECST. In this study surface irregularities, believed to arise from plaque rupture and ulceration, were found to predict an increased risk of arterial disease in other vascular beds, but not to depend on traditional vascular risk factors such as hyperlipidemia and hypertension. The authors propose the existence of, as yet undefined, systemic risk factors (74). It has been suggested that inflammation, and possibly chronic infection, could mediate this systemic activation. Epidemiological evidence suggests that low-grade systemic inflammation, as indicated by the acute phase reactant C-reactive protein (CRP), is associated with an increased risk of plaque destabilization. In the Bruneck study the natural history of carotid atherosclerosis was studied over a 5-year period by means of repeated high-resolution duplex ultrasound examination. Plaques with rapid growth (episodic marked increases in plaque size followed by long stable periods) were identified. This process was found not to be associated with baseline levels of traditional risk factors, but rather with increased thrombotic potential or impaired fibrinolysis. Peak levels of these risk variables appear to be more important than cumulative exposure (26).

Understanding the mechanisms of plaque activation has a major clinical importance. There are a number of therapeutic approaches which may intervene in the process. The use of statins have been proposed, as they appear to have plaque-stabilizing properties as well as cholesterol-lowering effects. Antibiotic therapy could reduce systemic infection and therefore inflammation although trials in coronary artery disease have not shown a consistent reduction in recurrent myocardial infarction rate.

REFERENCES

1. Lusis AJ. Atherosclerosis. Nature 2000; 407:233–241.
2. Glass CK, Witztum JL. Atherosclerosis: the road ahead. Cell 2001; 104: 503–516.
3. Libby P, Ridker PM, Maseri A. Inflammation and atherosclerosis. Circulation 2002; 105:1135–1143.
4. Celermajer DS. Endothelial dysfunction: Does it matter? Is it reversible? J Am Coll Cardiol 1997; 30:325–333.
5. Topper JN, Cai J, Falb D, Gimbrone MA. Identification of vascular endothelial genes differentially responsive to fluid mechanical stimuli: cyclooxygenase-2, manganese superoxide dismutase, and endothelial cell nitric oxide synthase are selectively up-regulated by steady laminar shear stress. Proc Natl Acad Sci USA 1996; 93:10417–10422.
6. Gimbrone MA. Vascular endothelium, hemodynamic forces, and atherogenesis. Am J Pathol 1999; 155:1–5.
7. Skalen K, Gustafsson M, Rydberg EK, Hulten LM, Wiklund O, Innerarity TL, Boren J. Subendothelial retention of atherogenic lipoproteins in early atherosclerosis. Nature 2002; 417:750–754.
8. Gu L, Okada Y, Clinton S, Gerand C, Sukhorn GK, Libby P, Rollins BJ. Absence of monocyte chemoattractant protein-1 reduces atherosclerosis in low-density lipoprotein-deficient mice. Mol Cell 1998; 2:275–281.
9. Smith JD, Trogan E, Ginsberg M, Grigaux C, Tian J, Miyata M. Decreased atherosclerosis in mice deficient in both macrophage colony-stimulating factor (op) and apolipoprotein E. Proc Natl Acad Sci USA 1995; 92:8264–8268.
10. Ridker PM, Cushman M, Stampfer MJ, Tracy RP, Hennekens CH. Inflammation, aspirin, and the risk of cardiovascular disease in apparently healthy men. N Eng J Med 1997; 336:973–979.
11. Grayston JT. Antibiotic treatment of atherosclerotic cardiovascular disease. Circulation 2003; 107:1228–1230.
12. Golledge J, Greenhalgh RM, Davies AH. The symptomatic carotid plaque. Stroke 2000; 31:774–781.
13. Loree HM, Kamm RD, Stringfellow RG, Lee RT. Effects of fibrous cap thickness on peak circumferential stress in model atherosclerotic vessels. Circ Res 1992; 71:850–858.

14. Seeger JM, Barratt E, Lawson GA, Klingman N. The relationship between carotid plaque composition, plaque morphology and neurologic symptoms. J Surg Res 1995; 58:330–336.
15. Sitzer M, Puac D, Buehler A, Steckel DA, von Kegler S, Markus HS, Steinmetz H. Internal carotid artery angle of origin. A novel risk factor for early carotid atherosclerosis. Stroke 2003; 34:950–955.
16. Malek AM, Alper SL, Izumo S. Hemodynamic shear stress and its role in atherosclerosis. JAMA 1999; 282:2035–2042.
17. Newby AC, Zaltsman AB. Molecular mechanisms in intimal hyperplasia. J Pathol 2000; 190:300–309.
18. Ojha M, Cobbold RS, Johnston KW. Influence of angle on wall shear stress distribution for an end-to-side anastomosis. J Vasc Surg 1994; 19:1067–1073.
19. Hazel AL, Pedley TJ. Alteration of mean wall shear stress near an oscillating stagnation point. J Biomech Eng 1998; 120:227–237.
20. Kornet L, Lambregts J, Hoeks AP, Reneman RS. Differences in near-wall shear rate in the carotid artery within subjects are associated with different intima-media thicknesses. Arterioscler Thromb Vasc Biol 1998; 18:1877–1884.
21. Jerrard-Dunne P, Markus HS, Steckel DA, Buehler A, von Kegler S, Sitzer M. Early carotid atherosclerosis and family history of myocardial infarction and stroke — specific effects on arterial sites have implications for genetic studies: The Carotid Atherosclerosis Progression Study (CAPS). Arterioscler Thromb Vasc Biol 2003; 23:302–306.
22. Jartti L, Ronnemaa T, Kaprio J, Jarvisalo MJ, Toikka JO, Marniemi J, Hammar N, Alfredsson L, Saraste M, Hartiala J, Koskenvuo M, Raitakari OT. Population-based twin study of the effects of migration from Finland to Sweden on endothelial function and intima-media thickness. Arterioscler Thromb Vasc Biol 2002; 22:832–837.
23. Bonithon-Kopp C, Touboul PJ, Berr C, Magne C. Ducimetiere P. Factors of carotid arterial enlargement in a population aged 59 to 71 years: the EVA study. Stroke 1996; 27:654–660.
24. Kiechl S, Willeit J. The natural course of atherosclerosis. I. Incidence and progression. Arterioscler Thromb Vasc Biol 2000; 20:529–537.
25. Kiechl S, Willeit J. The natural course of atherosclerosis. II. Vascular remodelling. Arterioscler Thromb Vasc Biol 2000; 20:529–537.
26. Willeit J, Kiechl S. Biology of arterial atheroma. Cerebrovasc Dis 2000; 10(suppl 5):1–8.
27. Brice JG, Dowsett DJ, Lowe RD. Hameodynamic effects of carotid artery stenosis. Brit Med J 1964; 2:1363–1366.
28. Virchow RLK. Ueber die akute entzündung der arterien. Archiv Pathologie Anatomie 1847; 1:272–378.
29. Chiari H. Über das verhalten des teilungswinkels des carotis communis bei endarteritis chronica deformans. Verhandlungen der Deutschen Pathologique Gessellschaft 1905; 9:326–330.
30. Fieschi C, Argentino C, Lenzi GL, Sacchetti ML, Toni D, Bozzao L. Clinical and instrumental evaluation of patients with ischemic stroke within the first six hours. J Neurol Sci 1989; 91:311–321.

31. Zanette EM, Roberti C, Mancini G, Pozzilli C, Bragoni M, Toni D. Spontaneous middle cerebral artery reperfusion in ischemic stroke. A follow-up study with transcranial Doppler. Stroke 1995; 26:210–213.

32. Fisher CM. Observations on the fundus oculi in transient monocular blindness. Neurology 1959; 9:333–347.

33. Ross Russell RW. Observations on the retinal blood-vessels in monocular blindness. Lancet 1961; 11:1422–1428.

34. Warlow CP, Dennis MS, van Gijn J, Hankey GJ, Sandercock PAG, Bamford JM, Wardlaw JM. Stroke. In: A Practical Guide to Management. 2nd ed. Oxford, UK: Blackwell Science, 2001:ch. 1, pp. 1–27.

35. Rothwell PM, Gibson R, Warlow CP. (on behalf of the European Carotid Surgery Trialists' Collaborative Group). Interrelation between plaque surface morphology and degree of stenosis on carotid angiograms and the risk of ischemic stroke in patients with symptomatic carotid stenosis. Stroke 2000; 31:615–621.

36. Markus HS. Monitoring embolism in real time. Circulation 2000; 102:826–828.

37. Markus HS, Tegeler C. Experimental aspects of high-intensity transient signals in the detection of emboli. J Clin Ultrasound 1995; 23:81–87.

38. Siebler M, Sitzer M, Rose G, Bendfeldt D, Steinmetz H. Silent cerebral embolism caused by neurologically symptomatic high-grade carotid stenosis. Event rates before and after carotid endarterectomy. Brain 1993; 116:1005–1015.

39. Markus HS, Thomson N, Brown MM. Asymptomatic cerebral embolic signals in symptomatic and asymptomatic carotid artery disease. Brain 1995; 118: 1005–1011.

40. Molloy J, Markus HS. Asymptomatic embolisation predicts stroke and TIA risk in patients with carotid artery stenosis. Stroke 1999; 30:1440–1443.

41. Georgiadis D, Lindner A, Manz M, Sonntag M, Zunker P, Zerkowski HR, Borggrege M. Intracranial microembolic signals in 500 patients with potential cardiac or carotid embolic source and in normal controls. Stroke 1997; 28:1203–1207..

42. MacKinnon AD, Aaslid R, Markus HS. Long term ambulatory monitoring for cerebral emboli using transcranial Doppler ultrasound. Stroke. 2004; 35: 73–78.

43. Heye N, Paetzold C, Steinberg R, Cervos-Navarro J. The topography of microthrombi in ischaemic brain infarct. Acta Neurol Scand 1992; 86:450–454.

44. Caplan LR, Hennerici M. Impaired clearance of emboli (washout) is an important link between hypoperfusion, embolism, and ischemic stroke. Arch Neurol 1998; 55:1475–1482.

45. Orlandi G, Parenti G, Bertolucci A, Puglioli M, Collavoli P, Murri L. Carotid plaque features on angiography and asymptomatic cerebral microembolism. Acta Neurol Scand 1997; 96:183–186.

46. Valton L, Larrue V, Arrue P, Geraud G, Bes A. Asymptomatic cerebral embolic signals in patients with carotid stenosis: correlation with the appearance of plaque ulceration on angiography. Stroke 1995; 26:813–815.

47. Sitzer M, Muller W, Siebler M, Hort W, Kniemeyer HW, Jancke L, Steinmetz H. Plaque ulceration and lumen thrombus are the main sources of cerebral microemboli in high-grade internal carotid artery stenosis. Stroke 1995; 26:1231–1233.

48. Forteza AM, Babikian VL, Hyde C, Winter M, Pochay V. Effect of time and cerebrovascular symptoms on the prevalence of microembolic signals in patients with cervical carotid stenosis. Stroke 1996; 27:687–690.
49. Siebler M, Nachtmann A, Sitzer M, Rose G, Kleinschmidt A, Rademacher J, Steinmetz H. Cerebral microembolism and the risk of ischaemia in asymptomatic high-grade internal carotid artery ischaemia. Stroke 1995; 26:2184–2186.
50. Valton L, Larrue V, Le Traon AP, Massabuau P, Gerard G. Microembolic signals and risk of early recurrence in patients with stroke or transient ischaemic attack. Stroke 1998; 29:2125–2128.
51. Censori B, Partziguian T, Castro L, Camerlingo M, Mamoli A. Doppler microembolic signals predict ischaemic recurrences in symptomatic carotid stenosis. Acta Neurol Scand 2000; 101:327–331.
52. Goertler M, Baeumer M, Kross R, Blaser T, Lutze G, Jost S, Wallesch CW. Rapid decline of cerebral microemboli of arterial origin after intravenous acetylsalicylic acid. Stroke 1999; 30:66–69.
53. Kaposzta Z, Martin JF, Markus HS. Switching off embolisation from the symptomatic carotid plaque using s-nitrosoglutathione. Circulation 2002; 105:1480–1484.
54. Goertler M, Blaser T, Krueger S, Hofmann K, Baeumer M, Wallesch CW. Cessation of embolic signals after antithrombotic prevention is related to reduced risk of recurrent arterioembolic transient ischaemic attack and stroke. J Neurol Neurosurg Psychiatr 2002; 72:338–342.
55. Mohr JP, Thompson JL, Lazar RM, Levin B, Sacco RL, Furie KL, Kistler JP, Albers GW, Pettigrew LC, Adams HP Jr, Jackson CM, Pullicino P. Warfarin-Aspirin Recurrent Stroke Study Group. A comparison of warfarin and aspirin for the prevention of recurrent ischemic stroke. N Engl J Med 2001; 345: 1444–1451.
56. Kendell RE, Marshall J. Role of hypotension in the genesis of transient focal cerebral ischaemic attacks. Brit Med J 1963; 2:344–348.
57. Morgenstern LB, Fox AJ, Sharpe BL, Eliasziw M, Barnett HJ, Grotta JC. [North American Symptomatic Carotid Endarterectomy Trial (NASCET) Group]. The risks and benefits of carotid endarterectomy in patients with near occlusion of the carotid artery. Neurology 1997; 48:911–915.
58. Ringelstein EB, Sievers C, Ecker S, Schneider PA, Otis SM. Noninvasive assessment of CO_2-induced cerebral vasomotor response in normal individuals and patients with internal carotid artery occlusions. Stroke 1988; 19:963–969.
59. Huber P, Handa J. Effect of contrast material, hypercapnia, hyperventilation, hypertonic glucose and papaverine on the diameter of cerebral arteries. Invest Radiol 1967; 2:17–32.
60. Kleiser B, Widder B. Course of carotid artery occlusions with impaired carbon dioxide reactivity. Stroke 1992; 23:171–174.
61. Webster MW, Makaroun MS, Steed DL, Smith HA, Johnson DW, Yonas H. Compromised cerebral blood flow reactivity is a predictor of stroke in patients with symptomatic carotid artery occlusive disease. J Vasc Surg 1995; 21: 338–344.

62. Markus H, Cullinane M. Severely impaired cerebrovascular reactivity predicts stroke and TIA risk in patients with carotid artery stenosis and occlusion. Brain 2001; 124:457–467.

63. Lunn S, Crawley F, Harrison MJH, Brown MM, Newman SP. Impact of carotid endarterectomy upon cognitive functioning. Cerebrovasc Dis 1999; 9: 74–81.

64. Visser GH, van der GJ, van Huffelen AC, Wieneke GH, Eikelboom BC. Decreased transcranial Doppler carbon dioxide reactivity is associated with disordered cerebral metabolism in patients with internal carotid artery stenosis. J Vasc Surg 1999; 30:252–260.

65. Lythgoe D, Perriera A, Cullinane M, Doyle V, Williams SCR, Markus HS. The relationship between N acetyl aspartate and impaired haemodynamics in patients with carotid artery disease. J Neurol Neurosurg Psychiatr 2001; 71:58–62.

66. European Carotid Surgery Trialists' Collaborative Group. Randomised trial of endarterectomy for recently symptomatic carotid stenosis: final results in the MRC European Carotid Surgery Trial (ECST). Lancet 1998; 351:1379–1387.

67. Barnett HJ, Taylor DW, Eliasziw M, Fox AJ, Ferguson GG, Haynes RB, Rankin RN, Clagett GP, Hachinski VC, Sackett DL, Thorpe KE, Meldrum HE. (for the North American Symptomatic Carotid Endarterectomy Trial Collaborators). Benefit of carotid endarterectomy in patients with symptomatic moderate or severe stenosis. N Eng J Med 1998; 339:1415–1425.

68. Johnston SC, Gress DR, Browner WS, Sidney S. Short-term prognosis after emergency department diagnosis of TIA. JAMA 2000; 284:2901–2906.

69. Lovett JK, Dennis MS, Sandercock PAG, Bamford J, Warlow CP, Rothwell PM. Very early risk of stroke after a first transient ischemic attack. Stroke 2003; 34:e139–e142.

70. Eliasziw M, Streifler JY, Fox AJ, Hachinski VC, Ferguson GG, Barnett HJ. Significance of plaque ulceration in symptomatic patients with high-grade carotid stenosis. North American Symptomatic Carotid Endarterectomy Trial. Stroke 1994; 25:304–308.

71. Rothwell PM, Gibson R, Warlow CP. Interrelation between plaque surface morphology and degree of stenosis on carotid angiograms and the risk of ischemic stroke in patients with symptomatic carotid stenosis. Stroke 2000; 31:615–621.

72. Benavente O, Eliasziw M, Streifler JY, Fox AJ, Barnett HJ, Meldrum H. (North American Symptomatic Carotid Endarterectomy Trial Collaborators). Prognosis after transient monocular blindness associated with carotid-artery stenosis. N Engl J Med 2001; 345:1084–1090.

73. Casscells W, Naghavi M, Willerson JT. Vulnerable atherosclerotic plaque. A multifocal disease. Circulation 2003; 107:2072–2075.

74. Rothwell PM, Villagra R, Gibson R, Donders R, Warlow CP. Evidence of a chronic systemic cause of instability of atherosclerotic plaques. Lancet 2000; 355:19–24.

4

Carotid Imaging—Is Angiography Still Needed?

David Pelz

Department of Diagnostic Radiology and Clinical Neurological Sciences, London Health Sciences Centre, University Campus, London, Ontario, Canada

1. INTRODUCTION

Digital subtraction angiography (DSA) is currently the gold standard for the accurate measurement of carotid artery bifurcation stenosis. The supremacy of this invasive technique is being strongly challenged as the quality, reliability, and validity of the less-invasive modalities such as duplex carotid ultrasound (DUS), magnetic resonance angiography (MRA), and computed tomographic angiography (CTA) steadily improve. This chapter will briefly review the current status of DSA for the investigation of carotid bifurcation stenosis, including the common angiographic appearances of atherosclerotic disease and the risks of the procedure. Magnetic resonance angiography and CTA will also be discussed, and their current relationship to DSA will be reviewed. Duplex carotid ultrasound is covered in another chapter. Finally, recommendations for carotid imaging in the future will be made.

2. DIGITAL SUBTRACTION ANGIOGRAPHY

2.1. Technique

The basic techniques of transfemoral catheterization have changed remarkably little since the original description by Seldinger in 1953 (1). Following a femoral puncture using an 18 or 19 gauge needle, a 5 or 6 French sheath is placed in the femoral artery. Most centers will administer an intravenous (IV) bolus of 2000 IU heparin for routine diagnostic studies, and use continuous heparinized saline flushes (3000 IU per 500 mL saline) for the catheters. Selective catheterizations of cerebral vessels are performed with guidewires (typically 0.035 in. diameter or smaller) and 4–6 French catheters, which come in a variety of shapes, with many having hydrophilic coatings. The use of non-ionic, low-osmolar contrast material and biplane DSA units with 1024×1024 matrix size are now routine, and computerized rotational angiography (CRA) is becoming commercially available for 3-dimensional (3D) vascular imaging. Selective common carotid artery injections of 8–12 cc are commonly used, and at least two orthogonal views of the carotid bifurcation are required, with oblique views often being helpful for complex lesions. Following the procedure, manual compression of the puncture site is recommended, although compression and closure devices are available. Supervised nursing observation is necessary for at least 1 h, and the patient must remain supine for 4–6 h. Transbrachial and transradial approaches using smaller catheters are gaining popularity (2,3).

2.2. Complications

The most common complication of DSA is stroke, usually caused by emboli related to clot formation on guidewires or catheters, or dislodgement of plaque or clot from the arterial wall, leading to distal branch occlusion. The risk of transient ischemic deficit has been reported to vary between 0.5 and 4.0% (4,5) with permanent deficits from 0.1 to 1.0% (6,7). Two prospective studies have shown stroke rates of 0.6–0.7% in patients being investigated for atherosclerotic disease, with hypertension, diabetes, longer procedure times, larger contrast dosages, and advanced age all being significant risk factors (6,7). There is a 5–10% risk of significant hematoma formation at the puncture site and 0.3–1.5% may need surgical evacuation (8). The incidence of life-threatening, anaphylactic reactions to the low-osmolar contrast agents is low, it being 0.04% in the largest series of patients (9).

2.3. Atherosclerotic Disease—Angiographic Appearance

2.3.1. Carotid Bulb

Carotid atherosclerosis has many angiographic manifestations, but the bulb is nearly always involved and is the source of 90% of thromboembolic strokes. Digital subtraction angiography most commonly shows irregularity and luminal stenosis of the bulb and proximal 2–3 cm of the internal carotid artery (ICA) (Fig. 1). The stenosis may be smooth, irregular, or ulcerated and usually involves the posterior wall. The lesion must be seen on at least two orthogonal views and oblique views or CRA may be necessary to avoid

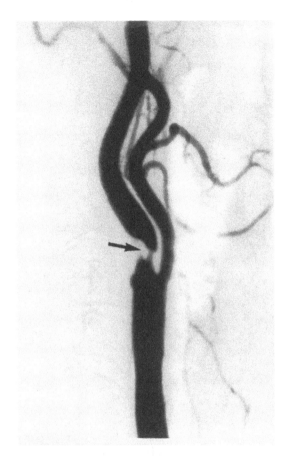

Figure 1 Common carotid DSA, lateral view. Severe atherosclerotic stenosis of the proximal ICA (arrow).

the stenosis measurement pitfalls of tortuosity, external carotid artery (ECA) overlap, web-like stenosis, and overhanging plaque. Ulceration is likely the commonest cause of emboli (10) and is seen as a classic ulcer niche in profile or as a double density en face (Fig. 2). However, DSA may be relatively insensitive for the detection of ulceration, missing between 14 and 47% of pathologically proven ulceration in post-operative specimens (11). Intraluminal thrombus, a relative contra-indication to immediate intervention, is seen as a polypoid or linear-filling defect, surrounded on three sides by contrast (12) (Fig. 3).

As the degree of stenosis increases, the diameter of the internal carotid artery beyond the lesion eventually decreases, thus invalidating most measurement schemes (see Sec. 2.3.2). In the early stages, this may be difficult to appreciate, but the term "approaching near-occlusion" has been used

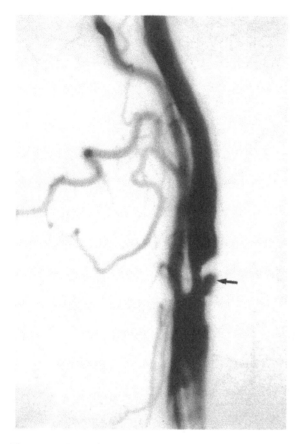

Figure 2 Common carotid DSA, oblique view. A classic ulcer niche is seen in the profile (arrow).

to describe this condition, which is arbitrarily assigned a severity of >95%. Angiographic clues include an ICA diameter less than or equal to the adjacent ECA (Fig. 4), filling of terminal ECA branches prior to pial cerebral vessels, and spontaneous filling of ipsilateral collateral channels (13).

Near-occlusion produces the classic "string" sign (Fig. 5), and a prolonged film run may be necessary to show slow, antegrade filling of the distal ICA and continuity with the intracranial circulation. Complete occlusion of the ICA may be blunt, rounded, or pointed, and a cone shape may be indistinguishable from dissection or tapered thrombus (Fig. 6).

2.3.2. Measurement of Carotid Stenosis

The three commonest methods are summarized in Fig. 7.

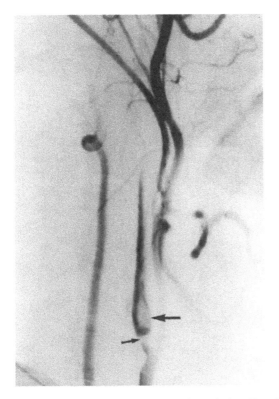

Figure 3 Common carotid DSA, lateral view. Intraluminal thrombus (large arrow) is seen just beyond a severe stenosis of the proximal ICA (small arrow).

i. *NASCET (North American Symptomatic Carotid Endarterectomy Trial) Method:* This method compares the linear measurement of the minimal residual lumen (MRL) on the view that shows the narrowest stenosis to the normal ICA, well beyond the bulb where the vessel walls are parallel (14).

ii. *ECST (European Carotid Surgery Trial) Method:* This method compares the MRL to the estimated normal diameter of the carotid bulb (15).

iii. *CSI (Carotid Stenosis Index or Common Carotid) Method:* This method compares the MRL to the diameter of the normal common carotid artery.

There have been criticisms of each of these schemes. Although it is likely the most commonly used (16), the NASCET method tends to underestimate disease severity by comparing the MRL of the bulb to the smaller distal ICA, not to the bulb itself. The ECST method is theoretically more

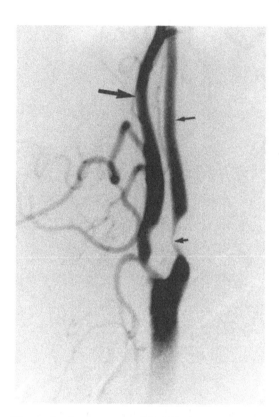

Figure 4 Common carotid DSA, lateral view. "Approaching" near-occlusion, or >95% stenosis. The ICA (small arrow) is decreased in caliber beyond a severe stenosis (arrowhead) and is smaller than the adjacent internal maxillary artery (large arrow).

valid, but depends on a hypothetical, subjective measurement of the normal bulb. The CSI method may be the most accurate, but it is not commonly used. The disparity between the NASCET and ECST measurement schemes was recently addressed (17). A re-measurement of all pre-randomization angiograms from the ECST and a re-definition of outcome events according to NASCET showed that the results of the two trials were consistent, i.e., surgery is beneficial for stenoses of 70–99%, with a moderate benefit in the 50–69% range. Surprisingly, there was no benefit for surgery in patients with near-, or "approaching" near-occlusion stenoses. This suggests that the discrimination of these patients from those with complete occlusion, a commonly cited failing of the less-invasive investigative modalities, may not be of any clinical significance. The authors recommend that the NASCET method be the universally accepted technique for measurement of carotid bifurcation stenosis.

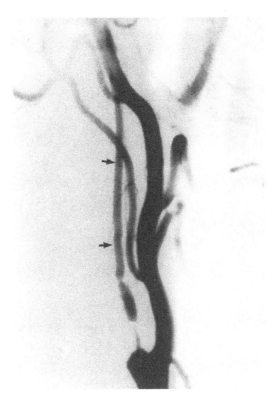

Figure 5 Common carotid DSA, lateral view. Near-occlusion of the ICA, producing the classic "string" sign (small arrows).

2.3.3. Magnetic Resonance Angiography

Magnetic resonance angiography is the result of the flow-sensitive nature of magnetic resonance imaging (MRI). The techniques are evolving and acquisition sequences are becoming shorter as technology improves. The two basic types of MRA are time-of-flight (TOF) and phase contrast (PC).

2.3.3.1. Time-of-Flight MRA: This technique is based on the principle of flow-related enhancement, or the difference in magnetization between flowing blood and adjacent stationary soft tissues. Flowing blood may be seen as a signal void ("black blood") or as a high signal in a vessel ("bright blood") due to the inflow of fully magnetized blood or intravenous contrast material [contrast-enhanced MRA (CEMRA)]. The acquisitions may be 2-dimensional (2D) or 3D. The 2D acquisitions are faster and more sensitive to slow flow, but the slice thickness is higher and the signal-to-noise ratio (SNR) is lower than in 3D (Fig. 8). The commonly used multiple overlapping thin slab angiography (MOTSA) sequence is a relatively fast 3D

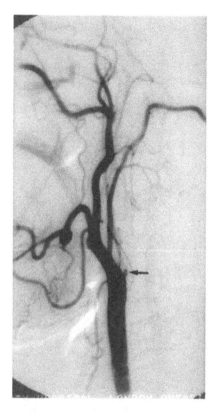

Figure 6 Common carotid DSA, lateral view. Complete occlusion of the ICA, with a small stump (arrow).

technique, which provides excellent rotational images of focal vascular regions (Fig. 9). The "black blood" techniques are not optimal for stenosis measurement, but may be better for actual tissue characterization of atherosclerotic plaque.

2.3.3.2. Phase Contrast MRA: This technique uses velocity-induced phase shifts to show blood flow. Gradient echo sequences are used to suppress background and to provide better characterization of both flow velocity and direction than TOF MRA. Both 2D and 3D acquisitions are used, and both arteries and veins are visualized (Fig. 10). Acquisition times are generally longer than for TOF techniques.

2.3.3.3. Contrast-enhanced MRA: This 3D-TOF technique, which uses a bolus of intravenous gadolinium to enhance the images, is rapidly gaining popularity for vascular imaging. The paramagnetic effects of gadolinium shorten the intravascular T1 relaxation time, thus increasing the

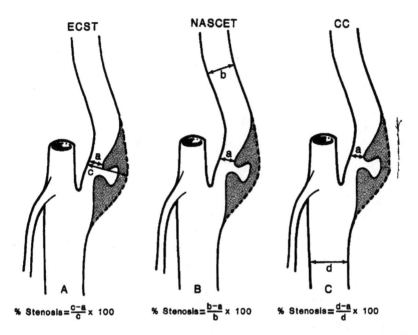

Figure 7 Measurement of carotid stenosis (from Osborn AG. Atherosclerosis and carotid stenosis. In: Diagnostic cerebral angiography. Philadelphia: Lippincott Williams & Wilkins, 1999:73.)

signal intensity of blood relative to surrounding soft tissues and decreasing acquisition times. The use of multiple overlapping (phased-array) coils allows routine visualization of the entire cerebral vasculature, from the aortic arch to the Circle of Willis and first-order branches (Fig. 11). The disadvantages of this technique include the increased cost of contrast material, the need for an intravenous injection, and the need for precise timing of image acquisition to the arrival of the contrast bolus in the vessels of interest.

All TOF and PC MRA images are post-processed, in which the vascular structures are isolated by maximum intensity pixel (MIP) detection, and then re-projected in a rotational format, which is more familiar to clinicians. Both the source images and re-projected datasets can be utilized for diagnostic purposes.

2.3.3.4. Limitations of MRA: The spatial resolution of most MRA techniques remains lower than that of DSA, by approximately 50%. There are many confusing artifacts, usually the result of slow flow and turbulence, which can lead to signal loss and over-estimation of stenosis. Post-processing artifacts from blood clots in a vessel, metal in dental work, or aneurysm clips can all cause image distortion. The vascular field of view may be relatively limited, unless phased array coils are used. Magnetic resonance angiography is exquisitely sensitive to motion, and most sequences take at least 2–10 min to

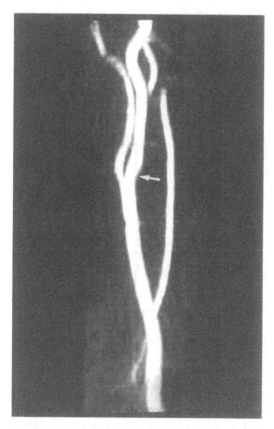

Figure 8 3D-TOF MRA, sagittal view, of a normal carotid bifurcation (arrow).

acquire data. As is generally the case with MRI, claustrophobia is a significant problem and patients with pacemakers and older aneurysm clips cannot be imaged.

2.3.3.5. Magnetic Resonance Angiography of Carotid Bifurcation Atherosclerotic Stenosis: Magnetic resonance angiography has been used to image carotid stenosis for over 13 years, and this technique can elegantly demonstrate severe atherosclerotic disease, including ulceration (Figs. 12–14). The sensitivity and specificity relative to the gold standard, DSA, have been steadily improving. A recent meta-analysis (18) of 126 papers published between 1990 and 1999 showed joint sensitivity and specificity of 99% for 70–79% stenosis by NASCET criteria, and 90% for 50–99% stenosis. Only four of these studies, however, included CEMRA, and many of the papers were of a low quality with heterogeneous patient groups, leading the authors to conclude that MRA is not yet good enough to replace DSA for the diagnosis

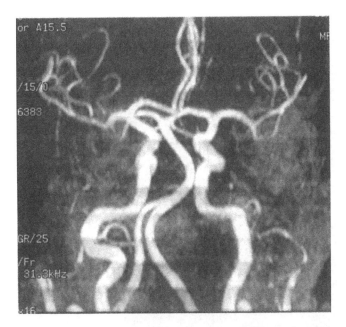

Figure 9 MOTSA MRA of the Circle of Willis, coronal view.

of 50–99% stenosis, and that studies which directly address clinical decision-making are needed. Contrast-enhanced MRA is rapidly gaining popularity as a follow-up procedure after screening DUS, yet a recent comparison study with DSA in 50 patients with carotid stenosis (19) showed that 24% would have been misclassified for carotid endarterectomy (CEA) on the basis of MRA alone. This rate decreased to 17% if the results of DUS were included. A more recent evaluation of CEMRA showed agreement with DSA in 89% of 240 imaged vessels (20). Another study of 167 consecutive symptomatic patients found that for the detection of severe stenosis, CEMRA had a sensitivity of 93.0% and a specificity of 80.6% with a misclassification rate of 15.0% (21). Other authors have recommended the DUS and MRA combination as a worthy alternative to DSA for deciding on the need for CEA (22–25) with misclassification rates as low as 8% (23). There is general agreement, however, that many of the early comparison studies are flawed (26,27), that MRA still tends to overestimate moderate disease, is not yet sensitive enough to distinguish complete from near-occlusion or reliably demonstrate collateral flow, and that this technique alone cannot yet replace DSA for accurate decision-making (28).

2.3.3.6. Magnetic Resonance Imaging of Carotid Bifurcation Plaque: Magnetic resonance imaging has the ability to image all three layers

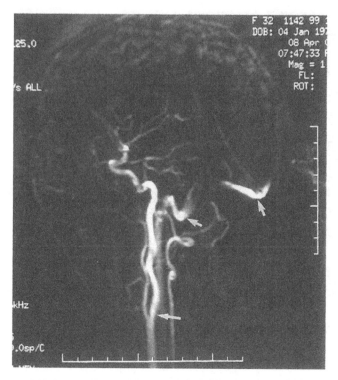

Figure 10 2D-PC MRA, sagittal view, of a normal carotid bifurcation (arrow). There is also a demonstration of normal dural venous sinuses (arrowheads).

of the vessel wall, and there is abundant animal evidence that all stages of plaque evolution can be characterized, from intimal thickening to intra-plaque hemorrhage (29). In vivo human plaque imaging using clinical 1.5 Tesla units and standard neck coils can differentiate the fibrous cap from the lipid core. Magnetic resonance imaging demonstrations of ulceration, intra-plaque hemorrhage, and calcification have all been shown to correlate well with post-operative specimens. It has been used to monitor the intimal response to balloon angioplasty of popliteal arteries. Active areas of research include the magnetic resonance features of plaque, which may be predictive of future rupture and embolus generation, and the use of gadolinium to better elucidate plaque structure (30). Carotid plaque burden may be the best indicator of the outcome for studies evaluating dietary and drug treatments for stroke, and high resolution MRI (to 250 μm) can accurately quantitate plaque progression and regression (31), geometry, and shear stress at the carotid bifurcation. In the near future, reliable measurements of plaque burden and composition will be standard additions to the morphologic data of MRA.

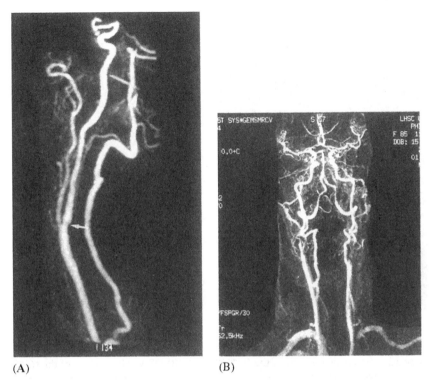

(A) (B)

Figure 11 (A) CEMRA, sagittal view, showing a normal carotid bifurcation (arrow). (B) CEMRA, coronal view, showing the cerebral vasculature from the aortic arch to the Circle of Willis.

2.3.4. Computer Tomography Angiography

Recent advances in rapid, multi-slice computer tomography (CT) technology have revolutionized the acquisition of vascular data. An intravenous bolus of contrast material is followed by a high-speed spiral CT scan that produces excellent, computer-generated images of large and medium-sized vessels (Fig. 15). For carotid imaging, approximately 120 mL of low-osmolar contrast material is injected at 3 mL/s, and 3 mm helical scans are performed from at least C6 or below to the skull base. Three-dimensional MIP images and shaded surface displays are generated at a computer workstation, with a processing time of ~20 min. The advantages of computer tomography angiography (CTA) over MRA are the relatively short acquisition times (~1 min), the accessibility of CT, and the lack of concern over claustrophobia, pacemakers, and metallic hardware. Theoretically, CTA should be free of the artifacts caused by slow flow or turbulence. The disadvantages are the use of iodinated contrast material and ionizing radiation, and the effects of calcification on bifurcation stenosis measurement.

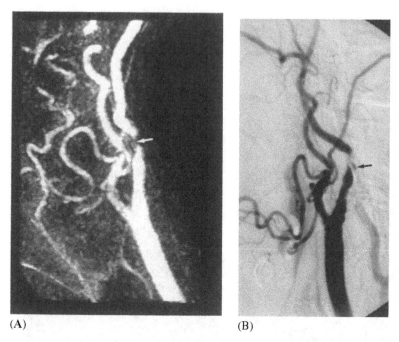

(A)   (B)

Figure 12 (A) CEMRA, sagittal view, of the right carotid bifurcation, showing a severe atherosclerotic stenosis of the ICA (arrow). (B) DSA, lateral view, of the same vessel, showing the severe stenosis with ulceration (arrow), which was not appreciated on the CEMRA.

2.3.4.1. Computer Tomography Angiography of Carotid Bifurcation Atherosclerotic Stenosis: The CTA of carotid atherosclerosis has been performed for approximately 10 years, and despite recent technologic advances, sensitivities and specificities of CTA relative to DSA have remained relatively static. Early studies, which relied more on the axial source imaging of bifurcation disease (32–34), showed variable results, with significant over-estimation of disease and insensitivity to ulceration (32), and reasonable accuracy (82%) relative to DSA (34). A more recent work (35) has shown a good correlation with DSA for mild diseases and complete ICA occlusion (Fig. 16), but difficulty in the reliable differentiation of moderate (50–69%) from severe (70–99%) stenosis (Fig. 17). Heavy bifurcation calcification can hinder stenosis measurement in up to 30% of cases (Fig. 18), and tandem stenoses can be missed due to obscuration of the carotid siphon by the skull base. Up to 21% of patients would have been misclassified for CEA on the basis of CTA alone in one series (34). Other groups have found better correlation with DSA in small numbers of patients (35–37). In a series in which 81 vessels were compared for CTA and DSA, CTA had an excellent negative predictive value

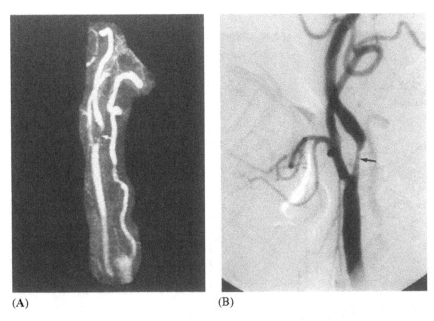

(A)   (B)

Figure 13 (A) CEMRA, sagittal view, showing a very severe stenosis of the proximal ICA (arrowhead). (B) DSA, lateral view, of the same vessel, again showing a severe stenosis that was overestimated by CEMRA.

(100%) for ruling out >70% stenosis, but there was a tendency for over-estimation of stenosis. In eight cases where CTA reported >70% stenosis, it was confirmed by angiography in only 63% (38). It is clear that at the present time, CTA alone cannot yet reliably select patients for carotid intervention, and that more work needs to be done to validate the technique relative to DSA.

2.3.4.2. Computer Tomography Angiography of Carotid Bifurcation Plaque: Considerable effort has been made to characterize the "vulnerable" plaque using CT. The ability to quantitate plaque content using Hounsfield numbers has allowed the demonstration of necrotic lipid debris, fibrosis, and calcification (39). Unfortunately, most comparison studies have shown that DUS is better at characterizing the histological components of bifurcation plaque, and there has as yet been no correlation between CT findings and clinical ischemic events. Problems include the timing of the contrast bolus, the distorting effects of calcification, difficulties identifying vessel wall components, and lengthy computer processing times.

2.3.5. Recommendations

Both MRA and CTA are promising techniques for the accurate depiction of carotid bifurcation stenosis, but the critical factor determining the utility of

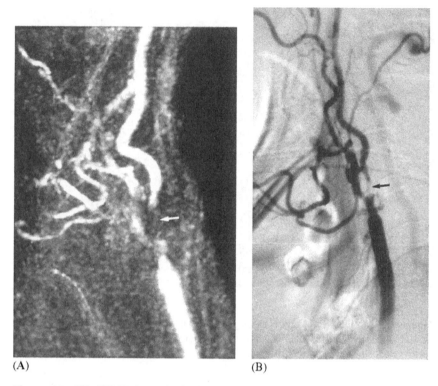

(A)   (B)

Figure 14 (A) CEMRA, sagittal view, of the left carotid bifurcation, showing a severe stenosis of the proximal ICA, manifested by a signal void in the stenotic segment (arrow). (B) DSA, lateral view, of the same vessel, showing the severe stenosis (arrow) which is actually "approaching" near-occlusion, or >95% in severity.

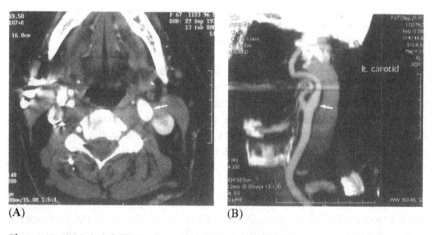

(A)   (B)

Figure 15 (A) Axial CTA of a normal left carotid bifurcation (arrow). (B) Sagittal computer reformatted image of the same vessel (arrow).

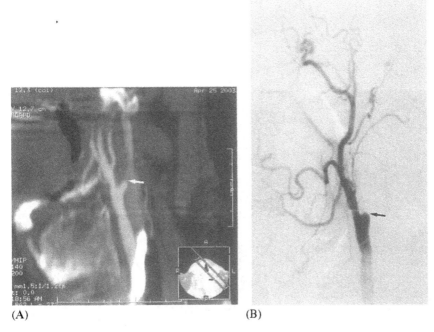

(A)   (B)

Figure 16 (A) CTA, sagittal reformation, showing a complete occlusion of the ICA (arrow). (B) DSA, lateral view, showing the complete ICA occlusion (arrow).

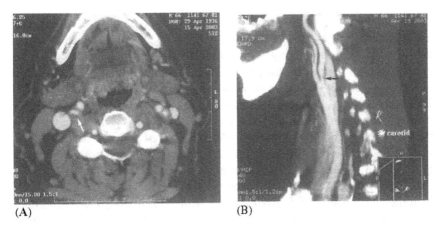

(A)   (B)

Figure 17 (A) CTA, axial projection, shows a severe stenosis of the right ICA (arrow). (B) CTA, sagittal computer reformation, shows the same lesion (arrow). Precise differentiation between moderate and severe (>70%) stenosis is difficult.

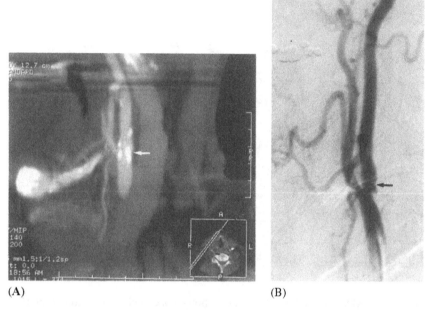

(A)   (B)

Figure 18   (A) CTA, sagittal reformation, showing a heavily calcified stenosis of the carotid bifurcation (arrow). Precise measurement of stenosis degree is difficult. (B) DSA, lateral view, in the same patient, showing only a mild degree of atherosclerotic stenosis (arrow).

an imaging modality in this condition is its ability to identify a lesion which needs either surgical or endovascular intervention. There is a body of literature gradually accumulating which shows that surgical decisions can be made in a high proportion of patients using a combination of less-invasive techniques, usually DUS with either MRA or CTA, eliminating the need for DSA (35,40,41). Yet even in these studies, up to 20% of the vessels were suboptimally imaged and the lack of congruence in stenosis estimation between the less-invasive modalities led to DSA in 10–15% of patients. Neither MRA nor CTA gives exact numerical stenosis measurements, and both have yet to be validated in the rigorous fashion achieved with DSA in NASCET. The risk of stroke by missing a severe stenosis using less-invasive modalities must be weighed against the low risk of stroke from a DSA study (28). The safety of a procedure must take into account the consequences of its accuracy. There is general agreement that the imaging investigation of symptomatic patients with carotid disease should begin with DUS. A consensus is building that if a good quality DUS shows evidence for a severe stenosis, MRA or CTA should follow. There is currently little evidence to favor one over the other with regard to diagnostic accuracy, although both techniques are in evolution. If there is congruence between the less-invasive modalities, then surgical decisions can be made in a high proportion of patients. If the studies are of sub-optimal quality, or there is significant disagreement between them, then DSA must be performed. Although the demise of arterial DSA for the diagnosis of atherosclerotic carotid stenosis has been predicted for decades, the moment has not yet arrived.

ACKNOWLEDGMENTS

The author thanks Dr. S.P. Lownie, Dr. A.J. Fox, and Cathy Lockhart.

REFERENCES

1. Seldinger SI. Catheter replacement of the needle in percutaneous arteriography: a new technique. Acta Radiol 1953; 39:368.
2. Barnett FJ, Lecky DM, Freiman DB, Montecalvo RM. Cerebrovascular disease: outpatient evaluation with selective carotid DSA performed via a transbrachial approach. Radiology 1989; 170:535–539.
3. Matsumoto Y, Hongo K, Toriyama T, Nagashima H, Kobayashi S. Transradial approach for diagnostic selective cerebral angiography: results of a consecutive series of 166 cases. AJNR Am J Neuroradiol 2001; 22:704–708.
4. Heiserman JE, Dean BL, Hodak JA, Flom RA, Bird CR, Drayer BP, Fram EK. Neurologic complications of cerebral angiography. AJNR Am J Neuroradiol 1994; 15:1401–1407.
5. Hankey GJ, Warlow CP, Sellar RJ. Cerebral angiographic risk in mild cerebrovascular disease. Stroke 1990; 21:209–222.
6. Dion JE, Gates PC, Fox AJ, Barnett HJ, Blom RJ. Clinical events following neuroangiography: a prospective study. Stroke 1987; 18:997–1004.
7. Earnest F, Forbes G, Sandok BA, Piepgras DG, Faust RJ, Ilstrup DM, Arndt LJ. Complications of cerebral angiography: prospective assessment of risk. AJR Am J Roentgenol 1984; 142:247–253.
8. Mani RL, Eisenberg RL. Complications of catheter cerebral angiography: analysis of 5000 procedures. AJR Am J Roentgenol 1978; 131:871–874.
9. Katayama H, Yamaguchi K, Kozuka T, Takashima T, Seez P, Matsuura K. Adverse reactions to ionic and nonionic contrast media. Radiology 1990; 175:621–628.
10. Sitzer M, Muller W, Seibler M, Hort W, Kniemeyer HW, Jacke L, Steinmetz H. Plaque ulceration and lumen thrombus are the main sources of cerebral microemboli in high-grade internal carotid artery stenosis. Stroke 1995; 26:1231–1223.
11. Streifler JY, Eliasziw M, Fox AJ, Benavente OR, Hachinski VC, Ferguson GG, Barnett HJ. Angiographic detection of carotid plaque ulceration. Stroke 1994; 25:1130–1132.

12. Pelz DM, Buchan A, Fox AJ, Barnett HJM, Vinuela F. Intraluminal thrombus of the internal carotid arteries: angiographic demonstration of resolution with anticoagulant therapy alone. Radiology 1986; 160:369–373.

13. Fox AJ, Sharpe BL, Wortzman G, Barnett HJM on behalf of the NASCET Investigators. The art of carotid stenosis measurement: recognition of "approaching" near occlusion (a) ASNR Proceedings, Chicago, April 23, 1995, p. 20.

14. North American Symptomatic Carotid Endarterectomy Trialists Collaborative Group. The final results of the NASCET trial. N Eng J Med 1998; 339: 1415–1425.

15. European Carotid Surgery Trialists Collaborative Group. Randomized trial of endarterectomy for recently symptomatic carotid stenosis: final results of the MRC European Carotid Surgery Trial (ECST). Lancet 1998; 351:1379–1387.

16. Chaturvedi S, Policherla P, Femino L. Cerebral angiography practices at US teaching hospitals. Stroke 1997; 28:1895–1897.

17. Rothwell PM, Gutnikov SA, Warlow CP. Reanalysis of the Final Results of the European Carotid Surgery Trial. Stroke 2003; 34:514–523.

18. Westwood ME, Kelly S, Berry E, Bamford JM, Gough MJ, Airey CM, Meaney JM, Davies LM, Cullingworth J, Smith MA. Use of magnetic resonance angiography to select candidates with recently symptomatic carotid stenosis for surgery: systematic review. Brit Med J 2002; 324:198–201.

19. Johnston DCC, Eastwood JD, Nguyen T, Goldstein LB. Contrast-enhanced magnetic resonance angiography of the carotid arteries: utility in routine clinical practice. Stroke 2002; 33:2834–2838.

20. Remonda L, Senn P, Barth A, Arnold M, Lovblad KO, Schroth G. Contrast-enhanced 3D MR angiography of the carotid artery: comparison with conventional digital subtraction angiography. AJNR Am J Neuroradiol 2002; 23: 213–219.

21. U-King-Im JM, Trivedi RA, Graves MJ, Higgins NJ, Cross JJ, Tom BD, Hollingworth W, Eales H, Warburton EA, Kirkpatrick PJ, Antoun NM, Gillard JH. Contrast-enhanced MR angiography for carotid disease: diagnostic and potential clinical impact. Neurology 2004; 62:1282–1290.

22. Cosottini M, Pingitore A, Puglioli M, Michelasi MC, Lupi G, Abbruzzese A, Calabrese R, Lombardi M, Parenti G, Bartolozzi C. Magnetic resonance angiography of atherosclerotic internal carotid stenosis as the noninvasive imaging modality in revascularization decision making. Stroke 2003; 34:660–664.

23. Johnston DCC, Goldstein LB. Clinical carotid endarterectomy decision making: noninvasive vascular imaging versus angiography. Neurology 2001; 56: 1009–1015.

24. Nederkoorn PJ, Mali WP, Eikelboom BC, Elgersma OE, Buskens E, Hunink M, Kappelle LJ, Buijis PC, Wust AF, van der Lugt A, van der Graaf Y. Preoperative diagnosis of carotid artery stenosis: accuracy of noninvasive testing. Stroke 2002; 33:2003–2008.

25. Long A, Lepoutre A, Corbillon E, Brancherau A. Critical review of non- or minimally invasive methods (duplex ultrasonography, MR- and CT-angiography) for evaluating stenosis of the proximal internal carotid artery. Eur J Vasc Endovasc Surg 2002; 24:43–52.

26. Rothwell PM, Pendlebury ST, Wardlaw J, Warlow CP. Critical appraisal of the design and reporting of studies of imaging and measurement of carotid stenosis. Stroke 2000; 31:1444–1450.

27. Patel SG, Collie DA, Wardlaw JM, Lewis SC, Wright AR, Gibson RJ, Sellar RJ. Outcome, observer reliability and patient preferences if CTA, MRA or Doppler ultrasound were used, individually or together, instead of digital subtraction angiography before carotid endarterectomy. J Neurol Neurosurg Psych 2002; 73:21–28.

28. Norris JW, Rothwell PM. Noninvasive carotid imaging to select patients for endarterectomy: Is it really safer than conventional angiography? Neurology 2001; 56:990–991.

29. Demarco JK, Rutt BK, Clarke SE. Carotid plaque characterization by magnetic resonance imaging: review of the literature. Top Magn Reson Imaging 2001; 12:205–217.

30. Weiss CR, Arai AE, Bui MN, Agyerman KO, Waclawiw MA, Balaban RS, et al. Arterial wall MRI characteristics are associated with elevated serum markers of inflammation in humans. J Magn Reson Imaging 2001; 14:698–704.

31. Corti R, Fayad ZA, Fuster V, Worthley SG, Helft G, Chesebro J, Mercuri M, Badimon JJ. Effects of lipid- lowering by simvastatin on human atherosclerotic lesions; a longitudinal study by high resolution non-invasive magnetic resonance imaging. Circulation 2001; 104:249–252.

32. Castillo M, Wilson JD. CT angiography of the common carotid artery bifurcation: comparison between two techniques and conventional angiography. Neuroradiology 1994; 36:602–604.

33. Cumming MJ, Morrow IM. Carotid artery stenosis: a prospective comparison of CT angiography and conventional angiography. AJR Am J Roentgenol 1994; 163:517–523.

34. Dillon EH, van Leeuwen MS, Fernandez MA, et al. CT angiography: application to the evaluation of carotid artery stenosis. Radiology 1993; 189:211–219.

35. Anderson GB, Ashforth R, Steinke DE, Ferdinandy R, Findlay JM. CT angiography for the detection and characterization of carotid artery bifurcation disease. Stroke 2000; 31:2168–2174.

36. Magarelli N, Scarabino T, Simeone AL, Florio F, Carriero A, Salvolini U, et al. Carotid stenosis: a comparison between MRA and spiral CT angiography. Neuroradiology 1998; 40:367–373.

37. Randoux B, Marro B, Koskas F, Duyme M, Sahel M, Zouaoui A, Marsault C. Carotid artery stenosis: prospective comparison of CT, three-dimensional gadolinium-enhanced MR, and conventional angiography. Radiology 2001; 220:179–185.

38. Josephson SA, Bryant SO, Mak HK, Johnston SC, Dillon WP, Smith WS. Evaluation of carotid stenosis using CT angiography in the initial evaluation of stroke and TIA. Neurology 2004; 63:457–460.

39. Gronholdt MLM. B-mode ultrasound and spiral CT for the assessment of carotid atherosclerosis. Neuroimag Clin N Am 2002; 12:421–435.

40. Friese S, Krapf H, Fetter M, Klase U, Skalej M, Kuker W. Ultrasonography and contrast-enhanced MRA in ICA stenosis: is conventional angiography obsolete? J Neurol 2001; 248:506–513.

41. Patel MR, Kuntz KM, Klufas RA, Kim D, Kramer J, Polak JF, Skillman JJ, Whittemore AD, Edelman RR, Kent KC. Preoperative assessment of the carotid bifurcation. Can magnetic resonance angiography and duplex ultrasonography replace contrast arteriography? Stroke 1995; 26:1753–1758.

5

Carotid Imaging: Use of Ultrasound

Michael G. Hennerici and Michael Daffertshofer
*Department of Neurology, University of Heidelberg,
Universitätsklinikum Mannheim, Germany*

1. INTRODUCTION

Although extensive research in atherosclerosis has been performed for more than a century, we still fail to understand the mechanisms causing atherogenesis, and believe that the disease has a discontinuous natural course with long asymptomatic stages until all of a sudden, symptoms due to local thrombosis or distal embolism occur. Distinction from normal aging has long been difficult, but seems to be facilitated by new ultrasound (US) investigations [intima-media thickness (IMT) imaging, plaque development, and vascular remodeling] (1). On the other end of the spectrum, compensatory mechanisms may be identified in patients with few symptoms but extensive cerebrovascular occlusive disease; in contrast to what has long been believed, these patients usually do not need any surgical or interventional treatment because of an associated developing collateral capacity of complex networks from large and small arteries.

Ischemic strokes and transient ischemic attacks (TIAs) are frequently caused by cerebral embolism from an atherothrombotic plaque, or cerebral artery atherothrombosis at the site of plaque rupture. Both mechanisms may be implicated when complex plaques are involved. The mechanisms that are responsible for these events include: rupture of the fibrous plaque surface, generation of an unstable plaque; exposure of thrombogenic parts of plaques; activation of the coagulation cascade and platelet adhesion, activation, and aggregation; and thrombosis and hemodynamic compromise (2).

Carotid atherosclerosis has been imaged by means of ultrasound since the late 1970s, with continuously improving technologies. Apart from diagnostic purposes in individual patients, carotid atherosclerosis has been investigated as the most appropriate model for its excellent accessibility in humans. Two major processes associated with the progression of atherosclerotic disease have been identified: (i) continuously increasing carotid artery intima–media thickness, which is an independent risk factor for myocardial infarction (MI) and stroke; and (ii) non-linear plaque development, with growing plaques from focal eccentric accumulation of lipid to late, obstructive lesions with different risks of hemodynamic and embolic complications (3).

Data from the ECST (European Carotid Surgery Trial) and NASCET (North American Symptomatic Carotid Endarterectomy Trial) have shown that plaque size and degree of lumen obstruction represent important indicators of the risk of stroke associated with carotid stenosis (4–6). These trials demonstrated the benefit of treating severe, symptomatic carotid stenoses with carotid endarterectomy, and suggested possible benefits of other methods (e.g., percutaneous transluminal angioplasty and stenting) that may be more widely available in the future (7). However, information on the extent of lumen obstruction is not sufficient to evaluate a patient's risk of recurrent cerebrovascular events with medical vs. surgical treatment. For example, analysis of data from NASCET has shown the protective effect of collateral circulation in patients with severe carotid artery stenosis. This protective effect was observed regardless of treatment (surgical or medical) and regardless of stroke etiology (8). Thus, the issue of whether differences in plaque characteristics beyond the size of lumen encroachment can distinguish between plaques that are likely to cause recurrent acute events and those that are likely to remain asymptomatic is an area of ongoing research.

2. ULTRASOUND TECHNOLOGY

2.1. Doppler Sonography

Ultrasound Doppler techniques are commonly used for examining the intra- and extracranial arteries supplying the brain. Interpretation of Doppler signals is based on the analysis of the audio signals and of the frequency spectrum. The Doppler effect is named after Christian Doppler, who described the effect of moving objects on the change in frequency of emitted light in 1842.

Continuous wave (CW) Doppler systems use two transducers, one of which emits while the other receives ultrasound continuously (9). While this

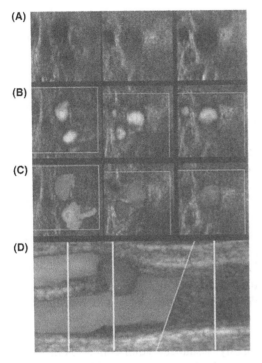

Figure 1 Color Doppler flow imaging assessing flow velocity (C) and amplitude (B) superimposed on B-mode images (A) in cross-sections of the carotid artery. Corresponding longitudinal section demonstrates different levels (indicated by lines) of cross-sections (D).

simple system is easily applicable for the detection of a broad range of flow velocity alterations including high blood flow velocities associated with severe stenosis, it provides only limited information about the topographic origin of the ultrasound-reflecting source. In contrast, pulsed wave (PW) Doppler systems, in which ultrasound is both emitted and received from a single piezoelectric crystal in the transducer, can provide a depth estimate of the site being insonated (9). This feature along with information on the direction of the Doppler frequency shift is used in transcranial PW–Doppler sonography to locate and differentiate intracranial cerebral arteries. Although CW and PW Doppler are simple, inexpensive screening procedures for the detection of stenoses and occlusions in large cerebral arteries, they have been replaced by more sophisticated ultrasound techniques offering real-time display of the vessel walls and lumen combined with color-coded visualization of blood flow (9) (Fig. 1).

2.2. Imaging Techniques

A number of complementary sonographic techniques are available for the evaluation of the intra- and extracranial arteries and for visualization of the brain parenchyma.

B-mode scanning displays the morphologic features of normal and pathological vessels (10–14). Since the extracranial carotid and vertebral arteries lie near the skin, linear array transducers are commonly used at ultrasound frequencies of 4.0–10.0 MHz.

Duplex sonography combines integrated PW Doppler spectrum analysis and B-mode sonography. In addition to providing information about the presence and morphology of arterial lesions, the B-mode image serves as a guide for the placement of the PW Doppler sample volume. Distinct criteria of the Doppler spectrum analysis are then used to evaluate hemodynamics and to categorize carotid artery stenoses. The common, internal, and external carotid arteries (CCA, ICA, and ECA, respectively) are usually characterized by a relatively distinct Doppler frequency spectrum, which allows their identification upon insonation with a Doppler system. The emission frequency of the integrated PW Doppler system ranges between 4 and 7 MHz.

Color Doppler flow imaging (CDFI) preserves the advantages of duplex sonography and additionally visualizes color-coded blood flow patterns superimposed on the gray-scale B-mode image (9,13–16). Using a defined color scale, the direction and the average mean velocity of moving blood cells within the sample volume at a given point in time is encoded. The generation of color signals is based on the detection of frequency and phase shifts by means of a multigate transducer. The technique of autocorrelation is used to obtain a real-time visualization of color-coded hemodynamics (Fig. 1C).

Power Doppler imaging (PDI) displays the amplitude of Doppler signals (Fig. 1B). The color and brightness of the signals are related to the number of blood cells producing the Doppler shift. Power Doppler imaging is more sensitive for the detection of blood flow than velocity imaging. This is because PDI is less angle-dependent, thus allowing better display of curving or tortuous vessels. This improves display of vessel wall pathology in areas of low or very high turbulent flow. This is a valuable technique for displaying plaque surface structure (17).

Real-time compound imaging is a new modality that enhances ultrasonographic visualization and characterization of carotid artery plaques (18,19). This technique uses ultrasound beams, which are steered off-axis from the orthogonal beams used in conventional ultrasound. The number of frames and steering angles varies, depending on the transducer characteristics. Frames acquired from sufficiently different angles contain independent random speckle patterns, which are averaged to reduce speckle and improve tissue differentiation.

Three-dimensional (3D) ultrasound can be used for both qualitative and quantitative analysis of plaques in the carotid artery. Surface features of carotid plaques, not readily appreciated in conventional two-dimensional (2D) B-mode scanning, can be clearly demonstrated by 3D ultrasound. In some cases, this may lead to a diagnosis not obtainable with other imaging techniques (20). New developments in 3D ultrasound image acquisition involve the use of position and orientation measurement (POM) devices capable of tracking scanheads in six degrees-of-freedom (6-DOF) (21–24). This approach allows "freehand" scanning to collect image data from different perspectives and potentially offers the ability to maximize tissue information that is not readily available from one imaging plane alone.

Contrast harmonic imaging (CHI) is based on the non-linear emission of harmonics by resonant microbubbles pulsating in an ultrasound field. The emission at twice the driving frequency, termed the second harmonic, can be detected and separated from the fundamental frequency. The advantage of the harmonic over the fundamental frequency is that contrast agent microbubbles resonate with harmonic frequencies, whereas adjacent tissues do so very little. In this way, CHI may enhance the signal-to-noise ratio and the ability of B-mode scanners to differentiate bubbles in the tissue vascular space from the echogenic surrounding vascular tissue.

3. NORMAL FINDINGS

3.1. Orbital Arteries

3.1.1. Principle and Findings

In the initial period of cerebrovascular ultrasonography insonation of the ophthalmic artery was used as an indirect test for the detection of significant carotid artery stenosis (25–27). This periorbital technique provides rapid information on the existence of collateral pathways. In the presence of severe stenosis or occlusion of the internal carotid artery, retrograde blood supply from the external carotid artery via the ophthalmic anastomosis can be easily detected with CW Doppler. However, with sufficient collateralization from the contralateral carotid or the vertebrobasilar systems, orthograde perfusion of the ophthalmic artery may persist. In this condition these indirect tests fail to detect even hemodynamically significant ipsilateral carotid obstructions. Thus while the detection of retrograde perfusion in the ophthalmic artery is a strong indicator of severe pathology within the ipsilateral extracranial carotid system (excellent >98% sensitivity), findings of normal perfusion of the ophthalmic branches cannot exclude severe carotid stenosis or occlusion (moderate <80% specificity).

4. NECK ARTERIES

4.1. Principle

Initially, Doppler sonography made it possible to assess the flow relationships in the neck arteries functionally and hemodynamically (27,28). Since the 1980s, blood vessels that are close to the surface have also been imaged using echotomograms (29–32).

    The display of both the arterial wall characteristics and the assessment of the extension of plaques and stenoses are possible. When combined with the color mode, it is possible to distinguish structure and flow conditions in the various arterial segments, which provides useful information to separate high- from low-risk plaques (Fig. 2). Computer-assisted image processing can now provide a 3D/4D display of the different sectional planes. This facilitates the evaluation and quantification of findings encountered during the examination, particularly when there are unusual anatomical relationships and pathological conditions (33–35). Spectral analysis is useful in

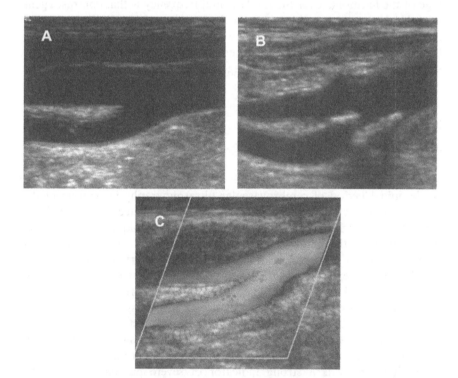

Figure 2 B-mode display of a normal carotid bulb (A). Identifying lack of flow velocity changes or turbulences nearby the plaque (C) is typical for a low-risk lesion: moderate hyperechoic plaque in the bulb at the entry into the ICA dorsal wall (B).

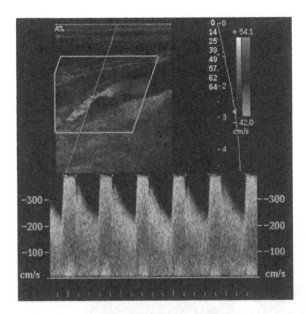

Figure 3 High-resolution B-mode image of a homogenous, asymptomatic anechoic plaque in the internal carotid artery. The display is superimposed with color Doppler flow imaging, showing a moderate 70% stenosis with increased flow velocity (>300 cm/s) and turbulent post-stenotic flow.

analyzing Doppler signals and provides semiquantitative numerical documentation of various parameters to evaluate the degree of stenosis (36,37) (Fig. 3).

4.2. Findings

4.2.1. Common Carotid Artery

Due to its superficial course in the neck, it is very easy to image the common carotid artery. The wall structure has the characteristic double reflection, with a hypoechoic zone lying in between (Fig. 4). This is termed the intima–media complex and the measurement of this parameter (IMT) is used in multicenter trials and in many standardized protocols as an indicator and prognostic parameter of atherosclerosis (progression vs. regression) (38). Normal values lie definitely below 1.5 mm (39) and, according to large series, range at 0.96 ± 0.19 mm in women and 1.04 ± 0.22 mm in men with risk factors of atherosclerosis. Intima-media thickness measurements have been agreed upon to represent independent risk factors of atherosclerosis by the American Heart Association (40). Furthermore IMT characterize a silent period of atherogenesis from infancy to senescence (41). If there is

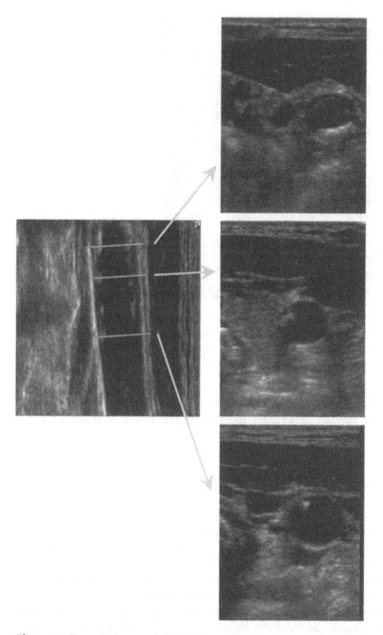

Figure 4 B-mode image of the intima-media complex and multiple small plaques within the common carotid artery. Longitudinal view (left side). Cross-sectional views (on the right side). The combination of both is needed to delineate and uncover plaques which may also be located outside a single longitudinal section.

associated coronary heart disease (CHD) or clinically manifest atherosclerosis, the IMTs increase (1.00 ± 0.22 mm and 1.10 ± 0.26 mm) (42).

Different methods of making quantitative measurements of the flow volume on the basis of duplex sonography have produced contradictory results (43–45). Without exactly reconstructing all ultrasound planes from several sections and measurements, it is not possible to correctly distinguish the laminar flow that takes place within the common carotid artery and the plug distortions near the arterial wall. Measurements using quantitative flow volumetry therefore have an error rate of between 10 and 40% (45–47). This is also true for commonly used angle-corrected color-coded duplex sonography measurements, which are provided in various versions by several manufactures. For routine or general clinical estimation of cerebrovascular blood flow volume, however, ultrasound methodology may be sufficient. Using standard techniques, flow volume measurements on the basis of color velocity imaging seem to be more accurate than those based on spectral Doppler imaging (48,49). Normal values depend on several variables, e.g., age, gender. More recently, sophisticated techniques utilizing 3D algorithms and gray-scale decorrelation were introduced (44,50) and may facilitate volume flow measurements.

4.2.2. Internal Carotid Artery

It is usually possible to image the internal carotid artery at its origin, since the widened sinus is clearly recognizable. According to Marosi and Ehringer (32), the width of the blood vessel at the sinus is 6.5–7.5 mm, and distal from this location it is 4.3–5.3 mm. Intima-media thickness values range at 1.35 ± 0.64 and 1.57 ± 0.67 mm for women and men, respectively, with the risk factor of atherosclerosis, and at 1.56 ± 0.70 and 1.87 ± 0.73 mm, respectively, in women and men with CHD and clinically manifest atherosclerosis, which is significantly associated with abnormal IMT values (42).

Depiction of the complex flow changes within the carotid sinus and in the proximal segment of the internal carotid artery is considerably better using the frequency mode of the color flow duplex sonography (51). Flow separation zones, variations in circulation, and cardiac cycle changes can be imaged in relation to the structural findings in at least two planes. It is only when the carotid sinus is absent that no flow separation zones are seen. Flow separation zones can usually be detected at the proximal origin of the internal carotid artery, and in almost one in two cases, they are also found at the origin of the external carotid artery and, during systole, they can be seen as a zone of clearly altered flow direction (against the axial or wall-directed flow) (52). A color signal is also sometimes missing if there is a clear decrease in the flow velocity. Experimental results show that changes in flow are usually not found directly at the location that causes the flow separation, but within the carotid sinus at the origin of the external carotid artery, and that they are distributed in a horseshoe shape around the flow separation point (52–54). The extent of the distribution of the flow separation is highly variable (52,55).

Doppler data analysis makes it easy to determine which of the arteries in the neck is being depicted, particularly when compression tests and vibration maneuvers (i.e., tapping) are registered at the same time.

Only two parameters in the Doppler spectrum are usually evaluated:

1. The systolic peak frequency.
2. The average mean frequency.

In addition, the diastolic frequency is sometimes important for side-to-side comparison. Asymmetries in the spectrum have so far been difficult to detect.

Many algorithms have been proposed to calculate the width of the spectrum or the systolic window, particularly in the carotid system, including comparisons of preceding and subsequent vascular segments. These investigations mostly date from the period when the quality of echotomographic imaging was still relatively poor. The aim was to detect early forms of arteriosclerosis by calculating this parameter. However, a systematic comparison of the structural and hemodynamic parameters shows that, even in completely normal situations, and particularly in younger patients with physiologic flow displacements and separation phenomena, there may be limitations. In doubtful cases, an unusual result obtained when analyzing the spectrum should subsequently be checked using duplex sonography, which is the ultimate diagnostic arbiter.

4.2.3. External Carotid Artery

In pure B-mode, there is often no difference between the origin of the external carotid artery and that of the internal carotid artery, although it is occasionally possible to use the origin of the superior thyroid artery to assist in the identification. Display of the typical flow signals in either color-coded mode is more reliable.

In contrast to what might be expected from experimental results, significant flow separation and even flow reversal zones are found at the origin of the external carotid artery too. This is due to the configuration of the carotid sinus and the variable branching of the carotid bifurcation (52).

The predictive value of the ultrasound method is significantly dependent on the quality of the examination procedure. Unfavorable conditions (e.g., an inability to study the arterial course in several sectional planes) can influence the specificity in individual cases. Also, isolated echotomographic imaging of the arteries of the neck, without additional examination of the hemodynamic findings using Doppler sonography, has a negative influence on the diagnostic predictive value (56) and should therefore be avoided. The advantage of color flow duplex sonography lies in the easy and quick simultaneous display of morphological and hemodynamic parameters. The specificity of the method ranges between 86 and 100% (15,57,58), similar to that of continuous wave and pulsed wave Doppler vs. angiography in the detection of carotid stenoses >50% (92–99 and 78–95%, respectively) in experienced hands. It may be improved by the combined use of color flow velocity and signal amplitude analysis (9).

5. INTIMA-MEDIA THICKNESS—THE INITIAL STAGE

Pignoli et al. (59) were the first to characterize a "double line" pattern of the normal carotid artery wall. They demonstrated that measurements of the IMT in tissue specimens from common carotid arteries correlated highly with the distance between these two echogenic lines (Fig. 5). Subsequently, several studies established associations between common carotid IMT, cardiovascular risk factors (60,61), and the prevalence of cardiovascular

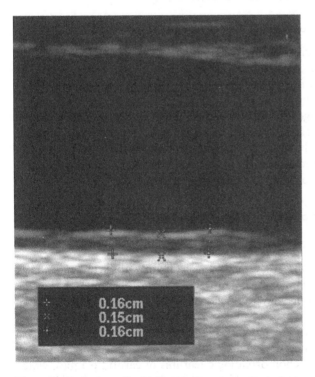

Figure 5 Intima-media thickness measurements at whatever locations in the carotid system should range >1.0 cm at the posterior wall vs. poor display at the near wall. Example of abnormally high IMT well displayed.

disease (42) using high-resolution ultrasonography. The increasing importance of the common carotid IMT is further reflected by its use as a surrogate end-point for determining the success of interventions that lower the
levels of low-density lipoprotein cholesterol. Azen et al. (61) used serial
measurements of IMT to assess the effect of supplementary vitamin E intake
in reducing the progression of atherosclerosis in subjects not treated with
lipid-lowering drugs, while the process is still confined to the arterial wall.
The results of several studies suggest an association between increased carotid IMT and myocardial infarction. A recent consensus (38) has confirmed
these findings and identified increased carotid artery IMT as a risk factor for
both myocardial infarction and stroke in older adults. In contrast, other studies questioned the clinical usefulness of measuring the carotid IMT,
because it was not specific or sensitive enough to identify patients with or
without significant coronary artery disease. Increasing age, male sex, and
the presence of diabetes were all associated with a significantly ($p < 0.01$)
higher coronary artery disease score than the average for any level of
carotid IMT, suggesting differential effects of these traditional risk factors
on the coronary and common carotid arteries (62).

5.1. Longitudinal Assessment

A major source of error in the longitudinal assessment of IMT is the
difficulty in retrieving the same echographic view of the vessel. While the
mean IMT might be considered a reproducible parameter to evaluate differences between populations exposed to diverse risk factors, evolutional or
therapy-induced changes in the individual may be better monitored on
predefined carotid artery sectors. External landmarks have been proposed
to increase the reproducibility (63). Another approach uses the discrete
Fourier transform to minimize the vessel contour after matching baseline
ultrasonographic images with a corresponding view (64).

6. PLAQUE DEVELOPMENT—THE INTERMEDIATE STAGE

6.1. Plaque Echogenicity

Plaques with homogenous echogenicity consist mainly of fibrotic tissue (12).
Ulceration is rare in homogenous plaques, perhaps accounting for the lack
of significant correlation with the occurrence of focal cerebral ischemia.
Heterogenous plaques represent matrix deposition, cholesterol accumulation, necrosis, calcification, and intraplaque hemorrhage (12,65). Several
studies have demonstrated that high-resolution B-mode scanning can allow
the characterization of echomorphologic features of carotid plaques, which
correlate with angiographic and histopathologic criteria (66). Although
echolucent areas within the plaque may represent thrombotic material or
hemorrhage, it has been recognized that lipid accumulation may produce

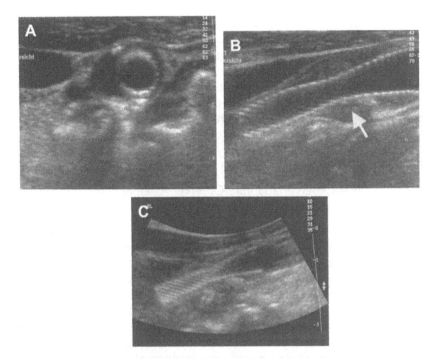

Figure 6 Display of carotid stents between 2 weeks and 2 months post-intervention in a cross-section (A) and a longitudinal-section using a linear probe (B) and a sector probe to better display the location of the stent (C). An often persisting mild residual stenosis does not indicate improper intervention (arrow).

similar echogenicity (67). Plaque calcification produces acoustic shadowing in echotomograms (Fig. 2B). Characteristic shadowing can also be demonstrated after stenting carotid lesions (Fig. 6). Depending on plaque location and the extent of calcification, this artifact can be a major obstacle for adequate visualization of the arterial wall as well as of the plaque itself.

Initial studies of plaque echogenicity with B-mode ultrasound reported an association between heterogenous plaques and the occurrence of cerebrovascular events (68–71). Support for this association was provided by several investigations of endarterectomy specimens which suggested a correlation between intraplaque hemorrhage and transient ischemic attacks or strokes (72–75). The issue on whether differences in plaque echogenicity can distinguish between symptomatic and asymptomatic plaques remained a subject of debate (76–78) until new ultrasonographic studies claimed again that heterogenous carotid plaques are more often associated with intraplaque hemorrhage and neurologic events, and concluded that the evaluation of plaque morphology may be helpful in selecting patients for carotid endarterectomy (79–81). Others argue that lipid-rich plaques are more prone to rupture and suggest that an association between intraplaque hemorrhage and a high lipid content as revealed in B-mode ultrasound may support this theory (82). These newer findings have been negated by other research groups finding little correlation between plaque morphology and histologic specimens (83). Recently, a definitive study on the significance of heterogenous plaque structure found differences in volume of intraplaque hemorrhage, lipid core, necrotic core, or plaque calcification in patients with highly stenotic carotid lesions undergoing endarterectomy, regardless of preoperative symptom status (84), although a large natural history study confirmed the capacity of plaque imaging to predict individual stroke risks associated herewith (85).

6.1.1. Inter-Observer and Intra-Observer Agreement on B-Mode Plaque Morphology

In the Tromsø Study in Norway, inter-observer and intra-observer agreement on plaque morphology classification was reported as being high, with κ values ranging between 0.54 and 0.73 (86). However, the majority of new studies on this subject report low inter-rater agreement indicating that unaided visual evaluation of static B-mode pictures for assessing plaque morphology in patients with carotid stenosis is not reliable (87). Reproducible grading of ultrasound images is not consistently achievable among experienced observers, and within-observer agreement may vary with time (88). In one study on subjective categorization of plaque types, the intra-observer agreement was moderate ($\kappa = 0.44$) and the inter-observer agreement low ($\kappa = 0.38$), emphasizing that subjective B-mode ultrasound categorization of atherosclerotic plaques cannot adequately determine the volume of fibrosis or lipids within plaques (89). These poor results on inter-observer and intra-observer agreement on B-mode plaque morphology may explain the discrepant findings of previous attempts to characterize carotid artery plaques in relation to clinical events. They also suggest that the current subjective ultrasound characterization of carotid plaque morphology used in clinical trials may be associated with unacceptable levels of reproducibility in some centers.

6.1.2. Computerized Evaluation of Plaque Echogenicity

Due to the poor inter-observer and intra-observer agreement in characterizing plaque morphology with ultrasound, several investigators have introduced various schemes for standardized assessment of carotid plaques. Linear scaling of the adventitia and blood with gray-scale medians has been proposed for quantifying echo intensity. Using this technique, decreased echogenicity in terms of gray-scale median and percentage of echolucent pixels has been reported for symptomatic plaques (90). Other groups have also used computer processing to yield a measure of plaque echogenicity (91). Spectral analysis of echo signals acquired from human carotid endarterectomy specimens has been performed to improve classification of fibrous, lipid pool, and thrombus constituents (92). By using three para-meters of the calibrated power spectrum (slope, intercept, and total power), the proportion of correctly classified tissue regions could be increased. These studies indicate that computer-aided analysis of ultrasonic B-mode features of carotid plaques may be valuable in multicenter clinical trials where different operators and equipment are used (85).

6.2. Plaque Surface Structure and Ulcerations

Attempts to characterize plaque surface structure with B-mode echotomo-graphy have been disappointing. Although a relatively good differentiation amongst smooth, irregular, and ulcerative plaque surfaces has been obtained for post-mortem carotid artery specimens, the in vivo accuracy as compared to findings at carotid endarterectomy has been considerably poorer (66,73,93,94). Surface defects showing a depth and a length of ≥ 2 mm with a well-defined base in the recess have been commonly used parameters for identifying plaque ulceration (95). Using these criteria, B-mode imaging has failed to provide a satisfactory diagnostic yield for ulcerative plaques with a sensitivity of only 47% (96). Other groups have been unable to distinguish between the presence and absence of intimal ulcerations with B-mode scans (97). Diagnostic sensitivity for detecting plaque ulceration with ultrasound is affected by the degree of carotid stenosis and increases to 77% in plaques associated with 50% or less stenosis (66). It is expected that power Doppler imaging could significantly improve the yield for reliable depiction of plaque ulcerations. Pathoanatomical comparisons with this technique, however, are lacking.

Conventional arteriography has likewise proven inadequate for defini-tion of ulcerative plaques, the sensitivity being approximately 53% (66). The angiographic detection of ulceration as compared to surgical specimens was equally poor in the NASCET study. A sensitivity of 45.9% and a specificity of 74.1% was found for 500 specimens, yielding a positive predictive value of only 71.8% (98). It has been demonstrated that angiographic assessment of plaque surface morphology may vary depending on the type of angiography and the quality of visualization of carotid stenosis (99). Whether plaque sur-face irregularities or ulcerations are useful parameters for defining patients at risk for carotid embolism is a matter of ongoing debate. Advocates of a pathophysiologic relationship maintain that ulcerations constitute a fertile ground for potential thrombosis and consequent embolic events. Indeed a recent report contends that the presence of an angiographically defined ulceration is associated with an increased risk of stroke in medically treated symptomatic patients (100). Notwithstanding the previous discussion on the poor sensitivity and specificity of arteriography for detecting plaque ulceration, it should be noted that many ulcers are smooth and thick, containing no thrombus at all (101) for putative plaque embolism.

Moreover, pathological studies have pointed out that in asymptomatic carotid plaques with stenosis exceeding 60%, there is an increased frequency of plaque hemorrhages, ulcerations, and mural thrombi, as well as of numerous healed ulcerations and organized thrombi (102). Likewise, comparisons of symptomatic with asymptomatic large and stenotic carotid endarterectomy plaques have revealed a high incidence of complex plaque structure and complications in each (76,103). There appears, therefore, to be little difference in plaque constituents or plaque surface structure between specimens from symptomatic and asymptomatic patients. These findings confirm that a traditional description of plaque structure or identification of plaque ulceration as depicted in current clinical imaging techniques, i.e., ultrasound, MRI, and angiography, are not sufficient for predicting individually which carotid plaques are susceptible to embolization (104).

6.3. Characterization of Plaque Motion

Experimental work has suggested that analysis of plaque motion, i.e., translational plaque movements coincident with those of arterial walls, plaque rotations, and local, plaque-specific deformations, may provide new insights into plaque modeling and mechanisms of plaque rupture with subsequent embolism. For example, in vitro observations on the relative position of markers placed along plaque specimens during pressure loading have demonstrated that prior to plaque fissuring, the markers display an asymmetrical movement. Such plaque surface movement may be attributable to deformations resulting from crack propagation of multiple local internal tears in the plaque. Identification of local variations in surface deformability could therefore provide information on the relative vulnerability to plaque fissuring or rupture.

An approach for studying plaque surface deformations has recently been reported (33). This technique uses four-dimensional (4D) ultrasonography to acquire temporal 3D ultrasound data of carotid artery plaques. The ultrasound data are then analyzed with motion detection algorithms to determine apparent velocity fields, also known as optical flow, of the plaque surface. Using this method, differences in plaque motion patterns between patients with symptomatic and asymptomatic carotid artery disease have been characterized. Asymptomatic plaques typically show a homogenous orientation and magnitude of computed surface velocity vectors, coincident with arterial wall movement. Analysis of symptomatic plaques, however, has demonstrated consistent evidence for plaque deformation, irrespective of arterial wall movements. Although analysis of plaque motion in patients with carotid artery stenosis facilitates detection of patterns likely to hint of an increased risk for plaque complications, plaque vulnerability is suggested to depend on a set-up of non-linearly active mechanisms rather than a simple abnormality.

6.4. Possible Mechanisms of Remodeling

A very well-known phenomenon in vascular medicine is the ability of blood vessels continually to adapt their cross-sectional size to the needs of dynamic downstream blood supply. This dynamic process, termed "arterial remodeling," came into the focus of vascular research when it became clear that remodeling and not plaque size was the primary determinant of lumen size in the presence of stable lesions. More recently, growing evidence seems to show an association of adequate outward remodeling with an increasing risk of plaque rupture as the underlying cause of acute coronary syndromes and sudden cardiac death.

6.5. Remodeling and Hemodynamic Stimuli

Under physiologic conditions, remodeling is a dynamic response to both flow changes to restore normal shear stress and to alterations of circumferential stretch to adjust the wall tension (105). Important factors that contribute to outward remodeling in response to increased flow are the shear-responsive endothelial production of nitric oxide (106) and of the matrix metalloproteinases (MMP) MMP-2 and MMP-9 (107). Nitric oxide seems to be crucial in this process, since it has the potential to induce MMPs (108), to inhibit proliferation, and to promote apoptosis of smooth muscle cells (109). On the other hand, in low-flow states, mitogenic and fibrogenic growth factors, such as platelet-derived growth factor and transforming growth factor-β, are preferably produced, which probably mediates inward remodeling by increasing smooth muscle cell proliferation and the deposition and cross-linking of collagen while MMP induction helps to reorganize vessel structure (96,110). The effect of stretch on remodeling is less clear. Many of the above-mentioned mediators are not only shear-sensitive but also stretch-responsive, so that a significant interaction between stretch and shear signals can be assumed (111). Most of the energy of pulsatile pressure is absorbed by elastin, whose production is highly stretch-responsive. This makes it quite probable that an alteration in elastin production may be important in remodeling, since vessel elasticity is the chief determinant of resting vessel size (112). How these molecular and cellular events are spatially coordinated to result in morphological change remains unclear. Possibly certain transmembrane proteins like the highly shear- and stretch-sensitive connexins, which have a rapid turnover, may play a role (113).

Theoretically, endothelial dysfunction and increasing plaque depth may prevent remodeling in response to hemodynamic stimuli, because under such conditions, effectors of remodeling must penetrate into atherosclerotic lesions. Furthermore, in focal lesions, the acceleration of flow both on the proximal and on the distal side of a protruding plaque is associated with a translesional deterioration in remodeling (114). At the same time, this leads to greater inflammatory infiltrate and less cellularity and collagen in the upstream side (115), and growth of angiographic stenosis downstream (116), indicative of persistent shear sensitivity.

6.6. Inflammation, Scarring, and Remodeling

Several mechanisms contribute to the dynamic processes finally leading to the atherosclerotic burden. Firstly, inflammatory cells, by producing MMPs, play a major role in atherosclerotic remodeling. Cell adhesion molecules such as ICAM-1 and VCAM have the ability to recruit monocytes and macrophages, which is a shear-sensitive process (117), partly explaining the predominance of this cell type in the upstream side of focal lesions (115). Secondly, the expression of MMPs by atherosclerotic lesions can be further promoted by an increasing infiltration of inflammatory cells due to hyperlipidemia. The reduction of MMP expression in plaques, mainly originating from macrophage foam cells, is a possible mechanism of action of lipid lowering and reduction in lipid oxidation (118,119). This may underlie the apparent stimulatory effect of hypercholesterolemia on outward remodeling response (120), which is reflected in ultrastructural changes in the internal elastic lamina (121), very similar to those induced by high blood flow (122). Both processes are MMP-dependent and can therefore lead to outward modeling.

The same local MMP activity provoked by hypercholesterolemia may explain why some eccentric plaques appear to initiate remodeling in the vessel wall directly beneath the plaque (123) and why medial thinning underlying a plaque is directly proportional to plaque burden (124). Outward remodeling may be prevented by excessive collagen deposition within a lesion. Under certain clinical conditions, such as after angioplasty (125) or plaque rupture, sudden or focal fibrotic responses are induced, and scar contracture may even result in inward remodeling.

6.6.1. Clinical Observations Regarding the Mechanisms of Atherosclerotic Remodeling

Whereas research on plaque formation has identified many factors that promote plaque growth, much less is known about possible determinants of remodeling. Obviously, some of the variation in remodeling response depends on the vascular bed involved, so that compensatory remodeling is frequently present in the carotid and coronary vessels, whereas ileofemoral arteries are prone to inadequate outward or to inward remodeling. In contrast, this process is uncommon in the renal arteries (126). These regional differences possibly reflect differences in endothelial responses to altered hemodynamics (127) or a variation in the underlying vessel structure, such as elastic vs. muscular (128). Other factors seem to influence remodeling patterns like systemic parameters [e.g., insulin-dependent vs. non-insulin dependent diabetes (129)] or the presence of risk factors like smoking, both of which make inadequate outward and inward remodeling more frequent, in contrast to hypercholesterolemia (121). Despite these factors, there is often a marked variability in remodeling response along the same artery (130,131). Some lesion specificity in remodeling response can be attributed to altered local hemodynamics such as in the inner curves of tortuous vessel segments, where low shear leads to a predisposition to atheroma (132) and may impair outward remodeling in a similar manner (133). This may be particularly important in the carotid bifurcation where outward remodeling is less frequent proximal to the bifurcation (134).

6.6.2. Remodeling and Plaque Rupture

Plaque ruptures are known to cause unstable angina, myocardial infarction, and sudden death from coronary artery disease and potentially stroke due to embolism (135). Most coronary lesions responsible for myocardial infarction were minimally occlusive prior to rupture as could be demonstrated by several angiographic studies. This is consistent with the fact that many patients had no prior history of ischemia. Post-mortem studies showed that patients who died with plaque rupture without a prior history of coronary disease had large lesions (136), suggesting that due to considerable outward remodeling, angiography would have failed to display any stenosis despite significant histological stenosis. This is in keeping with several recent studies showing an association between outward remodeling and plaque rupture in the coronary circulation. Earlier findings suggest that the remodeling response correlates with mechanical characteristics and the clinical presentation of the plaque. In this sense, calcified plaques are associated with inadequate outward or inward remodeling in patients presenting for angioplasty (131), whereas soft plaques exhibit better compensatory enlargement (137). The same is true for lesions responsible for unstable syndromes, which have larger, softer plaques with more outward remodeling compared to those in stable angina which are more fibrous and calcified (138–140).

The interaction of remodeling and plaque rupture can be understood through the involvement of MMPs and apoptosis in both processes. It remains uncertain, however, whether this interaction is causal or due to common mechanisms. In the case of a causal relationship, longitudinal rates of remodeling might be able to predict acute events. In contrast, if MMP inhibitors are used to prevent plaque rupture, this may be at the expense of increasing luminal compromise and the need for revascularization. In addition, if outward remodeling resulted in plaque rupture, it would also be interesting to know whether subsequent fibrous healing culminates in inward remodeling. Since inflammatory responses in the association between outward remodeling and plaque rupture are that important, anti-inflammatory and lipid-lowering agents might be useful agents via a decrease in outward remodeling responses. This may be a possible explanation for a relatively small regression in angiographic lumen stenosis compared to the reduction in clinical events in lipid-lowering trials (114).

6.7. Remodeling and Stroke—Specific Aspects

While the sequence of progressive fixed stenosis and resulting ischemia is very common in coronary and peripheral arterial disease, this does not necessarily hold true in the cerebral circulation due to the collateral circulation through the Circle of Willis, perhaps with the exception of basilar artery thrombosis. Nevertheless, carotid thrombosis, arterio-arterial embolism to intracranial endarteries leading to their occlusion, are far more important. Hence, the relationship between plaque rupture and remodeling is of great importance in the extra- and intracranial cerebral arteries. As plaque characteristics and local remodeling responses are extraordinarily well accessible in the carotid circulation, there is a great potential to quantitate the risk of plaque rupture both systemically (141) and locally (142), and to use statin therapy (143), anti-inflammatory drugs and metalloproteinase inhibitors (144) more selectively in the prevention of plaque rupture.

In addition, remodeling in the cerebral circulation may be promoted or attenuated by several local factors. As previously demonstrated in bifurcations of the coronary circulation, remodeling on the hips of the carotid bifurcation is reduced, leading to more severe luminal narrowing in the internal carotid following each increment in plaque mass (145). In addition, the finding that flow in the patent carotid increases as a compensatory response to contralateral occlusion is of clinical relevance since this leads to a greater local stimulation of the cascade of remodeling (114), inflammatory cell infiltration (115), and thus plaque rupture.

7. PLAQUE DEVELOPMENT—THE TERMINAL STAGE

Although ultrasound technology is continuously improving, diagnosis and vessel wall characterization of severe degrees of carotid stenoses are limited. In particular in cases with complex calcified plaques, a very high-grade stenosis may be mistaken for a complete occlusion, which has long been suggested as a major source of faulty therapeutic decisions. To overcome these limitations in about 15–20% of patients in large neurovascular centers (146), ultrasound contrast agents have been developed with the aim of improving diagnostic measures in cases that could not be sufficiently diagnosed by conventional means.

Such contrast agents were introduced almost a decade ago (147) and have been widely used in studies of peripheral vessels (148–150). They consist of microbubbles filled with air or gases, which depending on their size, are either filtered in the pulmonary capillary territories which makes them ideal to prove right-to-left shunting, e.g., to detect a patent foramen ovale, or survive the passage through the pulmonary capillary bed to enhance the signal-to-noise ratio during arterial ultrasound studies. This effect is due to the fact that the ultrasound reflectors (i.e., blood cells) in conventional Doppler/duplex scanning do not have ideal reflection characteristics. This is the main reason for the limitations of ultrasound techniques in differentiating (carotid artery) occlusion from high-grade stenosis, because under these circumstances, volume flow is maximally reduced, leading to a critical decrease in ultrasound reflectors. Addition of contrast agents will improve the ultrasound reflection characteristics of the compound and decrease the rate of false-negative results in the depiction of high-grade stenosis. Contrast agents, after intravenous injection, usually increase the Doppler signal by up to 30 dB, and depending on the concentration of the contrast agent and on the type of administration (perfusion vs. bolus) the enhancement usually occurs 30–60 s after injection with optimal contrast lasting approximately 3–6 minutes (151,152). Previously, the use of ultrasound contrast agents in small patient collectives led to controversial results being reported as to the usefulness of these agents in the differentiation of carotid occlusion from subtotal stenosis (1,153,154).

7.1. Assessment of Advanced Atherosclerotic Disease

An international consensus meeting has established the criteria for the quantification of internal carotid artery stenosis (155). Recommendations for interpretation of maximum Doppler shift velocities, systolic velocity ratios, and residual area are summarized in this report.

7.2. Non-atherosclerotic Vascular Disease

7.2.1. Carotid Inflammation

Figure 7 illustrates the contribution of ultrasound to other imaging modalities in the diagnosis of individual patients, such as large vessel arteritis.

7.2.2. Carotid Dissection

Ultrasound is useful for the diagnosis of carotid artery dissection, a cause of transient or permanent neurologic deficits, particularly in young patients. Internal carotid artery dissection usually occurs spontaneously and results in a typical syndrome of focal cerebral deficits, headache, neck pain, and ipsilateral Horner's syndrome.

Pathognomonic patterns can be observed in carotid dissection. Doppler flow studies can show marked flow reversal at the origin of the ICA in systole and absent or minimal blood flow in diastole corresponding to a high-resistance bidirectional Doppler signal (156). B-mode demonstrates a tapered lumen and occasionally a floating intimal flap. Narrowing of the true lumen by the false lumen thrombus can be associated with a

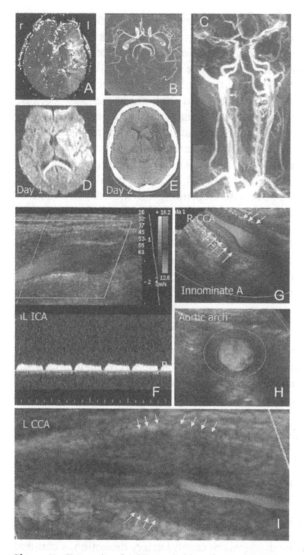

Figure 7 Example of a 22-year-old patient with Takayasu's arteritis who presented with an acute left hemispheric stroke. Initial PWI-MR (A) and DWI-MR (D) showed a pseudo-mismatch a few hours after the onset of symptoms with MCA-infant 24 hours later (E), despite normal MRA images of both MCAs (B) as a result of the markedly thinned left carotid arteries in the neck (C,F,I). Characteristic homogeneous thickening of all supra-aortic arteries (G,H,I) are pathognomonic.

low-velocity Doppler waveform. The direction of flow in a patent false lumen can vary from being forward, reversed, or bidirectional. The flow dynamics in carotid dissections are complex and are primarily dependent upon the presence of thrombus within the false lumen, the entry and exit flaps if the false lumen is patent, the motion of the flap wall, and the extent of the dissection (157). In some patients, the only finding may be a retromandibular high-velocity signal associated with a distal stenosis of the cervical carotid artery (158).

Follow-up examinations of carotid dissections demonstrate gradual normalization of the Doppler spectrum, indicating recanalization of the ICA within a few weeks to months in more than 2/3 of patients (159). Carotid aneurysms can occur as complications of ICA dissections. Their follow-up with angiography and MRA/MRI can be complemented with ultrasonography due to the development of broadband transducers with improved axial resolution and depth penetration.

8. PERSPECTIVES

The widening of therapeutic options and particularly the optimization of efficacy and safety of interventional procedures require pre- and post-procedure non-invasive testing. All available techniques can be used to minimize the disadvantages of an individual method in patients at risk of suffering a stroke, most with acute stroke symptoms and follow-up studies.

This ongoing research on the application of ultrasound for percutaneous and intra-luminal thrombolysis and plaque remodeling using molecular imaging is exciting. This is particularly promising for the prevention of plaque development in patients at risk of stroke who demonstrate clearly IMT changes in the absence of total atherosclerosis.

8.1. Molecular Imaging

Molecular imaging can be defined as the characterization and measurement of biological processes at the cellular and molecular level using remote imaging detectors. The goals of molecular imaging include non-invasive detection of pathology using disease-associated molecular signatures, in vivo delineation of complex molecular mechanisms of disease, and the detection of gene expression. Targeted ultrasound techniques combine ultrasound imaging technology with specific contrast agents for the assessment of molecular or genetic signatures of disease.

The addition of targeted ligands to microbubbles opens new avenues for the identification of vascular occlusion or areas of vascular injury. Adhesion molecules such as the integrin $\alpha_v \beta_3$, intercellular adhesion molecule-1 (ICAM-1), and fibrinogen receptor GPIIb/IIIa are over-expressed in regions of angiogenesis, inflammation, or thrombus, respectively.

Targeted microbubbles directed to the GPIIb/IIIa receptor of activated platelets have been developed for the visualization of thrombus (160,161), and leukocyte-targeted microbubbles can be used to characterize the severity of post-ischemic myocardial inflammation (162) and to identify inflamed plaques (163).

REFERENCES

1. Hennerici M, Bäzner H, Daffertshofer M. Ultrasound and arterial wall disease. Cerebrovasc Dis 2004; 17(suppl 1):19–33.
2. Hennerici M. The unstable plaque. Cerebrovasc Dis 2004; 17(suppl 3):17–22.
3. Hennerici M, Rautenberg W, Trockel U, Kladetzky RG. Spontaneous progression and regression of small carotid atheroma. Lancet 1985; 1(8443): 1415–1419.
4. Barnett HJ, Taylor DW, Eliasziw M, Fox AJ, Ferguson GG, Haynes RB, Rankin RN, Clagett GP, Hachinski VC, Sackett DL, Thorpe KE, Meldrum HE. Benefit of carotid endarterectomy in patients with symptomatic moderate or severe stenosis. North American Symptomatic Carotid Endarterectomy Trial Collaborators. N Engl J Med 1998; 339(20):1415–1425.
5. Schulz UG, Rothwell PM. Association between arterial bifurcation anatomy and angiographic plaque ulceration among 4,627 carotid stenoses. Cerebrovasc Dis 2003; 15(4):244–251.
6. Randomised trial of endarterectomy for recently symptomatic carotid stenosis: final results of the MRC European Carotid Surgery Trial (ECST). Lancet 1998; 351(9113): 1379–1387.
7. Endovascular versus surgical treatment in patients with carotid stenosis in the Carotid and Vertebral Artery Transluminal Angioplasty Study (CAVATAS): a randomised trial. Lancet 2001; 357(9270):1729–1737.
8. Henderson RD, Eliasziw M, Fox AJ, Rothwell PM, Barnett HJ. Angiographically defined collateral circulation and risk of stroke in patients with severe carotid artery stenosis. North American Symptomatic Carotid Endarterectomy Trial (NASCET) Group. Stroke 2000; 31(1):128–132.
9. Hennerici M, Neuerburg-Heusler D. Vascular Diagnosis with Ultrasound. Stuttgart: Thieme, 1998:1–499.
10. Hennerici MG, Steinke W. Carotid plaque developments—aspects of hemodynamic and vessel wall platelet interaction. Cerebrovasc Dis 1991; 1: 142–148.
11. Goes E, Janssens W, Maillet B, Freson M, Steyaert L, Osteaux M. Tissue characterization of atheromatous plaques: correlation between ultrasound image and histological findings. J Clin Ultrasound 1990; 18(8):611–617.
12. Wolverson MK, Bashiti HM, Peterson GJ. Ultrasonic tissue characterization of atheromatous plaques using a high resolution real time scanner. Ultrasound Med Biol 1983; 9(6):599–609.
13. Merritt CR. Doppler color flow imaging. J Clin Ultrasound 1987; 15(9): 591–597.
14. Middleton WD, Foley WD, Lawson TL. Color-flow Doppler imaging of carotid artery abnormalities. Am J Roentgenol 1988; 150:419–425.
15. Steinke W, Kloetzsch C, Hennerici MG. Carotid artery disease assessed by color Doppler flow imaging: correlation with standard Doppler sonography and angiography. Am J Neuroradiol 1990; 11:259–266.

16. Steinke W, Meairs S, Ries S, Hennerici MG. Sonographic assessment of carotid artery stenosis: comparison of power Doppler imaging and color Doppler flow imaging. Stroke 1996; 27:91–94.

17. Griewing B, Morgenstern C, Driesner F, Kallwellis G, Walker ML, Kessler C. Cerebrovascular disease assessed by color-flow and power Doppler ultrasonography. Comparison with digital subtration angiography in internal carotid artery stenosis. Stroke 1996; 27:95–100.

18. Kofoed SC, Gronholdt ML, Wilhjelm JE, Bismuth J, Sillesen H. Real-time spatial compound imaging improves reproducibility in the evaluation of atherosclerotic carotid plaques. Ultrasound Med Biol 2001; 27(10):1311–1317.

19. Kern R, Szabo K, Hennerici M, Meairs S. Characterisation of carotid plaques using real-time compound B-mode ultrasound. Stroke 2004; 35(4):870–875.

20. Meairs S, Timpe L, Beyer J, Hennerici M. Acute aphasia and hemiplegia during karate training. Lancet 2000; 356(9223):40.

21. Leotta DF, Detmer PR, Martin RW. Performance of a miniature magnetic position sensor for three-dimensional ultrasound imaging. Ultrasound Med Biol 1997; 23(4):597–609.

22. Detmer PR, Bashein G, Hodges T, Beach KW, Filer EP, Burns DH, Strandness DE Jr. 3D ultrasonic image feature localization based on magnetic scanhead tracking: in vitro calibration and validation. Ultrasound Med Biol 1994; 20(9):923–936.

23. Hodges TC, Detmer PR, Burns DH, Beach KW, Strandness DE Jr. Ultrasonic three-dimensional reconstruction: in vitro and in vivo volume and area measurement. Ultrasound Med Biol 1994; 20(8):719–729.

24. Barry CD, Allott CP, John NW, Mellor PM, Arundel PA, Thomson DS, Waterton JC. Three-dimensional freehand ultrasound: image reconstruction and volume analysis. Ultrasound Med Biol 1997; 23(8):1209–1224.

25. Büdingen HJ, Hennerici MG, Voigt K, Kendel K, Freund H-J. Die Diagnostik von Stenosen oder Verschlüssen der A carotis interna mit der direktionellen Ultraschall-Doppler-Sonographie der A supratrochlearis. Dtsch Med Wschr 1976; 101:269–275.

26. Maroon JC, Pieroni DW, Campbell RL. Ophthalmosonometry. An ultrasonic method for assessing carotid blood flow. J Neurosurg 1969; 30(3):238–246.

27. Büdingen HJ, von Reutern G-M. Ultraschalldiagnostik der hirnversorgenden Arterien. Stuttgart: Thieme, 1993.

28. Planiol T, Pourcelot L, Pottiers JM, Degiovanni E. Étude de la circulation carotidiénne par les methodes ultrasoniques et la thermographie. Rev Neurol 1972; 126:127–141.

29. Baker DW, Forster FK, Daigle RE. Doppler Principles and Techniques in Ultrasound: Its Application in Medicine and Biology. Amsterdam: Elsevier, 1978.

30. Hennerici MG. Nicht-invasive Diagnostik des Frühstadiums arteriosklerotischer Karotisprozesse mit dem Duplex-System. Vasa 1983; 12:228–232.

31. Comerota AJ, Cranley JJ, Katz ML. Real-time B-mode carotid imaging: a three-year multicenter experience. J Vasc Surg 1984; 1:85–95.

32. Marosi L, Ehringer H. Die extrakranielle Arteria carotis im hochauflösenden Ultraschallechtzeit-Darstellungssystem: Morphologische Befunde bei gesunden jungen Erwachsenen. Ultraschall 1984; 5:174–181.

33. Meairs S, Hennerici M. Four-dimensional ultrasonographic characterization of plaque surface motion in patients with symptomatic and asymptomatic carotid artery stenosis. Stroke 1999; 30:1807–1813.

34. Guo Z, Fenster A. Three-dimensional power Doppler imaging: a phantom study to quantify vessel stenosis. Ultrasound Med Biol 1996; 22:1059–1069.

35. Steinke W, Hennerici MG. Three-dimensional ultrasound imaging of carotid artery plaques. J Cardiovasc Technol 1989; 8:15–22.

36. Rittgers SE, Thornhill BM, Barnes RW. Quantitative analysis of carotid artery Doppler spectral waveforms: diagnostic value of parameters. Ultrasound Med Biol 1983; 9:255–264.

37. Spencer MP, Reid JM. Quantification of carotid stenoses with continuous wave (CW) Doppler ultrasound. Stroke 1979; 10:326–330.

38. Touboul P-J, Hennerici MG, Meairs S, Adams H, Amarenco P, Desvarieux M, Ebrahim S, Fatar M, Hernandez Hernandez R, Kownator S, Prati P, Rundek T, Taylor A, Bornstein N, Csiba L, Vicaut E, Woo KS, Zannad R. Mannheim intima-meida thickness consensus. Cerebrovasc Dis 2004; 18:346–349.

39. Riley WA, Barnes RW, Applegate W, Dempsey R, Hartwell T, Davis VG, Bond MG, Furberg CD. Reproducibility of noninvasive ultrasonic measurement of carotid atherosclerosis. The asymptomatic carotid artery plaque study. Stroke 1992; 23:1062–1068.

40. Smith SC Jr, Greenland P, Grundy SM. Prevention conference V: beyond secondary prevention: identifying the high-risk patient for primary prevention: executive summary. Circulation 2000; 101(1):111–116.

41. Hennerici M, Meairs S. Imaging arterial wall disease. Cerebrovasc Dis 2000; 10(suppl 5):9–20.

42. O'Leary DH, Polak JF, Kronmal RA, Manolio TA, Burke GL, Wolfson SK Jr. Carotid-artery intima and media thickness as a risk factor for myocardial infarction and stroke in older adults. Cardiovascular Health Study Collaborative Research Group. N Engl J Med 1999; 340(1):14–22.

43. Starmans-Kool MJ, Stanton AV, Zhao S, Xu XY, Thom SA, Hughes AD. Measurement of hemodynamics in human carotid artery using ultrasound and computational fluid dynamics. J Appl Physiol 2002; 92(3):957–961.

44. Li J, Li X, Mori Y, Rusk RA, Lee JS, Davies CH, Hashimoto I, El Sedfy GO, Li XN, Sahn DJ. Quantification of flow volume with a new digital three-dimensional color Doppler flow approach: an in vitro study. J Ultrasound Med 2001; 20(12):1303–1311.

45. Licht PB, Christensen HW, Roder O, Hoilund-Carlsen PF. Volume flow estimation by colour duplex. Eur J Vasc Endovasc Surg 1999; 17(3):219–224.

46. Müller HR, Radue EW, Saia A, Pallotti C, Buser M. Caroted blood flow measurement by means of ultrasonic techniques: limitations and clinical use. In: Hartmann A, Hoyer S, eds. Cerebral Blood Flow and Metabolism Measurement. Berlin: Springer, 1985.

47. Eicke BM, Tegeler CH, Dalley G, Myers LG. Angle correction in transcranial Doppler sonography. J Neuroimag 1994; 4:29–33.

48. Ho SS, Metreweli C. Preferred technique for blood flow volume measurement in cerebrovascular disease. Stroke 2000; 31(6):1342–1345.

49. Tan TY, Lien LM, Schminke U, Tesh P, Reynolds PS, Tegeler CH. Hemodynamic effects of innominate artery occlusive disease on anterior cerebral artery. J Neuroimag 2002; 12(1):59–62.
50. Rubin JM, Tuthill TA, Fowlkes JB. Volume flow measurement using Doppler and grey-scale decorrelation. Ultrasound Med Biol 2001; 27(1):101–109.
51. Schmid-Schönbein H, Perktold K. Physical factors in the pathogenesis of atheroma formation. In: Caplan LR, ed. Brain Ischemia. Basic Concepts and Clinical Relevance. Berlin: Springer, 1995.
52. Steinke W, Kloetzsch C, Hennerici MG. Variability of flow patterns in the normal carotid bifurcation. Atherosclerosis 1990; 84:121–127.
53. Karino T, Goldsmith HL. Particle flow behaviour in models of bending vessels. II. Effects of branching angle and diameter ratio on flow pattern. Biorheology 1985; 22:87–105.
54. Zierler RE, Philips DJ, Beach EW, Primozich JF, Strandness DE. Noninvasive assessment of normal carotid bifurcation hemodynamics with color-flow ultrasound imaging. Ultrasound Med Biol 1987; 13:471–476.
55. Middleton WD, Foley WD, Lawson TL. Flow reversal in the normal carotid bifurcation: color Doppler flow imaging analysis. Radiology 1988; 167:207–209.
56. Ricotta JJ, Bryan FA, Bond MG, Kurtz A, O'Leary D, Raines JK, Berson AS, Clouse ME, Calderon-Ortiz M, Toole JF, DeWeese JA, Smullens SN, Gustafson NF. Multicenter validation study of real-time (B-Mode) ultrasound, arteriography, and pathologic examination. J Vasc Surg 1987; 6:512–520.
57. Görtler M, Niethammer R, Widder B. Differentiating subtotal carotid artery stenoses from occlusions by colour coded duplex sonography. J Neurol 1994; 241:301–305.
58. Sitzer M, Fürst G, Fisher H, Siebler M, Fehlings T, Kleinschmidt A, Kahn T, Steinmetz H. Between-method correlation in quantifying internal carotid stenosis. Stroke 1993; 24:1513–1518.
59. Pignoli P, Tremoli E, Poli A, Oreste P, Paoletti R. Intimal plus medial thickness of the arterial wall: a direct measurement with ultrasound imaging. Circulation 1986; 74:1399–1406.
60. Poli A, Tremoli E, Colombo A, Sirtori M, Pignoli P, Paoletti R. Ultrasonographic measurement of the common carotid arterial wall thickness in hypercholesterolemic patients. Atherosclerosis 1988; 70:253–261.
61. Azen SP, Qian D, Mack WJ, Sevanian A, Selzer RH, Liu CR, Liu CH, Hodis HN. Effect of supplementary antioxidant vitamin intake on carotid arterial wall intima-media thickness in a controlled clinical trial of cholesterol lowering. Circulation 1996; 94(10):2369–2372.
62. Adams MR, Nakagomi A, Keech A, Robinson J, McCredie R, Bailey BP, Freedman SB, Celermajer DS. Carotid intima-media thickness is only weakly correlated with the extent and severity of coronary artery disease. Circulation 1995; 92(8):2127–2134.
63. Baldassarre D, Werba JP, Tremoli E, Poli A, Pazzucconi F, Sirtori CR. Common carotid intima-media thickness measurement. A method to improve accuracy and precision. Stroke 1994; 25(8):1588–1592.

64. Bruschi G, Cabassi A, Orlandini G, Regolisti G, Zambrelli P, Calzolari M, Borghetti A. Use of Fourier shape descriptors to improve the reproducibility of echographic measurements of arterial intima-media thickness. J Hypertens 1997; 15(5):467–474.

65. Bluth EI, Kay D, Merritt CRB, Sullivan MA, Farr G, Mills NG, Foreman M, Sloan K, Schlater M, Steward J. Sonographic characterization of carotid plaque: detection of hemorrhage. Am J Neuroradiol 1986; 7:311–315.

66. Comerota AJ, Katz ML, White JV, Grosh JD. The preoperative diagnosis of the ulcerated carotid atheroma. J Vasc Surg 1990; 11(4):505–510.

67. Bock RW, Lusby RJ. Carotid plaque morphology and interpretation of the echolucent lesion. In: Labs KH, Jäger KA, Fitzgerald DE, Woodcock JP, Neuerburg-Heusler D, eds. Diagnostic Vascular Imaging. London: Arnold, 1992:225–236.

68. Langsfeld M, Gray-Weale AC, Lusby RJ. The role of plaque morphology and diameter reduction in the development of new symptoms in asymptomatic carotid arteries. J Vasc Surg 1989; 9(4):548–557.

69. O'Donnell TF Jr, Erdoes L, Mackey WC, McCullough J, Shepard A, Heggerick P, Isner J, Callow AD. Correlation of B-mode ultrasound imaging and arteriography with pathologic findings at carotid endarterectomy. Arch Surg 1985; 120(4):443–449.

70. Sterpetti AV, Schultz RD, Feldhaus RJ. Ultrasonographic features of carotid plaque and the risk of subsequent neurological deficits. Surgery 1988; 104: 652–660.

71. Aldoori MI, Baird RN, Al-Sam SZ, Cole SE, Mera S, Davies JD. Duplex scanning and plaque histology in cerebral ischaemia. Eur J Vasc Surg 1987; 1(3):159–164.

72. Imparato AM, Riles TS, Mintzer R, Baumann FG. The importance of hemorrhage in the relationship between gross morphologic characteristics and cerebral symptoms in 376 carotid artery plaques. Ann Surg 1983; 197(2): 195–203.

73. Fisher M, Blumenfeld AM, Smith TW. The importance of carotid artery plaque disruption and hemorrhage. Arch Neurol 1987; 44(10):1086–1089.

74. Imparato AM, Riles TS, Gorstein F. The carotid bifurcation plaque: pathologic findings associated with cerebral ischemia. Stroke 1979; 10(3): 238–245.

75. Lusby RJ, Ferrell LD, Ehrenfeld WK, Stoney RJ, Wylie EJ. Carotid plaque hemorrhage. Its role in production of cerebral ischemia. Arch Surg 1982; 117(11):1479–1488.

76. Bassiouny HS, Davis H, Massawa N, Gewertz BL, Glagov S, Zarins CK. Critical carotid stenoses: morphologic and chemical similarity between symptomatic and asymptomatic plaques. J Vasc Surg 1989; 9(2):202–212.

77. Leen EJ, Feeley TM, Colgan MP, O'Malley MK, Moore DJ, Hourihane DO, Shanik GD. "Haemorrhagic" carotid plaque does not contain haemorrhage. Eur J Vasc Surg 1990; 4(2):123–128.

78. Lennihan L, Kupsky WJ, Mohr JP, Hauser WA, Correll JW, Quest DO. Lack of association between carotid plaque hematoma and ischemic cerebral symptoms. Stroke 1987; 18(5):879–881.

79. AbuRahma AF, Kyer PD 3rd, Robinson PA, Hannay RS. The correlation of ultrasonic carotid plaque morphology and carotid plaque hemorrhage: clinical implications. Surgery 1998; 124(4):721–726; discussion 726–728.
80. Park AE, McCarthy WJ, Pearce WH, Matsumura JS, Yao JS. Carotid plaque morphology correlates with presenting symptomatology. J Vasc Surg 1998; 27(5):872–878; discussion 878–879.
81. Golledge J, Cuming R, Ellis M, Davies AH, Greenhalgh RM. Carotid plaque characteristics and presenting symptom. Br J Surg 1997; 84(12):1697–1701.
82. Gronholdt ML, Wiebe BM, Laursen H, Nielsen TG, Schroeder TV, Sillesen H. Lipid-rich carotid artery plaques appear echolucent on ultrasound B-mode images and may be associated with intraplaque haemorrhage. Eur J Vasc Endovasc Surg 1997; 14(6):439–445.
83. Droste DW, Karl M, Bohle RM, Kaps M. Comparison of ultrasonic and histopathological features of carotid artery stenosis. Neurol Res 1997; 19(4): 380–384.
84. Hatsukami TS, Ferguson MS, Beach KW, Gordon D, Detmer P, Burns D, Alpers C, Strandness DE Jr. Carotid plaque morphology and clinical events. Stroke 1997; 28(1):95–100.
85. Nicolaides A, Kakkos S, Sabetal M, Griffin M, Loannidou E, Francis S, Kyriakou E. Asymptotic carotid stenosis and risk of stroke: natural history study. Stroke 2005; 36(2):424.
86. Joakimsen O, Bonaa KH, Stensland-Bugge E. Reproducibility of ultrasound assessment of carotid plaque occurrence, thickness, and morphology. The Tromso Study. Stroke 1997; 28(11):2201–2207.
87. Hartmann A, Mohr JP, Thompson JL, Ramos O, Mast H. Interrater reliability of plaque morphology classification in patients with severe carotid artery stenosis. Acta Neurol Scand 1999; 99(1):61–64.
88. Arnold JA, Modaresi KB, Thomas N, Taylor PR, Padayachee TS. Carotid plaque characterization by duplex scanning: observer error may undermine current clinical trials. Stroke 1999; 30(1):61–65.
89. Montauban van Swijndregt AD, Elbers HR, Moll FL, de Letter J, Ackerstaff RG. Ultrasonographic characterization of carotid plaques. Ultrasound Med Biol 1998; 24(4):489–493.
90. Elatrozy T, Nicolaides A, Tegos T, Griffin M. The objective characterisation of ultrasonic carotid plaque features. Eur J Vasc Endovasc Surg 1998; 16(3):223–230.
91. Gronholdt ML, Nordestgaard BG, Wiebe BM, Wilhjelm JE, Sillesen H. Echolucency of computerized ultrasound images of carotid atherosclerotic plaques are associated with increased levels of triglyceride-rich lipoproteins as well as increased plaque lipid content. Circulation 1998; 97(1):34–40.
92. Noritomi T, Sigel B, Swami V, Justin J, Gahtan V, Chen X, Feleppa EJ, Roberts AB, Shirouzu K. Carotid plaque typing by multiple-parameter ultrasonic tissue characterization. Ultrasound Med Biol 1997; 23(5):643–650.
93. Robinson ML, Sacks D, Perlmutter GS, Marinelli DL. Diagnostic criteria for carotid duplex sonography. Am J Roentgenol 1988; 151:1045–1049.

94. Widder B, Paulat K, Hachspacher J. Morphological characterisation of carotid artery stenoses by ultrasound duplex scanning. Ultrasound Med Biol 1990; 16:349–354.

95. Neuerburg-Heusler D, Hennerici M. Gefäßdiagnostik mit Ultraschall. New York: Thieme, 2000.

96. Mondy JS, Lindner V, Miyashiro JK, Berk BC, Dean RH, Geary RL. Platelet-derived growth factor ligand and receptor expression in response to altered blood flow in vivo. Circ Res 1997; 81(3):320–327.

97. Bluth EI, McVay LV 3rd, Merritt CR, Sullivan MA. The identification of ulcerative plaque with high resolution duplex carotid scanning. J Ultrasound Med 1988; 7(2):73–76.

98. Streifler JY, Eliasziw M, Fox AJ, Benavente OR, Hachinski VC, Ferguson GG, Barnett HJ. Angiographic detection of carotid plaque ulceration. Comparison with surgical observations in a multicenter study. North American Symptomatic Carotid Endarterectomy Trial. Stroke 1994; 25(6):1130–1132.

99. Rothwell PM, Gibson RJ, Villagra R, Sellar R, Warlow CP. The effect of angiographic technique and image quality on the reproducibility of measurement of carotid stenosis and assessment of plaque surface morphology. Clin Radiol 1998; 53(6):439–443.

100. Eliasziw M, Streifler JY, Fox AJ, Hachinski VC, Ferguson HB, Barnett HJM. Significance of plaque ulceration in symptomatic patients with high-grade carotid stenosis. Stroke 1994; 25(304):308.

101. Fischer CM, Ojemann RJ. A clinico-pathologic study of carotid endarectomy plaques. Rev Neurol 1986; 142:573.

102. Svindland A, Torvik A. Atherosclerotic carotid disease in asymptomatic individuals: an histological study of 53 cases. Acta Neurol Scand 1988; 78(6): 506–517.

103. Glagov S, Bassiouny HS, Giddens DP, Zarins CK. Intimal thickening: morphogenesis, functional significance and deterction. J Vasc Investig 1995; 1:2–14.

104. de Bray JM, Baud JM, Dauzat M, Glatt B. Consenus concerning the morphology and the risk of carotid plaques. Cerebrovasc Dis 1997; 7:289–296.

105. Langille BL. Arterial remodeling: relation to hemodynamics. Can J Physiol Pharmacol 1996; 74(7):834–841.

106. Tronc F, Wassef M, Esposito B, Henrion D, Glagov S, Tedgui A. Role of NO in flow-induced remodeling of the rabbit common carotid artery. Arterioscler Thromb Vasc Biol 1996; 16(10):1256–1262.

107. Abbruzzese TA, Guzman RJ, Martin RL, Yee C, Zarins CK, Dalman RL. Matrix metalloproteinase inhibition limits arterial enlargements in a rodent arteriovenous fistula model. Surgery 1998; 124(2):328–334; discussion 334–335.

108. Sasaki K, Hattori T, Fujisawa T, Takahashi K, Inoue H, Takigawa M. Nitric oxide mediates interleukin-1-induced gene expression of matrix metalloproteinases and basic fibroblast growth factor in cultured rabbit articular chondrocytes. J Biochem (Tokyo) 1998; 123(3):431–439.

109. Cooke JP, Dzau VJ. Derangements of the nitric oxide synthase pathway, L-arginine, and cardiovascular diseases. Circulation 1997; 96(2):379–382.

110. Bassiouny HS, Song RH, Hong XF, Singh A, Kocharyan H, Glagov S. Flow regulation of 72-kD collagenase IV (MMP-2) after experimental arterial injury. Circulation 1998; 98(2):157–163.
111. Lehoux S, Tedgui A. Signal transduction of mechanical stresses in the vascular wall. Hypertension 1998; 32(2):338–345.
112. Di Stefano I, Koopmans DR, Langille BL. Modulation of arterial growth of the rabbit carotid artery associated with experimental elevation of blood flow. J Vasc Res 1998; 35(1):1–7.
113. Cowan DB, Lye SJ, Langille BL. Regulation of vascular connexin43 gene expression by mechanical loads. Circ Res 1998; 82(7):786–793.
114. Ward MR, Jeremias A, Huegel H, Fitzgerald PJ, Yeung AC. Accentuated remodeling on the upstream side of atherosclerotic lesions. Am J Cardiol 2000; 85(5):523–526.
115. Dirksen MT, van der Wal AC, van den Berg FM, van der Loos CM, Becker AE. Distribution of inflammatory cells in atherosclerotic plaques relates to the direction of flow. Circulation 1998; 98(19):2000–2003.
116. Smedby O. Do plaques grow upstream or downstream? an angiographic study in the femoral artery. Arterioscler Thromb Vasc Biol 1997; 17(5):912–918.
117. Walpola PL, Gotlieb AI, Cybulsky MI, Langille BL. Expression of ICAM-1 and VCAM-1 and monocyte adherence in arteries exposed to altered shear stress. Arterioscler Thromb Vasc Biol 1995; 15(1):2–10.
118. Galis ZS, Asanuma K, Godin D, Meng X. N-acetyl-cysteine decreases the matrix-degrading capacity of macrophage-derived foam cells: new target for antioxidant therapy? Circulation 1998; 97(24):2445–2453.
119. Aikawa M, Rabkin E, Okada Y, Voglic SJ, Clinton SK, Brinckerhoff CE, Sukhova GK, Libby P. Lipid lowering by diet reduces matrix metalloproteinase activity and increases collagen content of rabbit atheroma: a potential mechanism of lesion stabilization. Circulation 1998; 97(24):2433–2444.
120. Tauth J, Pinnow E, Sullebarger JT, Basta L, Gursoy S, Lindsay J Jr, Matar F. Predictors of coronary arterial remodeling patterns in patients with myocardial ischemia. Am J Cardiol 1997; 80(10):1352–1355.
121. Kwon HM, Sangiorgi G, Spagnoli LG, Miyauchi K, Holmes DR Jr, Schwartz RS, Lerman A. Experimental hypercholesterolemia induces ultrastructural changes in the internal elastic lamina of porcine coronary arteries. Atherosclerosis 1998; 139(2):283–289.
122. Wong LC, Langille BL. Developmental remodeling of the internal elastic lamina of rabbit arteries: effect of blood flow. Circ Res 1996; 78(5):799–805.
123. Berglund H, Luo H, Nishioka T, Fishbein MC, Eigler NL, Tabak SW, Siegel RJ. Highly localized arterial remodeling in patients with coronary atherosclerosis: an intravascular ultrasound study. Circulation 1997; 96(5): 1470–1476.
124. Crawford T, Levene CI. Medial thinning in atheroma. J Pathol Bacteriol 1953; 66(1):19–23.
125. Zalewski A, Shi Y. Vascular myofibroblasts. Lessons from coronary repair and remodeling. Arterioscler Thromb Vasc Biol 1997; 17(3):417–422.
126. Pasterkamp G, Schoneveld AH, van Wolferen W, Hillen B, Clarijs RJ, Haudenschild CC, Borst C. The impact of atherosclerotic arterial remodeling

on percentage of luminal stenosis varies widely within the arterial system. A postmortem study. Arterioscler Thromb Vasc Biol 1997; 17(11):3057–3063.

127. Ferrer M, Encabo A, Conde MV, Marin J, Balfagon G. Heterogeneity of endothelium-dependent mechanisms in different rabbit arteries. J Vasc Res 1995; 32(5):339–346.

128. Ward MR, Kanellakis P, Ramsey D, Jennings GL, Bobik A. Response to balloon injury is vascular bed specific: a consequence of de novo vessel structure? Atherosclerosis 2000; 151(2):407–414.

129. Kornowski R, Mintz GS, Lansky AJ, Hong MK, Kent KM, Pichard AD, Satler LF, Popma JJ, Bucher TA, Leon MB. Paradoxic decreases in atherosclerotic plaque mass in insulin-treated diabetic patients. Am J Cardiol 1998; 81(11):1298–1304.

130. Pasterkamp G, Borst C, Post MJ, Mali WP, Wensing PJ, Gussenhoven EJ, Hillen B. Atherosclerotic arterial remodeling in the superficial femoral artery. Individual variation in local compensatory enlargement response. Circulation 1996; 93(10):1818–1825.

131. Mintz GS, Kent KM, Pichard AD, Satler LF, Popma JJ, Leon MB. Contribution of inadequate arterial remodeling to the development of focal coronary artery stenoses. An intravascular ultrasound study. Circulation 1997; 95(7):1791–1798.

132. Wensing PJ, Meiss L, Mali WP, Hillen B. Early atherosclerotic lesions spiraling through the femoral artery. Arterioscler Thromb Vasc Biol 1998; 18(10):1554–1558.

133. Krams R, Wentzel JJ, Oomen JA, Schuurbiers JC, Andhyiswara I, Kloet J, Post M, de Smet B, Borst C, Slager CJ, Serruys PW. Shear stress in atherosclerosis, and vascular remodelling. Semin Interv Cardiol 1998; 3(1):39–44.

134. Bonithon-Kopp C, Touboul PJ, Berr C, Magne C, Ducimetiere P. Factors of carotid arterial enlargement in a population aged 59 to 71 years: the EVA study. Stroke 1996; 27:654–660.

135. Fuster V, Badimon J, Chesebro JH, Fallon JT. Plaque rupture, thrombosis, and therapeutic implications. Haemostasis 1996; 26(suppl 4):269–284.

136. Qiao JH, Fishbein MC. The severity of coronary atherosclerosis at sites of plaque rupture with occlusive thrombosis. J Am Coll Cardiol 1991; 17(5): 1138–1142.

137. Kearney P, Erbel R, Rupprecht HJ, Ge J, Koch L, Voigtlander T, Stahr P, Gorge G, Meyer J. Differences in the morphology of unstable and stable coronary lesions and their impact on the mechanisms of angioplasty. An in vivo study with intravascular ultrasound. Eur Heart J 1996; 17(5): 721–730.

138. Smits PC, Pasterkamp G, de Jaegere PP, de Feyter PJ, Borst C. Angioscopic complex lesions are predominantly compensatory enlarged: an angioscopy and intracoronary ultrasound study. Cardiovasc Res 1999; 41(2):458–464.

139. Filardo SD, Schwarzacher SP, Lo ST, Herity NA, Lee DP, Huegel H, Mullen WL, Fitzgerald PJ, Ward MR, Yeung AC. Acute myocardial infarction and vascular remodeling. Am J Cardiol 2000; 85(6):760–762, A8.

140. Schoenhagen P, Ziada KM, Kapadia SR, Crowe TD, Nissen SE, Tuzcu EM. Extent and direction of arterial remodeling in stable versus unstable coronary

syndromes: an intravascular ultrasound study. Circulation 2000; 101(6): 598–603.

141. Ridker PM, Cushman M, Stampfer MJ, Tracy RP, Hennekens CH. Inflammation, aspirin, and the risk of cardiovascular disease in apparently healthy men. N Engl J Med 1997; 336(14):973–979.

142. Casscells W, Hathorn B, David M, Krabach T, Vaughn WK, McAllister HA, Bearman G, Willerson JT. Thermal detection of cellular infiltrates in living atherosclerotic plaques: possible implications for plaque rupture and thrombosis. Lancet 1996; 347(9013):1447–1451.

143. Ridker PM, Rifai N, Pfeffer MA, Sacks FM, Moye LA, Goldman S, Flaker GC, Braunwald E. Inflammation, pravastatin, and the risk of coronary events after myocardial infarction in patients with average cholesterol levels. Cholesterol and Recurrent Events (CARE) Investigators. Circulation 1998; 98(9):839–844.

144. de Smet BJ, de Kleijn D, Hanemaaijer R, Verheijen JH, Robertus L, van Der Helm YJ, Borst C, Post MJ. Metalloproteinase inhibition reduces constrictive arterial remodeling after balloon angioplasty: a study in the atherosclerotic Yucatan micropig. Circulation 2000; 101(25):2962–2967.

145. Crouse JR, Goldbourt U, Evans G, Pinsky J, Sharrett AR, Sorlie P, Riley W, Heiss G. Arterial enlargement in the atherosclerosis risk in communities (ARIC) cohort. In vivo quantification of carotid arterial enlargement. The ARIC Investigators. Stroke 1994; 25(7):1354–1359.

146. Ringelstein EB. Echocontrast agents in neurovascular ultrasound. Eur Heart J Suppl 2002; 4(suppl C):C48–C50.

147. Frush DP, Babcock DS, White KS, Barr LL. Quantification of intravenous contrast-enhanced Doppler power spectrum in the rabbit carotid artery. Ultrasound Med Biol 1995; 21(1):41–47.

148. Gebel M, Caselitz M, Bowen-Davies PE, Weber S. A multicenter, prospective, open label, randomized, controlled phase IIIb study of SH U 508 a (Levovist) for Doppler signal enhancement in the portal vascular system. Ultraschall Med 1998; 19(4):148–156.

149. Melany ML, Grant EG. Clinical experience with sonographic contrast agents. Semin Ultrasound CT MR 1997; 18(1):3–12.

150. Schwarz KQ, Becher H, Schimpfky C, Vorwerk D, Bogdahn U, Schlief R. Doppler enhancement with SH U 508A in multiple vascular regions. Radiology 1994; 193(1):195–201.

151. Bazzocchi M, Quaia E, Zuiani C, Moroldo M. Transcranial Doppler: state of the art. Eur J Radiol 1998; 27(suppl 2):S141–S148.

152. Deklunder G. Role of ultrasound and contrast-enhanced ultrasound in patients with cerebrovascular disease. Eur Heart J Suppl 2002; 27(suppl 2): S141–S148.

153. Elgersma OE, van Leeuwen MS, Meijer R, Eikelboom BC, van der Graaf Y. Lumen reduction measurements of the internal carotid artery before and after Levovist enhancement: reproducibility and agreement with angiography. J Ultrasound Med 1999; 18(3):191–201.

154. Sitzer M, Müller W, Siebler M, Hort W, Kniemeyer HW, Janke L, Steinmetz H. Plaque ulceration and lumen thrombus are the main sources of cerebral

microemboli in high-grade internal carotid stenosis. Stroke 1995; 26: 1231–1233.

155. de Bray JM, Glatt B. For the International Consensus Conference: Quantification of atheromatous stenosis in the extracranial internal carotid artery. Cerebrovasc Dis 1995; 5:414–426.

156. Hennerici MG, Steinke W, Rautenberg W. High-resistance Doppler flow pattern in extracranial carotid dissection. Arch Neurol 1989; 46:670–672.

157. Sidhu PS, Jonker ND, Khaw KT, Patel N, Blomley MJ, Chaudhuri KR, Frackowiak RS, Cosgrove DO. Spontaneous dissections of the internal carotid artery: appearances on colour Doppler ultrasound. Br J Radiol 1997; 70:50–57.

158. Sturzenegger M, Mattle HP, Rivoir A, Baumgartner RW. Ultrasound findings in carotid artery dissection: analysis of 43 patients. Neurology 1995; 45(4):691–698.

159. Steinke W, Rautenberg W, Schwartz A, Hennerici MG. Noninvasive monitoring of internal carotid artery dissection. Stroke 1994; 25:998–1005.

160. Schumann PA, Christiansen JP, Quigley RM, McCreery TP, Sweitzer RH, Unger EC, Lindner JR, Matsunaga TO. Targeted-microbubble binding selectively to GPIIb IIIa receptors of platelet thrombi. Invest Radiol 2002; 37(11):587–593.

161. Tardy I, Pochon S, Theraulaz M, Nanjappan P, Schneider M. In vivo ultrasound imaging of thrombi using a target-specific contrast agent. Acad Radiol 2002; 9(suppl 2):S294–S296.

162. Christiansen JP, Leong-Poi H, Klibanov AL, Kaul S, Lindner JR. Noninvasive imaging of myocardial reperfusion injury using leukocyte-targeted contrast echocardiography. Circulation 2002; 105(15):1764–1767.

163. Lindner JR. Detection of inflamed plaques with contrast ultrasound. Am J Cardiol 200; 90(10C):32L–35L.

6

Antithrombotic Therapy for Carotid Artery Stenosis

Seemant Chaturvedi

Department of Neurology, Detroit Medical Center, Wayne State University, Detroit, Michigan, U.S.A.

All patients with symptomatic internal carotid artery (ICA) stenosis should be placed on antithrombotic therapy. The major options for the clinician are antiplatelet agents or oral anticoagulants.

There is virtually no head-to-head data comparing individual antiplatelet agents or antiplatelet agents vs. warfarin for patients with ICA stenosis. Therefore, the clinician must rely on "global" stroke prevention studies, which typically include a combination of patients with large vessel atherosclerotic, lacunar, and cryptogenic stroke. In addition, many of the major trials conducted in the last three decades have enrolled both transient ischemic attack (TIA) and stroke patients.

In this chapter, individual antithrombotic agents for stroke prevention will be reviewed, in general, and if information is available, for stroke prevention in the setting of ICA stenosis.

1. EXTRACRANIAL SYMPTOMATIC CAROTID STENOSIS

1.1. Aspirin

As mentioned above, most clinical trials of antithrombotic agents for stroke prevention have been symptom-based, meaning patients were treated after they presented to medical attention with either a TIA or a stroke. The same applies to studies of aspirin for stroke prevention.

Aspirin is widely used for secondary prophylaxis in patients with symptomatic carotid stenosis. In a broad group of patients, the Antithrombotic Trialists' Collaboration found a 22% relative risk reduction with antiplatelet therapy, primarily aspirin (Fig. 1) (1). In the North American Symptomatic Carotid Endarterectomy Trial (NASCET), it was recommended that patients in the medically treated group receive 1300 mg/day of aspirin for stroke prevention (2). The treatment was not mandated by the protocol and, therefore, individual physicians in the study could prescribe lower doses of aspirin, other antiplatelet agents, or warfarin if they desired. Nevertheless, 1300 mg of aspirin was considered an element of "best medical therapy" when NASCET began in 1987. There was no protocol-mandated dose of aspirin in the European Carotid Surgery Trial (3).

In prior symptom-based trials such as the Canadian Cooperative Stroke Study, it was not reported as to whether aspirin was better than placebo for the subgroup of patients with extracranial carotid stenosis, nor is it likely that the study would have sufficient statistical power to answer this question (4). Other studies that have compared aspirin with placebo, such as the Swedish Aspirin Low Dose Trial (SALT), also cannot provide a definite conclusion regarding how beneficial aspirin is for the category of patients with symptomatic carotid atherosclerosis (5).

In the absence of studies focusing exclusively on carotid stenosis, we must rely on studies which include patients with non-cardioembolic stroke or TIA, which should account for approximately 80% of cerebral ischemic events. These studies, in aggregate, show an approximately 22% risk reduction conferred by aspirin for the prevention of the composite outcome stroke, myocardial infarction, or vascular death (1). It must be extrapolated, not

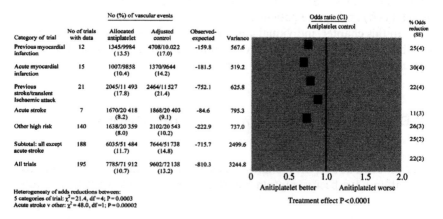

Figure 1 Overview of antiplatelet therapy. *Source*: Reproduced from Ref. 1.

unreasonably, that platelet inhibition with aspirin is useful for patients with symptomatic carotid stenosis, since the majority of patients with symptomatic disease will have artery-to-artery emboli of platelet–fibrin material as the mechanism for their symptoms. The benefits of aspirin in patients with symptomatic carotid stenosis is also supported by a transcranial Doppler (TCD) study in which microembolic signals (MES) in the middle cerebral artery were eliminated 2 h after the injection of 500 mg of intravenous aspirin in seven of nine patients with symptomatic disease (6).

The optimal dose of aspirin for stroke prevention has been a source of longstanding controversy. In this context, one usually considers high-dose aspirin as two or more adult aspirin (650–1300 mg/day). Low-dose aspirin is conventionally regarded as one adult aspirin or less (≤325 mg/day). There is no prospective, randomized data at present to establish that high-dose aspirin is more effective than low-dose aspirin. The proponents of high-dose aspirin use a variety of arguments drawing on physiologic factors and clinical trial data to support the assertion that high dose is superior. The physiologic factors include the fact that low-dose aspirin does not prevent platelet aggregation in all situations, such as conditions of high shear stress (7). In addition, laboratory data suggest that the dose of aspirin necessary to achieve full platelet inhibition may vary from person to person and may change over time. Helgason et al. demonstrated that 32.7% of stroke patients with complete platelet inhibition at the outset had lost part of the antiplatelet effect and had only partial platelet inhibition with the same aspirin dosage when the platelets of these patients were tested serially over 33 months (8). Some patients were able to achieve complete platelet inhibition with an increase in the aspirin dosage. These results suggest that a fraction of patients may develop "aspirin resistance" over a period of years and that, in general, those taking high-dose aspirin are likely to have more persistent platelet inhibition than those ingesting low-dose aspirin.

There is no standardized methodology at the current time to test for aspirin resistance (9). However, if aspirin resistance is identified, this may place patients at a higher risk for vascular events. In one study, 326 outpatients with a prior history of ischemic heart disease or stroke were evaluated for aspirin resistance with an optical platelet aggregation test (10). Patients were treated with 325 mg/day of aspirin. Aspirin resistance was defined as >70% aggregation with 10 μM ADP and >20% aggregation with 0.5 mg/mL arachidonic acid. Overall, 5.2% of patients were aspirin-resistant. During a mean follow-up of 679 days, there was an increased risk of stroke, myocardial infarction, or death in patients deemed to have aspirin resistance compared to aspirin-sensitive patients (24 vs. 10%, hazard ratio 3.12, $p = 0.03$). Platelet polymorphisms and genetic factors are likely to play a role in the variable clinical response to aspirin (11,12).

The clinical trial data supporting high-dose aspirin come from overview analyses of the major randomized trials. In one review, Dyken et al.

concluded that high-dose aspirin has been shown to provide a 25–42% risk reduction, compared to low-dose aspirin studies, where the risk reduction has been in the range of 3–18% (13). In addition, Bornstein et al. analyzed the timing of recurrent cerebral ischemic events in patients taking a variety of aspirin doses (14). This study found that patients taking 100–250 mg of aspirin had an episode of recurrent cerebral ischemia at an average of 10–11 months, compared to individuals on 500 mg of aspirin, where the recurrent event was observed at a mean time of 24 months.

On the other hand, recent clinical trials such as the European Stroke Prevention Study 2 (ESPS2) show that even 50 mg/day of aspirin does confer stroke protection (15). In this study, which is discussed further below, patients were enrolled after a TIA or stroke and treated with either placebo, aspirin alone (25 mg twice daily), extended-release dipyridamole (ERDP, 200 mg twice daily), or the combined aspirin/ERDP formulation (25 mg/ 200 mg twice daily). Over a subsequent 2-year follow-up period, aspirin alone had an 18% relative risk reduction compared to placebo. There was no information provided on the number of patients in ESPS2 with moderate-to-severe ICA stenosis.

Based on more recent clinical trial results, the American College of Chest Physicians is now recommending lower doses of aspirin (50–325 mg daily) for stroke prevention (16). In the absence of new data, this aspirin dose would appear to be sensible for patients with symptomatic ICA stenosis as well.

For patients with carotid stenosis undergoing carotid endarterectomy (CE), low-dose aspirin is preferred. The Aspirin and Carotid Endarterectomy (ACE) trial enrolled 2849 patients and randomly assigned them to either low-dose aspirin (81 or 325 mg/day) or high-dose aspirin (650 or 1300 mg/day) (17). For the outcome of stroke, myocardial infarction, or death, there was a lower endpoint rate in the low-dose aspirin group at both 30 days and 3 months. At 30 days, there was a trend favoring low-dose aspirin (5.4 vs. 7.0%, $p = 0.07$) and at 3 months it was significant (6.2 vs. 8.4%, $p = 0.03$). Thus, low-dose aspirin (81–325 mg/day) is recommended prior to CE and during the perioperative period.

Treatment with aspirin should continue following CE. In an overview of six trials that evaluated antiplatelet therapy vs. control following CE in which treatment duration was at least 30 days and follow-up was at least 3 months, 907 patients were identified (18). In these patients, a statistically significant benefit for the prevention of stroke was identified (odds ratio 0.58, 95% CI: 0.34–0.98, $p = 0.04$).

1.2. Ticlopidine

A second antiplatelet option is ticlopidine hydrochloride, a thienopyridine that inhibits adenosine diphosphate-induced fibrinogen binding to platelets, a necessary step in the platelet aggregation process. Two large trials (19,20) assessed ticlopidine for the prevention of stroke and other vascular events in patients presenting with cerebrovascular symptoms.

The Ticlopidine Aspirin Stroke Study (TASS) (20) studied 3069 patients following a minor stroke or TIA. There was a 21% relative risk reduction for stroke with ticlopidine compared with aspirin, and a 9% reduction for the combined endpoint of stroke, MI, or vascular death at 3 years. Noteworthy GI side-effects (e.g., ulcers and bleeding) were more common in the aspirin group (2.5 times higher). Severe neutropenia occurred in 0.9% of patients in the ticlopidine-treated group. Neutropenia was noted within the first 3 months of drug treatment and was usually reversible. For this reason, as well as for the risk of thrombotic thrombocytopenic purpura (TTP), blood counts are required at 2-week intervals for the first 3 months of ticlopidine therapy (i.e., six blood counts in 3 months).

Due to hematologic toxicity, ticlopidine is not in widespread use currently. A recent study which should decrease ticlopidine use even further is the African American Antiplatelet Stroke Prevention Study (AAASPS) (21). This was a randomized prospective study comparing 325 mg of aspirin twice per day to 250 mg of ticlopidine twice daily. The study protocol excluded patients with planned CE for a symptomatic ICA stenosis and, therefore, it is unlikely that many patients with >70% ICA stenosis were included, although it is possible that patients with symptomatic moderate stenoses or symptomatic intracranial ICA stenoses were enrolled. In general, however, the study was heavily weighted to lacunar stroke patients (67.5% of patients).

In the final analysis, AAASPS enrolled 1809 patients and follow-up was planned for 2 years. The study was stopped prematurely, however, when it was felt that ticlopidine would not emerge superior to aspirin. In fact, at the time the study was halted, there was a trend favoring aspirin over ticlopidine. For the primary outcome of stroke, MI, or vascular death, the hazard ratio for ticlopidine compared to aspirin was 1.22 (CI 0.94–1.57). For patients with stroke due to large vessel atherosclerosis, there was no definite evidence that ticlopidine was of greater benefit than aspirin.

1.3. Clopidogrel

Clopidogrel is also a thienopyridine derivative. The efficacy of clopidogrel was established in the Clopidogrel vs. Aspirin in Patients at Risk of Ischemic Events (CAPRIE) study (22). This was a randomized, blinded, multicenter trial which included the following three groups of patients: those with recent ischemic stroke, recent MI, and symptomatic peripheral vascular disease.

Patients were assigned to either clopidogrel (75 mg/day) or aspirin (325 mg/day). In 19,185 patients, it was found that there was an 8.7% relative risk reduction in favor of clopidogrel (95% CI, 0.3–16.5; $p = 0.043$), and an absolute risk reduction of 0.5%. An on-treatment analysis showed a relative risk reduction of 9.4%. The inclusion of major hemorrhages along with the primary endpoint led to a relative risk reduction with clopidogrel of 9.5% (95% CI, 1.2–18.5). There is no published data available regarding the comparative efficacy of clopidogrel vs. aspirin for patients with extracranial carotid stenosis.

Unlike ticlopidine, there was not an increased risk of neutropenia in association with clopidogrel. In the CAPRIE trial, major hemorrhages occurred at a slightly higher rate among patients taking aspirin (1.55 vs. 1.38%). A previous surveillance study found 11 cases of TTP associated with clopidogrel among >3 million patients who had been given this medication. The majority of these cases occurred within 2 weeks of starting clopidogrel treatment. Most cases improved with plasma exchange therapy. At the current time, routine blood monitoring for thrombocytopenia is not recommended since this side-effect is fortunately quite rare.

Post-hoc subgroup analyses have identified several groups in CAPRIE in which there was a magnified benefit from clopidogrel treatment as compared with aspirin. These subgroups include patients with a previous coronary artery bypass graft, patients with diabetes, and patients with disease in more than one vascular bed (Table 1) (23). These patients would be expected

Table 1 Enhanced Risk Reduction with Clopidogrel Therapy in High-Risk Patients in the CAPRIE' Study[a]

High-risk Populations	Clopidogrel ER, %	ASA ER, %	Clopidogrel		
			RRR, %	ARR, %	NNT
Total CAPRIE population	12.57	13.67	7.9	1.1	91
Patient with previous CABG	15.9	22.3	28.9	6.4	16
Patients with a history of ≥1 Ischemic event	18.4	20.4	10.0	2.0	50
Patients with involvement of multiple vascular beds	17.39	10.84	12.4	2.45	41
Patients with diabetes	15.6	17.7	12.5	2.1	48
Patients with hypercholesterolema	12.3	13.6	9.7	1.3	77

Abbreviations: ARR, absolute risk reduction; ASA, acetylsalicyclic acid; CABG, coronary artery bypass grafting; CAPRIE, Clopidogrel vs. Aspirin in Patients at Risk of Ischemic Events; ER, event rate; NNT, number of patients needed to treat to prevent an event; RRR, relative risk reduction.
[a]The average event rate of stroke, myocardial Infraction, vascular death, and rehospitalization for Ischemia or bleeding while receiving treatment with clopidogrel vs. ASA is depicted in various high-risk populations. Patients were followed up for 1.9 years.

to have a greater degree of carotid atherosclerosis compared to a broader group of patients where other mechanisms (small vessel occlusion, cryptogenic stroke) may be more common.

In other vascular beds, such as ischemic heart disease patients with a recent non-Q wave myocardial infarction or unstable angina, the addition of *clopidogrel to aspirin* was found to be superior to aspirin alone (24). In the CURE study, combination therapy for an average duration of 9 months decreased major vascular events by 20%. For patients with cerebrovascular disease, the Management of Atherothrombosis with Clopidogrel in High-risk patients with recent transient ischemic attack or ischemic stroke trial (MATCH) evaluated the addition of *aspirin to clopidogrel.*

In MATCH, 7599 patients were enrolled with either a TIA or a stroke plus an additional vascular risk factor such as a prior ischemic event or diabetes mellitus (25). All patients received 75 mg/day of clopidogrel and half of the patients received 75 mg/day of aspirin. Patients were treated for 18 months and were followed for the primary endpoint of stroke/MI/ vascular death or rehospitalization for a vascular ischemic event. The hypothesis of the study was that adding aspirin would decrease the primary endpoint by 14% but this was not demonstrated. Overall, 15.7% of the clopidogrel+aspirin patients had a primary endpoint event compared to 16.7% in the clopidogrel alone group (RRR 6.4%). Life-threatening bleeding was increased by 1.3% in absolute terms in the clopidogrel+aspirin group. Of the 7599 patients, 34% were described as having large vessel atherosclerosis as the cause of their qualifying cerebrovascular event, but the results for this subgroup were not reported separately. As pointed out in an accompanying editorial, the fact that >50% of the patients in MATCH had lacunar infarction may have altered the risk/benefit ratio and increased the cerebral hemorrhage rates (26).

Finally, an intriguing but relatively small study assessed the value of adding *clopidogrel to aspirin* in patients with symptomatic carotid stenosis using TCD-based methods. The Clopidogrel and Aspirin for the Reduction of Emboli in Symptomatic Carotid Stenosis (CARESS) study enrolled patients with a carotid territory TIA or stroke within the preceding 3 months who were positive for MES on TCD (27). Half of the patients received aspirin alone and half were given a 300 mg loading dose of clopidogrel followed by 75 mg/day plus daily aspirin. At 7 days, 37% of the aspirin patients remained MES-positive but this was reduced to 20% in the aspirin+ clopidogrel group ($p = 0.01$). There was no increase in major bleeding events with the addition of clopidogrel in this study. A larger study powered to evaluate clinical endpoints in patients with symptomatic carotid stenosis would be of interest.

1.4. Dipyridamole and Aspirin

The combination of aspirin, a cyclo-oxygenase inhibitor, and dipyridamole, a cyclic nucleotide phosphodiesterase inhibitor, theoretically offers a pharmacological advantage over each of these agents alone. The ESPS-2 study (15) was a multicenter, randomized, blinded, placebo-controlled study in 6602 patients with a preceding TIA or ischemic stroke. Patients were allocated to the following treatments: aspirin 25 mg bid; extended-release dipyridamole 200 mg bid; aspirin 25 mg plus extended-release dipyridamole 200 mg bid; and placebo. The primary endpoint was recurrent stroke (fatal and non-fatal). Both aspirin and extended-release dipyridamole were independently effective at reducing stroke risk (18 and 16% reductions, respectively). The combined agent had a 23% risk reduction over aspirin alone. This was the first demonstration in a primary stroke population that two antiplatelet agents with differing mechanisms of action were more effective than one medication alone. There is no published information available regarding aspirin and dipyridamole specifically for patients with carotid stenosis.

The most common side-effects of extended-release dipyridamole-containing preparations were headache and gastrointestinal disturbance. The aspirin group had an increase in bleeding, although the addition of dipyridamole did not lead to a significant increase in the bleeding events.

Since there are now three agents that have been proven to be more effective than aspirin, the question arises as to when the newer agents should be used as first line therapy. The most recent American College of Chest Physicians statement indicated that clopidogrel and aspirin/extended-release dipyridamole, in addition to aspirin, were reasonable first line therapy choices (16).

2. ORAL ANTICOAGULANTS

2.1. Anticoagulants in Non-cardioembolic Stroke

The success with warfarin in secondary stroke prevention in patients with atrial fibrillation led to trials evaluating warfarin in patients with non-cardioembolic stroke. The Warfarin Aspirin Recurrent Stroke Study (WARSS) was a large, multicenter trial which compared 325 mg/day of aspirin with warfarin (INR 1.4–2.8) in patients with non-cardioembolic stroke and no planned carotid endarterectomy (28). This trial did not show any difference between aspirin and warfarin in the prevention of stroke or death (there was a 11% trend in favor of aspirin) or in the rate of major hemorrhage. The rates of major hemorrhage were low (2.22 per 100 patient-years in the warfarin group and 1.49 per 100 patient-years in the aspirin group). In view of this data, anticoagulation is difficult to justify in patients with non-cardioembolic stroke and with the stroke subtypes seen in the WARSS trial.

In the WARSS trial, the most common stroke subtype at entry was lacunar stroke. In a subset of patients with large artery, severe stenosis, or occlusion, as the stroke subtype at entry, there was no evidence favoring warfarin over aspirin. In fact, there was an increased hazard ratio of 1.22 ($p = 0.51$) for the outcome of recurrent stroke or death at 2 years with warfarin treatment. The WARSS trial was not powered to determine the effectiveness of warfarin for particular stroke subtypes, but the trend favoring aspirin would suggest that antiplatelet therapy is preferable for patients with extracranial carotid stenosis.

Another trial, which evaluated warfarin vs. aspirin in patients with non-cardioembolic stroke, targeted a higher INR range of 3.0–4.5 (29). This study was prematurely stopped due to an excess in the number of cerebral hemorrhages in the warfarin group. In this study of 1316 patients, for each increase in the INR of 0.5, there was an increase in the rate of major hemorrhage by a factor of 1.4. Therefore, an INR of 3.0–4.5 in patients with arterial, non-cardioembolic cerebral ischemia does not appear to be safe and is not recommended.

Another arena in which warfarin is being tested is in patients with intracranial atherosclerotic occlusive disease. A previous retrospective, non-randomized study found that the recurrent stroke rate was lower in patients with intracranial stenosis treated with warfarin compared with those treated with aspirin (30). In this analysis, 88 patients treated with warfarin were followed for an average of 14.7 months and 63 patients on aspirin therapy were followed for a median duration of 19.3 months. The stroke rate per 100 patient-years was 3.6 in the warfarin group compared to 10.4 in the aspirin group. Even after including hemorrhage-related deaths as an end-point, patients given warfarin fared better ($p = 0.03$, log rank test). This retrospective study is not definitive, however. Further information is needed from the ongoing, prospective, randomized Warfarin Aspirin Symptomatic Intracranial Disease (WASID) trial to conclusively establish whether warfarin is superior to aspirin in patients with intracranial atherosclerosis (31). Preliminary results from WASID did not show an advantage for warfarin (INR 2–3) over aspirin (1300 mg/day). In 569 patients recruited, the rate of stroke or death at a mean of 1.8 years of follow-up was approximately 22% in both groups (32).

3. ONGOING STUDIES

There are a few ongoing trials which are examining alternative antithrombotic strategies for patients with stroke. These trials, like the studies mentioned above, include a heterogenous patient population and, therefore, they are unlikely to shed unequivocal light on the ideal antithrombotic regimen for patients with carotid stenosis as the cause of stroke.

One ongoing trial is the Prevention Regimen for Effectively Avoiding Second Strokes (PROFESS) study, which compares the aspirin/dipyridamole combination vs. clopidogrel. Patients with carotid stenosis are eligible for this stroke prevention trial.

Another ongoing study is the European/Australian Stroke Prevention in Reversible Ischemia Trial (ESPRIT) protocol, which is a three-arm comparison of aspirin, aspirin plus dipyridamole, and warfarin. This includes patients with non-cardioembolic stroke.

These studies may provide indirect evidence for clinicians on the preferred antithrombotic regimen for patients with carotid stenosis, although the statistical power for evaluating the carotid stenosis subgroup will be limited.

4. CONCLUSIONS

For patients with symptomatic extracranial carotid stenosis, either aspirin alone, clopidogrel, or aspirin+dipyridamole can be justified. Aspirin+clopidogrel can be supported if there is a recent acute coronary syndrome. For intracranial carotid stenosis, recently available data support the use of aspirin over warfarin as initial therapy in these patients.

REFERENCES

1. Antithrombotic Trialists Collaboration. Collaborative meta-analysis of randomized trials of antiplatelet therapy for prevention of death, myocardial infarction, and stroke in high-risk patients. Br Med J 2002; 324:71–86.
2. North American Symptomatic Carotid Endarterectomy Trial Collaborators. Beneficial effect of carotid endarterectomy in symptomatic patients with high-grade carotid stenosis. N Engl J Med 1991; 325:445–453.
3. European Carotid Surgery Trialists' Collaborative Group. Randomised trial of endarterectomy for recently symptomatic carotid stenosis: final results of the MRC European Carotid Surgery Trial (ECST). Lancet 1998; 351:1379–1387.
4. Canadian Cooperative Study Group. A randomized trial of aspirin and sulfinpyrazone in threatened stroke. N Engl J Med 1978; 299:53–59.
5. The SALT Collaborative Group. Swedish low-dose trial (SALT) of 75 mg aspirin as secondary prophylaxis after cerebrovascular ischemic events. Lancet 1991; 338:1345–1349.
6. Goertler M, Baeumer M, Kross R. Rapid decline of cerebral microemboli of arterial origin after intravenous acetylsalicylic acid. Stroke 1999; 30:66–69.
7. Ratnatunga CP, Edmondson SF, Rees GM, Kovacs IB. High-dose aspirin inhibits shear-induced platelet reaction involving thrombin generation. Circulation 1992; 85:1077–1082.
8. Helgason CM, Bolin KM, Hoff JA. Development of aspirin resistance in persons with previous ischemic stroke. Stroke 1994; 25:2331–2336.

9. Eikelboom JW, Hankey GJ. Aspirin resistance: a new independent predictor of vascular events? J Am Coll Cardiol 2003; 41:966–968.

10. Gum PA, Kottke-Marchant K, Welsh PA, White J, Topol EJ. A prospective, blinded determination of the natural history of aspirin resistance among stable patients with cardiovascular disease. J Am Coll Cardiol 2003; 41:961–965.

11. Macchi L, Christiaens L, Brabant S, Sorel N, Ragot S, Allal J, Mauco G, Brizard A. Resistance in vitro to low-dose aspirin is associated with platelet Pl (GP IIIa) polymorphism but not with C807T and C-5T Kozak Polymorphisms. J Am Coll Cardiol 2003; 42:1115–1119.

12. Schafer AI. Genetic and acquired determinants of individual variability of response to antiplatelet drugs. Circulation 2003; 108:910–911.

13. Dyken ML, Barnett HJM, Easton JD. Low-dose aspirin and stroke, "it ain't necessarily so." Stroke 1992; 23:1395–1399.

14. Bornstein NM, Karepov VG, Aronovich BD. Failure of aspirin treatment after stroke. Stroke 1994; 25:275–277.

15. Diener HC, Cunha L, Forbes C, Sivenius J, Smets P, Lowenthal A. European Stroke Prevention Study 2. Dipyridamole and acetylsalicylic acid in the secondary prevention of stroke. J Neurol Sci 1996; 143:1–13.

16. Albers GW, Amarenco P, Easton JD, Teal P. Antithrombotic and thrombolytic therapy for ischemic stroke. Chest 2001; 119(suppl 1):300S–320S.

17. Taylor DW, Barnett HJM, Haynes RB, Ferguson GG, Sackett DL, Thorpe KE, Simard D, Silver FL, Hachinski V, Clagett GP, Barness R, Spence JD, for the ASA and Carotid Endarterectomy Trial Collaborators. Low-dose and high-dose acetylsalicylic acid for patients undergoing carotid endarterectomy: a randomised controlled trial. Lancet 1999; 353:2179–2184.

18. Engelter S, Lyrer P. Antiplatelet therapy for preventing stroke and other vascular events after carotid endarterectomy. Stroke 2004; 35:1227–1228.

19. Gent M, Blakely JA, Easton JD. Canadian American Ticlopidine Study in thromboembolic stroke. Lancet 1989; I:1215–1220.

20. Hass WK, Easton JD, Adams HP. A randomized trial comparing ticlopidine hydrochloride with aspirin for the prevention of stroke in high-risk patients. N Engl J Med 1989; 321:501–507.

21. Gorelick PB, Richardson D, Kelly M, Ruland S, Hung E, Harris Y, Kittner S, Leurgans S, for the African American Antiplatlet Stroke Prevention Study Investigators. Aspirin and ticlopidine for prevention of recurrent stroke in black patients. JAMA 2003; 289:2947–2957.

22. CAPRIE Steering Committee. A randomised, blinded, trial of clopidogrel versus aspirin in patients at risk of ischaemic events (CAPRIE). Lancet 1996; 348:1329–1339.

23. Hirsh J, Bhatt DL. Comparative benefits of clopidogrel and aspirin in high-risk patient populations: lessons from the CAPRIE and CURE studies. Arch Intern Med 2004; 164:2106–2110.

24. The Clopidogrel in Unstable Angina to Prevent Recurrent Events Trial Investigators. Effects of clopidogrel in addition to aspirin in patients with acute coronary syndromes without ST-segment elevation. N Engl J Med 2001; 345:494–502.

25. Diener HC, Bogousslavsky J, Brass LM, Cimminiello C, Csiba L, Kaste M, Leys D, Matias-Guiu J, Rupprecht H, on behalf of the MATCH Investigators.

Aspirin and clopidogrel compared with clopidogrel alone after recent stroke or transient ischemic attack in high-risk patients (MATCH): randomised, double-blind, placebo-controlled trial. Lancet 2004; 364:331–337.

26. Rothwell PM. Lessons from MATCH for future randomised trials in secondary prevention of stroke. Lancet 2004; 364:305–306.

27. Markus H. Clopidogrel and aspirin for the reduction of emboli in symptomatic carotid stenosis. Cerebrovasc Dis 2004.

28. Mohr JP, Thompson JLP, Lazar RM, A comparison of warfarin and aspirin for the prevention of recurrent ischemic stroke. N Engl J Med 2001; 345:1444–1451.

29. The Stroke Prevention in Reversible Ischemia Trial (SPIRIT) Study Group. A random trial of anticoagulants versus aspirin after cerebral ischemia of presumed arterial origin. Ann Neurol 1997; 42:857–865.

30. Chimowitz MI, Kokkinos P, Strong J, Brown MB, Levine SR, Silliman S, Pessin MS, Weichel E, Sila CA, Furian AJ, (for the Warfarin-Aspirin Symptomatic Intracranial Disease Study Group). The warfarin-aspirin symptomatic intracranial disease study. Neurology 1995; 45:1488–1493.

31. The Warfarin-Aspirin Symptomatic Intracranial Disease (WASID) Trial Investigators. Design, progress and challenges of a double-blind trial of warfarin versus aspirin for symptomatic intracranial arterial stenosis. Neuroepidemiology 2003; 22:106–117.

32. Chimowitz MI, Lynn MJ, Howlett-Smith H, Stern BJ, Hertzberg VS, Frankel MR, Levine SR, Chaturvedi S, Kasner SE, Benesch CG, Sila CA, Jovin TG, Romano JG. Warfarin-Aspirin Symptomatic Intracranial Disease Trial Investigators. N Engl J Med 2005; 352: 1305–16.

7

Stroke Prevention, Blood Cholesterol, and Statins

Pierre Amarenco, Philippa Lavallée, and Pierre-Jean Touboul

Department of Neurology and Stroke Centre, Bichat, Claude Bernard University Hospital and Medical School, Denis Diderot University, Paris VII and Formation de Recherche en Neurologie Vasculaire (Association Claude Bernard), Paris, France

Before the statin era, any attempt to reduce total blood cholesterol levels, either by a diet approach or by a fibric acid agent-based lipid-lowering therapy, failed to significantly reduce the incidence of stroke (1). Indeed, although blood cholesterol has been closely associated with carotid atherosclerosis, which causes atherothrombotic strokes, paradoxically, the link between serum cholesterol level and all strokes has never been fully established (2). Consequently, reducing cholesterol levels after a stroke was not often considered a valuable objective by most clinicians.

In the past decade, nine large-scale trials have demonstrated that cholesterol-lowering treatment using HMG-CoA reductase inhibitors (statins) significantly reduces vascular events in primary as well as secondary prevention of myocardial infarction (MI) (3–11). All these studies but three (6,7,9) also showed a reduction in the risk of strokes, including brain infarctions, transient ischemic attacks, and brain hemorrhages, as a secondary end-point in the population studied.

1. ARE BLOOD LIPIDS A RECOGNIZED RISK FACTOR FOR STROKE?

The meta-analysis of 45 prospective cohorts including 450,000 subjects, a follow-up of 16 years on average (a total of 7.3 million patient-years), and 13,000 incident strokes found no association between total cholesterol and stroke (2). These cohorts were primarily designed to study the incidence of coronary heart disease, and therefore included middle-aged subjects at risk of myocardial infarction; thus, since brain infarction occurs far later than myocardial infarction, at a mean age of 70 years (compared with 55–60 years for MI), these subjects presented a higher risk of having fatal recurrent MI before a stroke; however, they were more likely to have aggressive risk factor management, which may have accounted for a lower incidence of stroke, and cerebrovascular events were not analyzed according to stroke subtypes (e.g., hemorrhagic vs. ischemic strokes). In particular, atherothrombotic brain infarction may have been under-represented in these studies.

The MRFIT study showed that the risk of death from non-hemorrhagic (i.e., ischemic) stroke increased in proportion to serum cholesterol in 351,000 men aged 35–57 years (12). Conversely, there was a negative association with hemorrhagic stroke for cholesterol levels under 200 mg/dL: the lower the total cholesterol levels, the higher the risk of hemorrhagic stroke, thus suggesting a U-shaped relationship between cholesterol and stroke. Therefore, in the cohorts examined in the Prospective Study Collaboration, counting hemorrhagic strokes together with ischemic strokes may have masked a small, true relationship with ischemic stroke.

In the Copenhagen City Heart Study, total cholesterol was positively associated with the risk of non-hemorrhagic stroke, but only for levels above 8 mmol/L (320 mg/dL), corresponding to the upper 5% of the distribution in the study population (13). Another prospective community-based study found a significant relationship between low-density lipoprotein (LDL) cholesterol levels and dementia with stroke in 1111 people without initial dementia (average age, 75 years) (14).

To sum up, most prospective observational cohorts were not representative of the whole population at risk for stroke, and did not identify blood cholesterol as a risk factor for all strokes, except those which considered stroke subtypes, particularly ischemic and atherothrombotic strokes. No epidemiological studies have considered the relationship between blood cholesterol as a continuous variable and the risk of incident strokes in a high-risk cohort selected on the basis of global cardiovascular risk approaches (high Framingham or PROCAM risk score, increased carotid IMT, or presence of carotid artery atherosclerotic plaques).

2. USE OF STATINS IN STROKE PREVENTION

The randomized controlled trials of statins have revolutionized our management of lipids in patients at risk of stroke (15–25).

2.1. The Scandinavian Simvastatin Survival Study (4-S) Trial

This secondary prevention trial showed that simvastatin 10–40 mg/day given 6 months after a myocardial infarction or unstable angina in men with serum total cholesterol above 270 mg/dL reduced mortality by 30% (15–42%; $P = 0.0003$) and major coronary events by 34% (25–41%; $P < 0.00001$) after 5 years (3). Post-hoc analysis showed that the incidence of strokes was reduced by 30% (4–48%; $P = 0.024$), but this was mainly due to the reduction in transient ischemic attacks (TIAs), which is considered a rather soft secondary end-point because of the difficulties in differential diagnosis with other transient neurological conditions (migraine attack, focal epilepsy, hypoglycemia, etc.). When TIAs were excluded from the analysis, the difference was no longer significant (3).

2.2. The Cholesterol and Recurrent Event (CARE) Study

The CARE trial was a secondary prevention trial using pravastatin 40 mg/ day in patients with myocardial infarction (4). The results were similar to those of the 4-S trial. However, the CARE patients had cholesterol levels within the normal range or moderately elevated (total cholesterol < 240 mg/dL and LDL cholesterol between 115 and 174 mg/dL). Among the 2078 patients in the placebo group and 2081 in the pravastatin group who had suffered a myocardial infarction between 3 and 20 months before randomization, the relative risk reduction of a fatal coronary event or non-fatal myocardial infarction was 24% in the pravastatin group after 5 years of treatment (4). On the basis of this combined criterion, event reduction was greatest in women (45%) and in elderly subjects aged 60–75 years, representing a total of 2129 patients (26%).

In CARE, a stroke occurred in 78 patients in the placebo group (3.7%) and 54 patients in the pravastatin group (2.5%), yielding a relative risk reduction of 31% (3–52%; $P = 0.03$) with $P = 0.03$. In a second analysis, the CARE investigators found a 27% reduction in stroke or TIA, and that all categories of stroke were reduced, although there was inadequate power to detect a significant result in each class (15). For example, there was a 21% reduction -20–48%, $P = 0.268$) for atherothrombotic strokes. Unlike the 4-S trial, in which only 37% of patients received aspirin, 85% of the CARE patients received antiplatelet therapy, so that the stroke risk reduction achieved by pravastatin was added to that obtained by the antiplatelet agents.

2.3. The Long-Term Intervention with Pravastatin in Ischemic Disease (LIPID) Trial

The LIPID trial confirmed the efficacy of pravastatin 40 mg/day after MI and unstable angina occurring between 3 and 36 months before entry to the study, in patients who had a total cholesterol level between 155 and 271 mg/dL, i.e., a broad spectrum including high-risk and low-risk patients. After a 6-year period, the relative reduction in risk of death from coronary heart disease was 24% in the pravastatin group (5).

The special design of the LIPID trial was that cerebrovascular events were pre-specified and analyzed and validated by an end-point committee composed of vascular neurologists. The results for brain infarction were a relative risk reduction of 19% and an absolute risk reduction of 0.8% over a 6-year period of treatment with pravastatin (5,16). These results were obtained in all ischemic stroke subtypes (lacunar, cardioembolic, and atherothrombotic strokes), mainly in the group of patients with low LDL (<138 mg/dL) and low high-density lipoprotein (HDL)(<39 mg/dL).

2.4. WOSCOP and AFACPS/TexCAPS Trials

These were primary prevention trials, one in high-risk (WOSCOP) and another in low-risk patients (AFCAPS/TexCAPS). The first trial demonstrated that pravastatin reduced the incidence of fatal and non-fatal coronary events by 31%, all cardiovascular deaths by 32%, and death from any cause by 22% in hypercholesterolemic men (272 ± 23 mg/dL on average) (6). In the other trial, lovastatin reduced major coronary events (fatal and non-fatal MI, unstable angina, and sudden cardiac death) by 27% in men and women with average total and LDL-cholesterol levels and below-average HDL cholesterol levels (7).

AFCAPS/TexCAPS did not report on stroke end-point. In WOSCOP, there was no significant reduction in the incidence of stroke. However, the mean age of the patients included was low, accounting for a low incidence of stroke and consequently for lack of power to detect a significant difference (6,7).

2.5. The Heart Protection Study (HPS) Trial

The HPS trial included 10,269 patients receiving simvastatin 40 mg/day and 10,267 patients receiving a placebo (8). This trial included 13,379 patients with established coronary heart disease (CHD) (65%), and 3280 patients with stroke prior to randomization (no TIAs), including 1822 strokes without established CHD. There was a 24% relative risk reduction for major vascular events (major coronary events, stroke, and revascularization), and the incidence of ischemic stroke was reduced by 25% (4.3% in the simvastatin group and 5.7% in the placebo group), yielding an absolute stroke risk reduction of 1.4%, which essentially confirmed the results of the other three statin trials. Reduction of stroke incidence was observed with the same magnitude in diabetic patients (20). Furthermore, in 3280 patients with stroke prior to randomization, there was a 19% relative risk reduction for major vascular events [HR = 0.81 (0.71–0.93)], and in the 1822 stroke patients without an established CHD, the reduction in major vascular events was 23% [HR = 0.77 (0.63–0.94)]. However, this effect was due mainly to a reduction in major coronary events and revascularization, with no effect on stroke itself, although the confidence intervals of the effect of treatment did not exclude a clinically important reduction (21). Among patients with pre-existing cerebrovascular disease as a whole, there was also no apparent reduction in the stroke rate, but there was a highly significant 20% (8–29) reduction in the rate of any major vascular event [406 (24.7%) vs. 488 (29.8%); $P = 0.001$].

2.6. The Prospective Study of Pravastatin in the Elderly at Risk (PROSPER) Trial

The PROSPER trial included 5804 elderly men and women (52%) aged 70–82 years with a total cholesterol level between 155 and 350 mg/dL, receiving pravastatin 40 mg/day or a placebo (9). Half were selected on the basis of a high-risk profile (62% were hypertensives, 11% diabetics, and 28% current smokers), and half on the presence of established vascular disease (44% had a cardiovascular disease and 11% had stroke prior to randomization). After a mean follow-up of 3.2 years, there was a significant 15% reduction in the primary composite end-point (CHD death, non-fatal MI, fatal, and non-fatal strokes) with 16.2% events in the placebo group and 14.1% in the pravastatin group ($P = 0.014$). However, there was no effect on stroke incidence, with 4.5% strokes (131/2913) in the placebo group and 4.7% strokes (135/2891) in the pravastatin group. In addition, the cognitive functions declined at the same rate in both treatment arms, as in the HPS trial (in which the MMS was only evaluated at the end of the trial).

In summary, PROSPER confirmed that statins could be used in elderly patients, as in younger patients, to prevent any cardiovascular events, but did not confirm a favorable effect on the incidence of stroke in this population.

Why did PROSPER fail to show a reduction in stroke and cognitive impairment?

1. One explanation may be the duration of the trial, which lasted only for 3 years. If the stroke end-point in earlier pravastatin trials (CARE and LIPID) is considered, the Kaplan–Meier curves started to diverge *after* the third year, and if the analyses had been performed after 3 years, these trials would also have had a neutral effect on the incidence of stroke (15,16).

2. Another explanation is lack of power, since the hypothesis was an 8% stroke rate in the placebo group (22), whereas the actual rate was 4.5%. Although this is a rather soft end-point, it may be worth noting that there was a trend towards a reduction in TIAs ($P = 0.051$).

3. A third factor is the design of the trial and the population selected which, as in the HPS trial, was based on "no true indication for a statin". The patients were selected in the primary care setting. We have no information about important baseline characteristics such as the presence of carotid stenosis, which are important for evaluation of the risk of stroke in the population included (22); as a result, it is not known whether this population was really representative of the entire elderly population at risk for stroke. Only 11% of patients had had a stroke at least 6 months before randomization. No documentation of carotid/vertebral atherosclerosis was required (22).

4. In this trial, pravastatin 40 mg/day was used; once again, a higher dosage might have worked better, as suggested by the results of the ARBITER trial, which showed a regression of carotid atherosclerosis with atorvastatin 80 mg and progression of carotid atherosclerosis with pravastatin 40 mg/day (23).

2.7. The Antihypertensive and Lipid-Lowering Treatment to Prevent Heart Attack Trial—Lipid-Lowering Treatment (ALLHAT-LLT)

The ALLHAT-LLT trial included 40,000 hypertensive patients aged 55 or older (24). Those with an LDL cholesterol level of 120–189 mg/dL (100 and 129 mg/dL if known CHD) and a triglyceride level of < 350 mg/dL were randomized to pravastatin 40 mg/day ($n = 5170$) or usual care ($n = 5135$). After a mean follow-up of 4.8 years, there was no significant difference in all-cause mortality, CHD mortality, the CHD event rate, or stroke incidence [4.07% in the pravastatin group and 4.5% in the usual arm group, RR = 0.91 (0.75–1.09); $P = 0.31$].

However, (i) this trial was not placebo-controlled; (ii) the power calculation was based on the inclusion of 20,000 patients to detect a 12.5% reduction in mortality rate that provided 80% power, and only 10,000 were randomized; (iii) 26.1% of patients in the usual care arm were treated with statins by the end of the trial; and finally (iv) the confidence interval did not exclude a powerful effect of pravastatin in stroke prevention.

2.8. The KYUSHU Lipid Intervention Study (KLIS)

The KLIS trial is the only large statin trial ever conducted on a Japanese population (25). It included men aged 45–74 years with a total cholesterol level > 220 mg/dL and without a history of myocardial infarction or coronary revascularization. Of the 3061 subjects assigned to pravastatin 10–20 mg/day and 2579 assigned to usual care, 2219 and 1634 respectively were analyzed. After a 5-year follow-up, the primary end-point (fatal and non-fatal MI, CABG, PTCA, cardiac death, and sudden and unexpected death) occurred in 2.9% of patients. There was a non-significant reduction of 14% in the pravastatin group [0.86 (0.61–1.20)], and a non-significant 22% stroke risk reduction [0.78 (0.54–1.13)].

The non-significant effects in the KLIS trial were due to (i) the absence of a placebo group and of intention-to-treat analysis due to a failure in the randomization process; (ii) the fact that the power calculation was based on the inclusion of 3000 patients in each group to detect a 30% reduction in coronary events that provided 80% power with an estimated rate of 3.5% of coronary events in the usual care group after 5 years; (iii) only 2219 patients in the pravastatin arm and 1634 in the usual care arm were analyzed, because many patients were excluded a posteriori (because of a total cholesterol level ≥ 300 mg/dL, protocol violations such as the use of lipid-lowering agents, a history of end-point disease, consent withdrawn, no contract with participants or missing data); (iv) the coronary event rate was 2.9% in both groups, and (v) the low pravastatin dosage used (10–20 mg/day) accounted for an LDL reduction of only 15% in the pravastatin group.

2.9. The Greek Atorvastatin and Coronary Heart Disease Evaluation (GREACE) Trial

The GREACE trial randomized 1600 patients with an established coronary heart disease and LDL > 100 mg/dL to atorvastatin or usual care (10). The patients on atorvastatin (10–80 mg, mean 24 mg/day) were titrated to the NECP goal of LDL < 100 mg/dL. After a 3-year follow-up, the primary end-point (death, non-fatal MI, UA, CHF, revascularization, or stroke) was reduced by 51% [0.49 (0.27–0.73)], and all components of the primary end-point were significantly reduced; stroke in particular was reduced by 47%. By the end of the follow-up, 26% of patients in the usual care arm were receiving some form of lipid-lowering therapy.

2.10. The Anglo-Scandinavian Collaborative Trial (ASCOT)

In this primary prevention trial, 19,342 hypertensive patients [systolic blood pressure (SBP) > 160 or diastolic blood pressure (DBP) > 100 mmHg] who also had at least three risk factors (LVH, ECG abnormalities, non-insulin dependent diabetes mellitus, PVD, TIA, man > 55 years, microalbuminuria, smoker, TC/HDL > 6, early CHD) were randomized to ß-blockers $\pm$ diuretics or amlodipine $\pm$ ACE inhibitor (11). The patients who had a total cholesterol level of < 6.5 mmol/dL were offered randomization in a factorial design t0 either atorvastatin 10 mg or placebo. A total of 10,297 patients were randomized in the lipid arm, and the follow-up was scheduled to be 5 years. However, on the recommendation of the independent DSMB committee of the study, the lipid arm was stopped early because of the great efficacy of the atorvastatin group on the primary end-point. Stroke reduction was 27%, and the Kaplan–Meier curves diverged very early and constantly during the follow-up. This stroke reduction was obtained in addition to the 40% stroke reduction obtained in a population of patients who are well controlled for their hypertension after the blood pressure goal (<140/90 mmHg) is achieved. This trial emphasizes the need for a global cardiovascular risk approach, since statin treatment of these patients, who had "normal" cholesterol levels but were hypertensives, was very effective.

2.11. Summary

Of the 70,020 patients so far randomized in the 4-S, CARE, LIPID, HPS, PROSPER, ALLHAT, KLIS, GREACE, and ASCOT trials, an incident stroke occurred in 1500/34,684 patients (4.32%) randomized in the control groups and 1208/35,331 patients (3.42%) randomized in the statin groups, yielding a 21% relative risk reduction, and a modest 0.9% absolute risk reduction of stroke, i.e., approximately nine strokes prevented per 1000 patients who would be treated during a 5-year period (Table 1). By comparison, meta-analyses have shown that in similar patients with known CHD, antiplatelet agents prevent 17.3 strokes and ramipril prevents 17 strokes per 1000 patients treated for 5 years; in patients with prior stroke, antiplatelet agents prevent 27 strokes per 1000 patients treated for 29 months (136 projected at 5 years) (26).

3. SAFETY

3.1. Cancer

One concern with the statin trials has been the incidence of cancer, particularly after the PROSPER trial in which 245 (8.5%) patients on pravastatin and 199 (6.8%) patients on placebo had a cancer which was statistically significant [RR = 1.25 (1.04–1.51)]. Addition of incident cancer in all pravastatin trials (27) including PROSPER and ALLHAT, gives a cancer in 1290/17,956 (7.18%) patients randomized to pravastatin and in 1234/17,971 (6.87%) randomized to control group, i.e., a reassuring non-significant relative risk of 1.05 (0.97–1.14).

3.2. Hemorrhagic Stroke

One concern, because of the observational cohort data mentioned above, was an increased risk of hemorrhagic strokes with lipid-lowering therapy. In the Honolulu Heart Program, during an average 18-year follow-up of

Table 1 Major Statin Trials (70,070 Patients Randomised): Stroke End-Point

Trials[a]	Statin used (Dosage)	LDL reduction (mean between group difference)	No. Follow-Up (yrs)	Control	Statin	RRR	95% CI	ARR	No. of events prevented / 1000
SSSS	Simvastatin	35%	4444	95/2223 4.3%[c]	61/2221 2.7%	30%	04 to 48%	1.6%	16
CARE	10–40 mg Parvastatin	(68 mg) 32%	5.4 4159	76/2078 3.7%[c]	52/2081 2.5%	32%	04 to 52%	1.2%	12
LIPID	40 mg Pravastatin	(38 mg) 23%	5.0 9014	204/4502 4.5%[c]	169/4513 3.7%	19%	00 to 34%	0.8%	8
HPS	40 mg Simvastatin	(39 mg[b])	6.0 20,536	585/10267 5.7%[c]	444/10269 4.3%	25%	15 to 34%	1.4%	14
PROSPER	40 mg Pravastatin	(39 mg) 27%	5.3 5804	131/2913 4.5%[c]	135/2891 4.7%	3%	−31% to 19%	—	—
ALLHAT-LLT	40mg Pravastatin	(40 mg[e]) 27.7%	3.2 10,355	231/5185 4.5%[d]	209/5170 4.1%	9%	−14 to 21%	0.4%	4
KLIS	20–40 mg Pravastatin	(24 mg) 20%	4.8 3853	41/1643 2.5%[d]	47/2219 2.1%	22%	−13 to 46%	0.4%	4

(Continued)

Table 1 Major Statin Trials (70,070 Patients Randomised): Stroke End-Point (*Continued*)

Trials[a]	Statin used (Dosage)	LDL reduction (mean between group difference)	No. Follow-Up (yrs)	Control	Statin	RRR	95% CI	ARR	No. of events prevented / 1000
GREACE	10–20 Atorvastatin	(11 mg) 46%	5.0 1600	17/800 2.1%[d]	9/800 1.1%	47%	b	1.0%	10
ASCOT	10–80(24) Atorvastatin	(70 mg) 35%	3.0 10,305	121/5137 2.4[c]	89/5168 1.7%	27%	04 to 44%	0.7%	7
Combined total[a]		(37 mg)	3.3 70,070	4.32%	3.44%	21%	15 to 27%	0.9%	9

[a]Number of controls = 1501/34,739; number of patients receiving statin = 1215/35,331; *P* = 0.034.
[b]Data not provided.
52.31% (36,627 of 70,020 patients) had established coronary artery disease.
[c]Placebo.
[d]Usual care, no placebo.
[e]Assuming that LDL did not change in placebo group (LDL reduction not reported in that group).

7850 Japanese-American men living in Hawaii, 116 hemorrhagic strokes occurred, and there was an inverse relationship between serum cholesterol and the risk of intracerebral hemorrhage, with a higher incidence rate only for the men with total cholesterol in the lowest quintile (< 189 mg/dL) (28). The relative risk in this group, compared with the other four quintiles, was 2.55 (1.58–4.12) after controlling for some confounding risk factors (age, blood pressure, serum uric acid, cigarette smoking, and alcohol consumption) (28). In 172 patients from Korea who underwent brain MRI to test for microbleeds (on $T2^*$-weighted gradient-echo imaging, which shows the multifocal signal loss lesions that are believed to represent microbleeds histopathologically), the LDL concentrations were significantly lower in patients with a severe degree of microbleeding (29). Multivariate analysis showed that microbleeds were significantly correlated with hypertension, leukoaraiosis, the lowest quartile of serum total cholesterol (< 4.27 mmol/dL), and the highest quartile of HDL (>1.47 mmol/dL) (29). However, such a potentially increased risk of hemorrhagic stroke was not observed overall in long-term clinical trials that looked at this secondary end-point. In the PPP project (30) combining the LIPID and CARE data, there were 19 hemorrhagic strokes (0.5%) in the pravastatin group and 15 (0.4%) in the placebo group [HR $= 1.25$ (0.63–2.46)]. In HPS, there were 51 hemorrhagic strokes (0.5%) in the simvastatin group and 53 (0.5%) in the placebo group (8). These results, together with the nil increase in hemorrhagic strokes in the elderly population of the PROSPER trial, are reassuring. It is noteworthy that low cholesterol levels are frequent in patients in poor conditions such as loss of weight, severe handicap, severe illness, and chronic illness, which may have constituted confounding factors for the relationship between the occurrence of a hemorrhagic stroke and low total cholesterol in observational studies. In a recent evaluation of all-cause mortality over 20 years in 3572 Japanese-Americans aged 71–93 years included in the Honolulu Heart Program, mean cholesterol fell significantly with increasing age (31). Only the group with a low cholesterol concentration < 4.65 mmol/dL at both examinations (20 years apart) had a significant association with mortality [RR $= 1.64$ (1.13–2.36)] (31). One explanation is that the patients with high cholesterol died before the age of 75; weight loss $\geq 10\%$ and poor physical function were more frequent in patients with a low serum cholesterol concentration.

3.3. Muscle and Nerves

Muscle pain and rhabdomyolysis are well-known and very rare occurrences in patients treated by statins. It is worth noting that in the PROSPER trial in elderly patients, the rate of reported muscle pain was similar in the pravastatin and placebo groups (36 and 32 instances in the pravastatin and placebo arms, respectively) and there was no case of rhabdomyolysis.

Four cases of peripheral neuropathy have been reported associated with simvastatin treatment (32). In a population-based study, the first-time-ever case of idiopathic polyneuropathy was registered in a 5-year period (1994–1998) (33). For each case validated, 25 control subjects were randomly selected and matched for age, sex, and calendar time within the background population. Idiopathic polyneuropathy was diagnosed in 166 cases, 35 being definite, 54 probable, and 77 probable. There was a strong association with the use (current or ever) of statin with an odds ratio of 3.7 (1.8–7.6), particularly when the idiopathic polyneuropathy was definite [OR = 14.2 (5.3–38)], and when patients were exposed to a statin during 2 years or more [OR = 26.4 (7.8–45.4)] (33). However, in the large-scale and long-term clinical trials reviewed above, there was no concern about an increased risk of polyneuropathy in patients on statin therapy. This case-control study thus must be confirmed by a prospective study.

4. THE USE OF FIBRIC ACID AGENTS AND STROKE PREVENTION

Until recently, the meta-analysis of cholesterol-lowering trials before the era of statins, including modified diet, use of vegetable oil, or medications such as colestipol, niacin, clofibrate, cholestyramine, and gemfibrozil, failed to show a significant reduction of stroke incidence (34).

4.1. The Veterans Administration HDL Intervention Trial (VA-HIT)

Recently, one fibrate (gemfibrozil) has proved to be effective in reducing clinical events, particularly myocardial infarction and death from coronary heart disease in the VA-HIT study (35). This trial included patients with a past history of coronary events (MI, coronary revascularization—PTCA or CABG—or documented coronary artery stenosis ≥50%). In this study, treatment with gemfibrozil reduced the risk of stroke, TIA, and carotid endarterectomy.

Patients had rather low serum cholesterol levels since they were included with LDL cholesterol < 140 mg/dL. One can estimate that roughly 40% of patients suffering from coronary heart disease have LDL cholesterol <140 mg/dL, that is even lower than most of the patients included in the 4-S, CARE, LIPID, and HPS trials. Among these patients, more than half have low levels of HDL cholesterol (the "good" cholesterol). Thus, 25% of patients with coronary heart disease have low LDL-and HDL-cholesterol levels. When screened systematically with ultrasound, it has been shown that these patients have a high frequency of carotid stenosis (36). The VA-HIT has thus included patients with LDL <140 mg/dL and HDL < 40 mg/dL.

The result was a relative risk reduction of non-fatal myocardial infarction or death from coronary causes of 22% after 5 years of treatment (35). In this study, cerebrovascular events were all adjudicated by a committee composed of three vascular neurologists, on predefined criteria. There was a 24% risk reduction of confirmed strokes (6% in the placebo group and 4.6% in the gemfibrozil group, $P < 0.10$), a 59% reduction of TIAs (4.2% in the placebo group vs. 1.7% in the gemfibrozil group; $P < 0.001$), and a 65% reduction in carotid endarterectomy (3.5 vs. 1.3%; $P < 0.001$). These results are somewhat provocative, since they are in contradiction with all other previous trials with fibrates including the Bezafibrate Infarction Prevention (BIP) trial using bezafibrate and four others with clofibrate, one with colestipol, one with cholestyramin, and one with gemfibrozil (in patients aged 40–55 years who had an elevated average cholesterol level of 270 mg/dL), three studies with low saturated fat and high polyunsaturated fat diet, and two meta-analyses of these studies which showed no reduction in stroke events among 46,000 and 36,000 participants who had 430 and 435 strokes, respectively (1,34).

It should be pointed out that in the VA-HIT, LDL cholesterol levels did not change in both groups and the mean total cholesterol level was 4% lower in the gemfibrozil group. Only HDL level increased by 6% and triglyceride level decreased by 31% in the gemfibrozil group. Therefore, the reduction obtained on clinical events as well as the dramatic one on the number of carotid endarterectomy performed, seems to have mainly involved pleiotropic or antiatherogenic effects of gemfibrozil on atherosclerotic plaques, including increased reverse cholesterol transport, decreased dense oxidizable LDL particles, and improvement of clearance of triglyceride-rich lipoproteins including VLDL and chylomicrons (37). Moreover, hypertriglyceridemia may well be a neglected risk factor, frequently forgotten mainly because of difficulties to interpret results due to its link with HDL-cholesterol level (38–43). An association with stroke has been reported in two series (13,44).

4.2. The BIP Registry

In the BIP trial, 3122 patients were included among 15,524 screened with a diagnosis of symptomatic CHD between 6 months and 5 years before randomization. Patients had to have total cholesterol < 270 mg/dL, HDL cholesterol < 45 mg/dL, and serum triglycerides < 300 mg/dL. The effect on the primary end-point was not positive, but in the sub-group of patients with triglyceride levels > 200 mg/dL, there was a significant reduction of fatal and non-fatal MI or sudden death. No information is available on the occurrence of stroke in this subgroup (45). The patients not included in the study were followed in a registry during a 6- to 8-year period. After exclusion of patients with stroke/TIAs at randomization, 11,117 patients were analyzed. During the follow-up period there were 487 verified ischemic strokes or TIAs. The relative risk of stroke/TIA was 1.27 (1.01–1.60) for triglyceride levels >200 mg/dL and 0.87 for HDL, the higher risk of stroke (6.4%) being for patients with triglycerides >200 mg/dL and in the lowest tertile of %HDL as compared to the risk of patients in the highest tertile of %HDL irrespective of the triglycerides being less (3.7% of stroke) or greater (3.8% of stroke) than 200 mg/dL (46).

4.3. Summary

Fibric acid agents, now popularized as PPAR activators, used in a selected population of patients with moderately elevated triglycerides, low HDL levels, and LDL within the normal range, a frequent profile in the stroke population, may be as effective as statins in preventing stroke, and this deserves to be tested in randomized control trials.

5. USE OF LIPID-LOWERING AGENTS IN STROKE PREVENTION, IMPORTANT SUBGROUPS

5.1. Elderly

Although PROSPER showed no effect on stroke incidence, the effect on the primary end-point (CHD death, non-fatal MI, and fatal and non-fatal stroke) was positive. In patients older than 70 years, HPS also showed a benefit in the simvastatin group with 690/2919 (23.6%) major vascular events in the simvastatin group and with 829/2887 (28.7%) in the placebo group, yielding a 23% relative risk reduction [0.77 (0.68–0.86)], which was highly significant and similar to the effect observed in other age sub-groups of 65–70 years and <65 years ($P = 0.73$ for heterogeneity). No data are available concerning the different parts of the composite end-point, including stroke.

5.2. Diabetics

Pravastatin in both the CARE and the LIPID studies had a non-significant reduction of ischemic stroke in diabetic patients (16,47). In CARE, the reduction of stroke in diabetics was 14% which was not significant with 24/284 (8%) strokes in the placebo group and 19/282 (6.7%) strokes in the pravastatin group. In LIPID, there were 40 strokes (10.4%) in 386 diabetics in the placebo group and 31 strokes (7.8%) in 396 diabetics in the pravastatin group, yielding a non-significant 27% relative risk reduction (−17–54%) (16).

The HPS trial showed for the first time a significant relative risk reduction of incident strokes in diabetic patients. There were 5.0% strokes in the 2978 diabetics patients on simvastatin and 6.6% strokes in the 2985 diabetic

Table 2 Populations in Which Statins have been Studied

Coronary heart disease [SSSS[a](3), CARE[a](4), LIPID[a](5), GREACE[a](10), HPS[a](8), and KLIS (25)]
Hypercholesterolemia [WOSCOP(6)]
Normocholesterolemic [AFCAPS/TEXCAPS[b](7)]
Hypertensives [ALLHAT (24), HPS[a](8), and ASCOT[a](11)]
Diabetics [CARE(4), LIPID(5), HPS[a](8), and CARDS[d]];
Elderly [PROSPER(9) and HPS[a](8)]
Stroke/TIA [HPS[c](8), and SPARCL[d](61)].

[a]Positive results on stroke end-point.
[b]Stroke end point not reported.
[c]Positive on combined primary end-point (major coronary events, stroke, revascularization) but stroke recurrence not yet reported.
[d]Pending results.

patients on placebo [RR = 0.74 (0.60–0.92)]. This was also true in diabetic patients without established CHD [4.0% strokes in 2006 diabetics on simvastatin and 5.8% strokes in 1976 diabetics on placebo, RR = 0.67 (0.51–0.89)] (48) (Table 2)..

6. THE USE OF LIPID-LOWERING AGENTS IN STROKE PREVENTION, PENDING QUESTIONS

6.1. Why Did Statins Show a Stroke Reduction? The Stroke Paradox

Since observational studies have failed to find a clear association between cholesterol levels and stroke, it may seem paradoxical that cholesterol-lowering agents reduced the risk of suffering a stroke (Table 3).

Table 3 Potential Mechanism of Benefit of Statin in Preventing Stroke

LDL cholesterol reduction
Reduction in brain embolism in CHD patients (reduction of left ventricular thrombus with less myocardial infarction)
Blood pressure lowering effect
Regression of carotid/vertebral artery atherosclerosis and intima-media thickness
Anti-inflammatory effect
Plaque stabilization (pleiotropic effects)
Improved endothelial dysfunction (with improved cerebral vasoreactivity)
Positive effect on fibrinolytic system and platelet function
Neuroprotection (with up regulation of eNOS activity)

(1) *In reducing incident MI, statins reduced the occurrence of left ventri-cular mural thrombus and subsequent thromboembolic complications in the brain:*

In the Myocardial Ischemia Reduction with Aggressive Cholesterol Lowering (MIRACL) trial, conducted on patients with unstable angina or non-Q-wave MI immediately after the qualifying event (49), a total of 3086 patients were randomized to atorvastatin 80 mg/day or placebo and treated for 4 months. After 4 months, the composite end-point (death, non-fatal MI, resuscitated cardiac arrest, or recurrent symptomatic myocar-dial ischemia requiring emergency rehospitalization) was reduced from 17.4 to 14.8%, a relative risk reduction of 16% ($P=0.048$) in the atorvastatin group. As secondary end-point, there were 12 fatal and non-fatal strokes in 1538 (0.8%) patients in the atorvastatin group and 24 in 1548 (1.6%) patients in the placebo group, with all three hemorrhagic strokes occurring in the placebo group. The risk reduction was 51% (2–76%, $P=0.04$).

Similarly, in the Sibrafiban Vs. Aspirin to Yield Maximum Protection from Ischemic Heart Events Post-Acute Coronary Syndromes (SYMPH-ONY) 1 and 2 post-hoc analyses, in which a total of 15,904 patients with an acute coronary syndrome were randomized, there were 12,365 not taking a statin before randomization (50). Among those who survived more than 5 days, 3952 received early statin therapy and 8413 never received a statin. Death, MI, and stroke occurred in 6.9% of the statin group and in 7.5% of the non-statin group [unadjusted $HR=0.90$ (0.78–1.04), covariate and propensity adjusted $HR=1.05$ (0.88–1.24)]. But of interest was the risk reduction of stroke incidence with 20 (0.5%) strokes in the statin group and 76 (0.9%) strokes in the non-statin group, a significant relative risk reduction of 47% [unadjusted $HR=0.53$ (0.32–0.89), adjusted $HR=0.54$ (0.30–0.97), $P=0.04$] (50).

As regards the stroke mechanism in MIRACL, there were 20 throm-boembolic strokes in the placebo group compared with 10 in the atorvastatin group (51). However, only nine of the 36 strokes were preceded by a non-fatal MI, with the stroke occurring between 2 and 86 days after the MI (51). Therefore, although the prevention of MI may in part prevent stroke by reducing the incidence of left ventricular thrombi, this is obviously not the only explanation.

(2) *Statins may reduce the incidence of stroke by reducing blood pressure* (52,53): Lowering cholesterol may reduce the blood pressure by between 2 and 5 mmHg (54). It is known that any blood pressure reduction results in a reduced incidence of stroke (55). Even a difference of 2 mmHg could account for a 15% difference in the risk of stroke (56).

After an 8-week placebo and diet run-in period, 30 patients with mod-erate hypercholesterolemia (total cholesterol 6.29 ± 0.52 mmol/L) and untreated hypertension ($149 \pm 6/97 \pm 2$ mmHg) were randomized to either placebo or pravastatin 20–40 mg/day in a cross-over design. Of the

25 participants who completed the 32-week trial, there was a reduction of systolic/diastolic blood pressure of $-8/-5$ mmHg ($P = 0.001$) and of pulse pressure (-3 mmHg, $P = 0.011$) (52).

However, a careful post-hoc analysis of the LIPID trial (16) and the PPP (30) somewhat contradict this hypothesis. It is worth noting that in these pravastatin trials, the patients were not hypertensive at baseline, while the patients in the Glorioso et al. study (52) were hypertensive. Further studies, especially analyses of the ASCOT trial results, in which all patients included were hypertensives, will shed light on this important, potent action mechanism of statin treatment.

(3) *Another explanation is that statins reduce stroke simply by reducing cholesterol levels:* A recent meta-analysis showed that stroke risk reduction in all lipid-lowering trials depends on the extent of the reduction of LDL and total cholesterol levels (57). Table 1 shows that positive studies have been those with a between-group difference in LDL cholesterol of at least 37 mg (except for PROSPER in which mean LDL reduction in the placebo group is not available in the publication). In the Framingham study there was a positive association between carotid stenosis, hypercholesterolemia, and coronary heart disease (58). In the same epidemiological study of 449 men and 661 women who underwent B-mode ultrasound measurements of the carotid artery, with a mean age of 75 years, moderate stenosis >25% was present in 189 men and 226 women. The baseline characteristics had been recorded 34 years earlier. Compared with minimal stenosis (< 25%), moderate stenosis in men was associated with an increase of 20 mmHg in SBP [2.11 (1.51–2.97)], 10 mg/dL in total cholesterol level [1.10 (1.03–1.16)], and five pack-years of smoking [1.08 (1.03–1.13)], a result which was similar in women (59). These results clearly suggested that the cumulative effects of these important risk factors interfere with the development of carotid stenosis, and further argued for a global cardiovascular risk approach, based on the Framingham or PROCAM score, to prevent the development of atherothrombotic disease, even for carotid atherothrombosis.

(4) *Statins may also directly act on atherosclerotic plaques in the carotid and vertebral basilar arteries:* This is reflected in the slow progression or even regression of the carotid wall thickness in the ACAPS study with lovastatin (60,61), the PLAC-II, KAPS, and LIPID ancillary studies with pravastatin (62–64), the ASAP trial with atorvastatin and simvastatin (65), and the ARBITER trial (66) with atorvastatin and pravastatin. The last two trials showed that aggressive cholesterol reduction has a greater and more rapid effect on the development of carotid atherosclerosis than a more "standard" dosage of statin therapy.

(5) *The pleiotropic effect of statins on atherosclerotic plaques acting on biological promoters of plaque instability* (67–71)*:*

The magnitude of atherosclerotic plaque regression has never appeared parallel to the amplitude of the clinical benefit. This fact forms the basis for the hypothesis that statins may work through an action on other biological parameters within plaques, making them less active. A positive effect by statins on all these factors has been demonstrated in vitro (71). It has also been shown in humans with pravastatin after a short-term lipid-lowering intervention. Of 24 patients scheduled for carotid endarterectomy, 11 were randomized to pravastatin and 13 to placebo. Carotid endarterectomy was performed after 3 months of treatment, and the material removed was analyzed. A positive effect of pravastatin was found on all biological parameters studied, including macrophage count, oxidized LDL, apoptotic cell count, metalloproteinases, and smooth muscle cell proliferation (72).

(6) *Statins may also have an impact on cerebral vasoreactivity* (73):

In 16 patients with lacunar strokes, cerebral vasomotor reactivity was examined using transcranial Doppler at baseline and after a 2-month treatment with pravastatin 20 mg/day. After injection of a bolus of 1 g of acetazolamide, the cerebral blood flow velocity increased better after pravastatin treatment (41.9 ± 23.7 vs. $55.7 \pm 18.3\%$; $P = 0.04$) (73).

Endothelial function is important for vasoreactivity, which may be impaired in small vessel disease. Arteriolar occlusions are often preceded by transient deficits, sometimes in cluster, which have been hypothesized to have a vasospastic origin on indirect evidence (74). This could reflect, at least in part, disturbances in the NO pathway. Due to their pleiotropic effects on inflammatory processes, proliferation of smooth muscle cells, macrophage activation, NO, oxidized LDL, and extracellular matrix, statins may interact with the endothelial function and modify vasoreactivity of small arteries $< 300 \, \mu m$ as it has been shown for coronary arteries in angina pectoris. Pravastatin, lovastatin, and simvastatin have proved to reduce the vasoconstriction response to acetylcholine (75–78). Fluvastatin inhibits tissue factor expression. Simvastatin and lovastatin increase endothelial constitutive nitric oxide synthase (ecNOS) expression (79). This question is specifically addressed in the Lacunar Brain Infarction, Cerebral Hyperreactivity, and Atorvastatin Trial (Lacunar-BICHAT) study in which 128 lacunar stroke patients are being randomized between atorvastatin 80 mg/day or placebo during 3 months with cerebral, carotid, and humeral vasoreactivity being the primary end-point.

(7) *Statins may have neuroprotective effects, mainly through the upregulation of endothelial NO synthase* (80,81):

There is mounting evidence that statins may have a neuroprotective effect in animal models, reducing the size of brain infarct, and augmenting cerebral blood flow with mevastatin which upregulates eNOS (80). It has also been shown with rosuvastatin (81). The clinical effect of this potential neuroprotective effect will be assessed in the Stroke Prevention with Aggressive Reduction of Cholesterol Levels (SPARCL) trial, since the severity of handicap and disability has been carefully evaluated throughout the trial and after a new stroke.

(8) *Impact on cognitive impairment?*

Decreased neuronal cholesterol levels inhibit the Aß-forming amyloidogenic pathway possibly by removing APP from cholesterol- and sphingolipid-enriched membrane microdomains. Depletion of cellular cholesterol levels reduces the ability of Aß to act as a seed for further fibril formation, which raises the hope that cholesterol-lowering strategies may positively influence the progression of Alzheimer disease (82).

There has been mounting evidence that statin therapy may reduce the incidence of vascular dementia as well as Alzheimer disease and mild cognitive impairment.

In a cross-sectional analysis comparing the prevalence of Alzheimer's disease in the computer databases of three different hospitals during a 2-year period, the prevalence was 60–73% lower in patients on statin therapy compared to the total population or to patients taking other treatments such as antihypertensive drugs (83).

In the UK-based General Practice Research Database, patients aged over 50 years were individuals who received lipid-lowering therapy, those hyperlipidemic who did not receive such a treatment, and controls. There were 284 cases of dementia and 1080 controls. The adjusted relative risk for those who were prescribed a statin was 0.29 (0.13–0.63; $P = 0.002$), thus suggesting a lower risk of dementia (Alzheimer's disease or vascular dementia) for those on statin treatment (84).

In a nationally representative population-based survey of 2305 Canadians aged 65 or older, there were 492 incident cases of dementia including 326 Alzheimer's disease, which were compared to 823 persons who had no cognitive impairment. Use of statins and other lipid-lowering agents in subjects aged < 80 years reduced the risk of Alzheimer's disease [OR = 0.26 (0.08–0.88)] after adjustment for sex, educational level, and self-rated health (85).

In a randomized trial of 44 patients with Alzheimer's disease allocated to either simvastatin 80 mg/day or placebo during 26 weeks, there was no significant effect on cerebrospinal fluid (CSF) levels of Aß40 and Aß42. However, in a post-hoc analysis of mildly affected subjects, there was a significant decrease of Aß40 CSF levels with a reduction of 24S-hydroxycholesterol (86).

Unfortunately, the two large-scale long-term clinical trials that looked at some cognitive functions (PROSPER and HPS) failed to show a positive effect on the incidence of dementia. New large specific trials are absolutely warranted to evaluate whether statin therapy may reduce the incidence of mild cognitive impairment or even Alzheimer's disease.

6.2. What are the Effects of Statins in Secondary Prevention of Stroke?

While HPS provided important information about the effect of simvastatin in patients with stroke prior to randomization, with a significant 19% reduction in major vascular events (major coronary events, revascularization, and stroke) in this population, this reduction was almost entirely due to the reduction in coronary events, and not to the reduction in stroke recurrence (20,21). What is reassuring in HPS is that of the 10,269 patients receiving simvastatin, 42 (0.4%) had a carotid endarterectomy or angioplasty, as against 79 (0.8%) of the 10,267 patients receiving the placebo, a significant relative risk reduction of 46% [0.54 (0.38–0.77)] (8). It is thus obvious that simvastatin had a clear impact by reducing the progression of carotid stenosis to surgical indication, and hence had the potential to reduce stroke recurrence.

Only a study dedicated to the secondary prevention of stroke/TIA (in patients without a past history of coronary events) can answer the question of the efficacy of statin therapy in preventing recurrent stroke (87). The SPARCL trial is ongoing, with 4700 stroke/TIA patients randomized to either atorvastatin 80 mg or placebo (88). The strengths of this study are that the patients were recruited in stroke departments (ensuring good representation of the entire population of stroke patients, as well as a good diagnosis of TIAs), the follow-up is 5 years, the primary end-point is fatal and non-fatal stroke, but the power calculation has been effected so as to ensure a positive effect on the secondary end-point (stroke, MI, or vascular death), and the presence of carotid stenosis has been recorded (88). The results should be available by 2005.

7. CURRENT GUIDELINES

In 2001, the National Cholesterol Education Program (NCEP) recognized symptomatic carotid stenosis as a coronary risk equivalent and recommended a target LDL of <100 mg/dL for these patients (89). The accumulating data regarding the benefits of statins in patients with vascular disease led to a broadening of this recommendation in 2004. In the most recent NCEP update, it was commented that coronary risk equivalents could include patients with TIA or stroke of carotid origin or >50% obstruction of a carotid artery (90). Similarly, in view of the expanding data on the benefits of statins, the American Stroke Association issued an advisory in 2004 commenting that clinicians should consider initiating statin treatment in the hospital for patients with stroke of atherosclerotic origin (91).

8. CONCLUSIONS

Statins have a good overall safety profile to date, with no increase in hemorrhagic stroke or cancer. They have favorable effects in the primary prevention of cardiovascular disease in high-risk young as well as elderly populations. Statins reduce the incidence of stroke in high-risk populations (mainly CHD patients, diabetics, and hypertensives) even with a normal baseline blood cholesterol level, which argues for a global cardiovascular risk-based treatment strategy. As for CHD, stroke reduction was mainly observed in studies with large between-group LDL cholesterol differences. In patients with prior strokes, statins probably reduce the incidence of coronary events, but it is not yet proven that they actually reduce the incidence of recurrent strokes in secondary prevention.

From a practical point of view, pending the results of ongoing trials specifically devoted to patients with a TIA or a stroke, it seems reasonable to treat stroke patients with carotid atherosclerosis, diabetes mellitus, previous coronary heart disease, hypertension, hypercholesterolemia, or cigarette smoking and LDL cholesterol >100 mg/dL with statins.

REFERENCES

1. Atkins D, Psaty BM, Koepsell TD, Longstreth WT Jr, Larson EB. Cholesterol reduction and the risk for stroke in men. A meta-analysis of randomized, controlled trials. Ann Intern Med 1993; 119:136–145.
2. Prospective Studies Collaboration. Cholesterol, diastolic blood pressure, and stroke: 13,000 strokes in 450,000 people in 45 prospective cohorts. Lancet 1995; 346:1647–1653.
3. Scandinavian Simvastatin Survival Study Group. Randomised trial of cholesterol lowering in 4444 patients with coronary heart disease: the Scandinavian Simvastatin Survival Study (4S). Lancet 1994; 344:1383–1389.
4. Sacks FM, Pfeffer MA, Moye LA, Rouleau JL, Rutherford JD, Cole TG, Brown L, Warnicka JW, Arnold JMO, Wun CC, Davis BR, Braunwald E (for the Cholesterol and Recurrent Events Trial Investigators). The effect of pravastatin on coronary events after myocardial infarction in patients with average cholesterol levels. N Engl J Med 1996; 336:1001–1009.
5. The Long-Term Intervention with Pravastatin in Ischemic Disease (LIPID) Study Group. Prevention of cardiovascular events and death with pravastatin in patients with coronary heart disease and a broad range of initial cholesterol levels. N Engl J Med 1998; 339:1349–1357.
6. Shepherd J, Cobbe SM, Ford I, Isles CG, Lorimer AR, Macfarlane PW, McKillop JH, Packard CJ (for the West of Scotland Coronary Prevention Study Group). Prevention of coronary heart disease with pravastatin in men with hypercholesterolemia. N Engl J Med 1995; 333:1301–1307.
7. Downs JR, Clearfield M, Weis S, Whitney E, Shapiro DR, Beere PA, Langendorfer A, Stein EA, Kruyer W, Gotto AM (for the AFACTS/TesxCAPS Research Group). Primary prevention of acute coronary events with lovastatin in men and women with average cholesterol levels. JAMA 1998; 279:1615–1622.

8. Heart Protection Study Collaborative Group. MRC/BHF Heart Protection Study of cholesterol lowering with simvastatin in 20536 high-risk individuals: a randomised placebo-controlled trial. Lancet 2002; 360:7–22.

9. Shepherd J, Blauw GJ, Murphy MB, Bollen ELEM, Buckley BM, Cobbe SM, Ford I, Gaw A, Hyland M, Julema JW, Kamper AM, Macfarlane PW, Meinders AE, Norrie J, Packard CJ, Perry IJ, Stott DJ, Sweeney BJ, Twonmey C, Westendorp RGJ (on behalf of the PROSPER study group). Pravastatin in elderly individuals at risk of vascular disease (PROSPER): a randomised controlled trial. Lancet 2002; 360:1623–1630.

10. Athyros VG, Papageorgiou AA, Mercouris BR, Athyrou VV, Symeonidis AN, Basayannis EO, Demitriadis DS, Kontopoulos AG. Treatment with atorvastatin to the National Cholesterol Educational Program goal versus "usual" care in secondary coronary heart disease prevention. The GREek Atorvastatin and Coronary-heart-disease Evaluation (GREACE) Study. Curr Med Res Opin 2002; 18:220–228.

11. Sever PS, Dahlöf B, Poulter NR, Wedel H, Beevers G, Claufield M, Collins R, Kjeldsen SE, Kristinsson A, McInnes GT, Mehlsen J, Nieminen M, O'Brien E, Östergren J (for the ASCOT Investigators). Prevention of coronary and stroke events with atorvastatin in hypertensive patients who have average or lower-than-average cholesterol concentrations, in the Anglo-Scandinavian Cardiac Outcomes Trial—Lipid-lowering Arm (ASCT-LLA): a multicentre randomized controlled trial. Lancet 2003; 361:1149–1158.

12. Iso H, Jacobs DR, Wentworth D, Neaton JD, Cohen JD (for the MRFIT Research Group). Serum cholesterol levels and six-year mortality from stroke in 350,977 men screened for the multiple risk factor intervention trial. N Engl J Med 1989; 320:904–910.

13. Lindenstrøm E, Boysen G, Nyboe J. Influence of total cholesterol, high density lipoprotein cholesterol, and triglycerides on risk of cerebrovascular disease: the Copenhagen city heart study. Br Med J 1994; 309:11–15.

14. Moroney JT, Tang M-X, Berglund L, Small S, Merchant C, Bell K, Stern Y, Mayeux R. Low-density lipoprotein cholesterol and the risk of dementia with stroke. JAMA 1999; 282:254–260.

15. Plehn JF, Davis BR, Saks FM, Rouleau JL, Pfeffer MA, Bersntein V, Cuddy E, Moyé LA, Piller LB, Rutherford J, Simpson LM, Braunwald E (for the CARE Investigators). Reduction of stroke incidence after myocardial infarction with pravastatin. The Cholesterol and Recurrent Events (CARE) Study. Circulation 1999; 99:216–223.

16. White HD, Simes RJ, Anderson NE, Hankey GJ, Watson JDG, Hunt D, Colouhoun DM, Glasziou P, MacMahon S, Kirby AC, West MJ, Tonkin AJ. Pravastatin therapy and the risk of stroke. N Engl J Med 2000; 343: 317–326.

17. Crouse JR III, Byington RP, Hoen HM, Furberg CD. Reductase inhibitor monotherapy and stroke prevention. Arch Intern Med 1997; 157:1305–1310.

18. Hebert PR, Gaziano JM, Chan KS, Hennekens CH. Cholesterol-lowering with statin drugs, risk of stroke, and total mortality. An overview of randomized trials. JAMA 1997; 278:313–321.

19. Amarenco P. Hypercholesterolemia, lipid-lowering agents, and the risk for brain infarction. Neurology 2001; 57(suppl 2):S35–S44.
20. Heart Protection Study Collaborative Group. MRC/BHF Heart Protection Study of cholesterol-lowering with simvastatin in 5963 people with diabetes: a randomized placebo-controlled trial. Lancet 2003; 361:2005–2016.
21. Collins R, Armitage J, Parish S, Sleight P, Peto R (Heart Protection Study Collaborative Group). Effects of cholesterol-lowering with simvastatin on stroke and other major vascular events in 20536 people with cerebrovascular disease or other high-risk conditions. Lancet 2004; 363:757–767.
22. Shepherd J, Blauw GJ, Murphy MB, Cobbe SM, Bollen ELEM, Buckley BM, Ford I, Jukema JW, Hyland M, Gaw A, Lagaay AM, Perry IJ, Macfarlane PW, Meinders AE, Sweeney BJ, Packard CJ, Westendorp RGJ, Twomey C, Stott DJ (on behalf of the Prosper Study Group). The design of a prospective study of pravastatin in the elderly at risk (PROSPER). Am J Cardiol 1999; 84: 1192–1197.
23. Taylor AJ, Kent SM, Flaherty PJ, Coyle LC, Markwood TT, Vernalis MN. ARBITER: Arterial Biology for Investigation of the Treatment Effects of Reducing Cholesterol. A randomized trial comparing the effects of atorvastatin and pravastatin on carotid intima-medial thickness. Circulation 2002; 106:2055–2060.
24. The ALLHAT Officers and Coordinators for the ALLHAT Collaborative Research Group. Major outcomes in moderately hypercholesterolemic, hypertensive patients randomized to pravastatin vs usual care. The Antihypertensive and Lipid-Lowering Treatment to Prevent Heart Attack Trial (ALLHAT-LLT). JAMA 2002; 288:2998–3007.
25. The Kyushu Lipid Intervention Study Group. Pravastatin use and risk of coronary events and cerebral infarction in Japanese men with moderate hypercholesterolemia: the Kyushu Lipid Intervention Study. J Atheroscler Thromb 2000; 7:110–121.
26. Antithrombotic Trialists' Collaboration. Collaborative meta-analysis of randomised trials of antiplatelet therapy for prevention of death, myocardial infraction, and stroke in high risk patients. Br Med J 2002; 324:71–86.
27. Pfeffer MA, Keech A, Sacks FM, Cobbe SM, Tonkin A, Byington RP, Davis BR, Friedman CP, Braunwald E. Safety and tolerability of pravastatin in long-term clinical trials. Prospective Pravastatin, Pooling (PPP) Project. Circulation 2002; 105:2341–2346.
28. Yano K, Reed DM, McLean CJ. Serum cholesterol and hemorrhagic stroke in the Honolulu Heart Program. Stroke 1989; 20:1460–1465.
29. Lee S-H, Bae H-J, Yoon B-W, Kim H, Kim D-E, Roh J-K. Low concentration of serum total cholesterol is associated with multifocal signal loss lesions on gradient-echo magnetic resonance imaging. Analysis of risk factors for multifocal signal loss lesions. Stroke 2002; 33:2845–2849.
30. Byington RP, Davis BR, Plehn JF, White HD, Baker J, Cobbe SM, Shepherd J (for the PPP Investigators). Reduction of stroke events with pravastatin. The Prospective Pravastatin Pooling (PPP) Project. Circulation 2001; 103: 387–392.

31. Schatz IJ, Masaki K, Yano K, Chen R, Rodriguez BL, Curb JD. Cholesterol and all-cause mortality in elderly people from the Honolulu Heart Program: a cohort study. Lancet 2001; 358:351–355.

32. Phan T, McLeod JG, Pollard JD, Peiris O, Rohan A, Halpern J-P. Peripheral neuropathy associated with simvastatin. J Neurol Neurosurg Psychiatr 1995; 58:625–628.

33. Gaist D, Jeppesen U, Andersen M, Garcia Rodriguez LA, Hallas J, Sindrup SH. Statins and risk of polyneuropathy. A case-control study. Neurology 2002; 58: 1333–1337.

34. Hebert PR, Gaziano JM, Hennekens CH. An overview of trials of cholesterol lowering and risk of stroke. Arch Intern Med 1995; 155:50–55.

35. Bloomfield Rubins H, Robins SJ, Collins D, Fye CL, Anderson JW, Elam MB, Faas FH, Linares E, Schaefer EJ, Schectman G, Wilt TJ, Wittes J (for the Veterans Affairs High-Density Lipoprotein Cholesterol Intervention Trial Study Group). Gemfibrozil for the secondary prevention of coronary heart disease in men with low levels of high-density lipoprotein cholesterol. N Engl J Med 1999; 341:410–418.

36. Wilt TJ, Rubins HB, Robins SJ, Riley WA, Collins D, Elam M, Rutan G, Anderson JW. Carotid atherosclerosis in men with low levels of HDL cholesterol. Stroke 1997; 28:1919–1925.

37. Staels B, Dallongeville J, Auwerx J, Schoonjans K, Leitersdorf E, Fruchart J-C. Mechanism of action of fibrates on lipid and lipoprotein metabolism. Circulation 1998; 98:2088–2093.

38. Gotto AM Jr. Triglyceride. The forgotten risk factor. Circulation 1998; 97: 1027–1028.

39. Jeppesen J, Hein HO, Suadicani P, Gyntelberg F. Triglyceride concentration and ischemic heart disease. An eight-year follow-up in the Copenhagen Male Study. Circulation 1998; 97:1029–1036.

40. Garber AM, Lavins A. Triglyceride concentration and coronary heart disease. Not yet proved of value as a screening test. Br Med J 1994; 309:2–3.

41. Fontbonne A, Eschwege E, Cambien F, Richard J-L, Ducimetière P, Thibult N, Warnet J-M, Claude J-R, Rosselin G-E. Hypertriglyceridemia as a risk factor of coronary heart disease mortality in subjects with impaired glucose tolerance or diabetes. Results from the 11-year follow-up of the Paris Prospective Study. Diabetologia 1989; 32:300–304.

42. Hokanson JE, Austin MA. Plasma triglyceride level is a risk factor for cardiovascular disease independent of high-density lipoprotein cholesterol level: a meta-analysis of population-based prospective studies. J Cardiovasc Risk 1996; 3:213–219.

43. Haim M, Benderly M, Brunner D, Behar S, Graff E, Reicher-Reiss H, Goldbourt U (for the BIP Group). Elevated serum triglyceride levels and long-term mortality in patients with coronary heart disease. The Bezafibrate Infarction Prevention (BIP) Registry. Circulation 1999; 100:475–482.

44. Lehto S, Ronnemaa T, Pyorala K, Laakso M. Predictors of stroke in middle-aged patients with non-insulin-dependent diabetes. Stroke 1996; 27:63–68.

45. The BIP Study Group. Secondary prevention by raising HDL cholesterol and reducing triglycerides in patients with coronary artery disease. The Bezafibrate Infarction Prevention (BIP) Study. Circulation 2000; 102:21–27.

46. Tanne D, Koren-Morag N, Graff E, Goldbourt U (for the BIP Study Group). Blood lipids and first-ever ischemic stroke/transient ischemic attack in the Bezafibrate Infarction Prevention (BIP) Registry. High triglycerides constitute an independent risk factor. Circulation 2001; 104:2892–2897.

47. Goldberg RB, Mellies MJ, Saks FM, Moyé LA, Howard BV, Howard WJ, Davis BR, Cole TG, Pfeffer MA, Braunwald E. Cardiovascular events and their reduction with pravastatin in diabetic and glucose-intolerant myocardial infarction survivors with average cholesterol levels. Subgroup analyses in the Cholesterol And Recurrent Events (CARE) trial. Circulation 1998; 98:2513–2519.

48. MRC/BHF Heart Protection Study of cholesterol-lowering with simvastatin in 5963 people with diabetes: a randomised placebo-controlled trial. Lancet 2003; 361:2005–2016.

49. Schwartz GG, Olsson AG, Ezekowitz MD, Ganz P, Oliver MF, Waters D, Zeiher A, Chaitman BR, Leslie S, Stern T [for the Myocardial Ischemia Reduction with Aggressive Cholesterol Lowering (MIRACL) Study Investigators]. Effects of atorvastatin on early recurrent ischemic events in acute coronary syndromes. The MIRACL Study: a randomized controlled trial. JAMA 2001; 285:1711–1718.

50. Newby LK, Kristinsson A, Bhapkar MV, Aylward PE, Dimas AP, Klein WW, McGuire DK, Moliterno DJ, Verheugt FWA, Weaver WD, Califf RM (for the SYMPHONY and 2nd SYMPHONY Investigators). Early statin initiation and outcomes in patients with acute coronary syndromes. JAMA 2002; 287: 3087–3095.

51. Waters DD, Schwartz GG, Olsson AG, Zeiher A, Oliver MF, Ganz P, Ezekowitz M, Chaitman BR, Leslie SJ, Stern T (for the MIRACL Study Investigators). Effects of atorvastatin on stroke in patients with unstable angina or non-Q-wave myocardial infarction. A Myocardial Ischemia Reduction with Aggressive Cholesterol Lowering (MIRACL) substudy. Circulation 2002; 106:1690–1695.

52. Glorioso N, Troffa C, Filigheddu F, Dettori F, Soro A, Parpaglia PP, Collatina S, Pahor M. Effect of the HMG-CoA reductase inhibitors on the blood pressure in patients with essential hypertension and primary hypercholesterolemia. Hypertension 1999; 34:1281–1286.

53. Wilkinson IB, Cockcroft JR. Pravastatin, blood pressure, and stroke. Hypertension 2000; 36:e1.

54. Goode T, Miller JP, Heagerty AM. Hyperlipidaemia, hypertension, and coronary heart disease. Lancet 1995; 354:362–364.

55. Staessen JA, Wang JG, Thijs L. Cardiovascular protection and blood pressure reduction: a meta-analysis. Lancet 2001; 358:1305–1315.

56. Cook NR, Cohen J, Hekbert PR, Taylor JO, Henneckens CH. Implications of small reductions in diastolic blood pressure for primary prevention. Arch Intern Med 1995; 155:701–709.

57. Corvol JC, Bouzamondo A, Sirol M, Hulot S, Sanchez P, Lechat P. Differential effects of lipid-lowering therapy on stroke prevention. Arch Intern Med 2003; 163:669–676.

58. Wolf PA, D'Agostino RB. Epidemiology of Stroke. In: Barnett HJM, Mohr JP, Stein BM, Yatsu FM (eds), Stroke: Pathophysiology, Diagnosis, and Management, 3d ed. New York: Churchill Livingstone, 1998; Ch. 1:3–28.

59. Wilson PWF, Hoeg JM, D'Agostino RB, Silbershatz H, Belanger AM, Poehlmann H, O'Leary D, Wolf PA. Cumulative effects of high cholesterol levels, high blood pressure, and cigarette smoking on carotid stenosis. N Engl J Med 1997; 337:516–522.

60. Furberg CD, Adams HP, Applegate WB, Byington RP, Espeland MA, Hartwell T, Hunninghake DB, Lefkowitz DS, Probstfield J, Riley WA, Young B [for the Asymptomatic Carotid Artery Progression Study (ACAPS) Research Group]. Effect of lovastatin on early carotid atherosclerosis and cardiovascular events. Circulation 1994; 90:1679–1688.

61. Adams HP, Byington RP, Hoen H, Dempsey R, Furberg CD. Effect of cholesterol-lowering medications on progression of mild atherosclerotic lesions of the carotid arteries and on the risk of stroke. Cerebrovasc Dis 1995; 5:171–177.

62. Crouse JR, Byington RP, Bond MG, Espeland MA, Craven TE, Sprinkle JW, McGovern ME, Furberg CD. Pravastatin, Lipids, and Atherosclerosis in the Carotid Arteries (PLAC-II): a clinical trial with atherosclerosis outcome. Am J Cardiol 1995; 75:455–459.

63. Salonen R, Nyyssönen K, Porkkala E, Rummukainen J, Belder R, Park J-S, Salonen JT. Kuopio Atherosclerosis Prevention Study (KAPS): a population-based primary prevention trial of the effect of LDL lowering on atherosclerotic progression in carotid and femoral arteries. Circulation 1995; 92:1758–1764.

64. MacMahon S, Sharpe N, Gamble G, Hart H, Scott J, Simes J, White H (on behalf of the LIPID Trial Research Group). Effects of lowering average or below-average cholesterol levels on the progression of carotid atherosclerosis. Results of the LIPID atherosclerosis substudy. Circulation 1998; 97:1784–1790.

65. Smilde TJ, van Wissen S, Wollersheim H, Kastelein JJP, Stalenhoef AFH. Effect of aggressive versus conventional lipid lowering on atherosclerosis progression in familial hypercholesterolemia (ASAP): a prospective, randomised, double-blind trial. Lancet 2001; 357:577–581.

66. Taylor AJ, Kent SM, Flaherty PJ, Coyle LC, Markwood TT, Vernalis MN. ARBITER: Arterial Biology for Investigation of the Treatment Effects of Reducing Cholesterol. A randomized trial comparing the effects of atorvastatin and pravastatin on carotid intima-medial thickness. Circulation 2002; 106:2055–2060.

67. Levine GN, Keaney JF Jr, Vita JA. Cholesterol reduction in cardiovascular disease. Clinical benefits and possible mechanisms. N Engl J Med 1995; 332:512–521.

68. Vaughan CJ, Murphy MB, Buckley BM. Statins do more than just lower cholesterol. Lancet 1996; 348:1079–1082.

69. Delanty N, Vaughan CJ. Vascular effects of statins in stroke. Stroke 1997; 28:2315–2320.

70. Rosenson RS, Tangney CC. Antiatherothrombotic properties of statins. Implications for cardiovascular event reduction. JAMA 1998; 279:1643–1650.

71. Takemoto M, Liao JK. Pleiotropic effects of 3-hydroxy-3-methylglutaryl coenzyme A reductase inhibitors. Arterioscler Thromb Vasc Biol 2001; 21:1712–1719.

72. Crisby M, Nordin-Fredricksson G, Shah PK, Yano J, Zhu J, Nilsson J. Pravastatin treatment increases collagen content and decreases lipid content, inflam-

mation, metalloproteinases, and cell death in human carotid plaques. Implications for plaque stabilization. Circulation 2001; 103:926–933.

73. Sterzer P, Meintzschel F, Rösler A, Lanfermann H, Steinmetz H, Sitzer M. Pravastatin improves cerebral vasomotor reactivity in patients with subcortical small-vessel disease. Stroke 2001; 32:2817–2820.

74. Pullicino PM. Pathogenesis of lacunar infarcts and small deep infarcts. Adv Neurol 1993; 62:125–140.

75. Anderson TJ, Meredith IT, Yeung AC, Frei B, Selwyn AP, Ganz P. The effects of cholesterol-lowering and antioxidant therapy on endothelium-dependent coronary vasomotion. N Engl J Med 1995; 332:488–493.

76. Treasure CB, Klein JL, Weintraub WS, Talley JD, Stillabower ME, Kosinski AS, Zhang J, Boccuzzi SJ, Cedarholm JC, Alexander RW. Beneficial effects of cholesterol-lowering therapy on the coronary endothelium in patients with coronary artery disease. N Engl J Med 1995; 332:481–487.

77. Dupuis J, Tardif J-C, Cernacek P, Théroux P. Cholesterol reduction rapidly improves endothelial function after acute coronary syndromes. The RECIFE (Reduction of Cholesterol in Ischemia and Function of the Endothelium) Trial. Circulation 1999; 99:3227–3233.

78. Baller D, Notohamiprodjo G, Gleichmann U, Holzinger J, Weise R, Lehmann J. Improvement in coronary flow reserve determined by positron emission tomography after 6 months of cholesterol-lowering therapy in patients with early stages of coronary atherosclerosis. Circulation 1999; 99:2871–2875.

79. Laufs U, La Fata V, Plutzky, Liao JK. Upregulation of endothelial nitric oxide synthase by HMG CoA reductase inhibitors. Circulation 1998; 97:1129–1135.

80. Amin-Hanjani S, Stagliano NE, Yamada M, Huang PL, Liao JK, Moskowitz MA. Mevastatin, an HMG-CoA reductase inhibitor, reduces stroke damage and upregulated endothelial nitric oxide synthase in mice. Stroke 2001; 32:980–986.

81. Laufs U, Gertz K, Dirnagl U, Bohm M, Nickenig G, Endres M. Rosuvastatin, a new HMG-CoA reductase inhibitor, upregulates endothelial nitric oxide synthase and protects from ischemic stroke in mice. Brain Res 2002; 942:23–30.

82. Simons M, Keller P, Dichgans J, Schulz JB. Cholesterol and Alzheimer's disease. Is there a link? Neurology 2001; 57:1089–1093.

83. Wolozin B, Kellman W, Ruosseau P, Celesia GG, Siegel G. Decreased prevalence of Alzheimer disease associated with 3-hydroxy-3-methyglutaryl coenzyme A reductase inhibitors. Arch Neurol 2000; 57:1439–1443.

84. Jick H, Zornberg GL, Jick SS, Seshadri S, Drachman DA. Statins and the risk of dementia. Lancet 2000; 356:1627–1631.

85. Rockwood K, Kirkland S, Hogan DB, MacKnight C, Merry H, Verreault R, Wolfson C, McDowell I. Use of lipid-lowering agents, indication bias, and the risk of dementia in community-dwelling elderly people. Arch Neurol 2002; 59:223–227.

86. Simons M, Schwärzler F, Lütjohann D, von Bergmann K, Beyreuther K, Dichgans J, Wormstall H, Hartmann T, Schlz JB. Treatment with simvastatin in normocholesterolemic patients with Alzheimer's disease: a 26-week randomized, placebo-controlled double-blind trial. Ann Neurol 2002; 52: 346–350.

87. Goldstein LB, Amarenco P, Bogousslavsky J, Callahan AS, Hennerici MG, Welch KM, Zivin J, Sillesen H. The SPARCL Steering Committee. Statins for secondary stroke prevention in patients without known coronary heart disease: the jury is still out. Cerebrovasc Dis 2004; 18:1–2.
88. The SPARCL Investigators. Design and baseline characteristics of the stroke prevention by aggressive reduction in cholesterol levels (SPARCL). Cerebrovasc Dis 2003; 16:389–395.
89. Executive summary of the third report of the national cholesterol education program (NCEP) expert panel on detection, evaluation, and treatment of high blood cholesterol in adults (adult treatment panel III). JAMA 2001; 285: 2486–2497.
90. Grundy SM, Cleeman JI, Merz NB, et al. Implications of recent clinical trials for the National Cholesterol Education Program Adult Treatment Panel III Guidelines. Circulation 2004; 110: 227–239.
91. The Stroke Council. Statins after ischemic stroke and transient ischemic attack. Stroke 2004; 35:1023.

8

Management of Hypertension in Carotid Stenosis

J. David Spence

Stroke Prevention and Atherosclerosis Research Centre, Robarts Research Institute, London, Ontario, Canada

Patients with carotid stenosis are at a high risk not only of stroke, but also of myocardial infarction (MI); indeed they can have a higher risk of MI than do patients with a history of coronary disease. Chimowitz et al. (1) reported that in the Veterans' Administration Asymptomatic Carotid Surgery Trial, patients with no history of coronary artery disease (CAD) had a 33% 4-year risk of MI, and those with both carotid stenosis and a history of CAD had a 40% 4-year risk of MI. In contrast, patients with CAD in the placebo arm of the Scandinavian Simvastatin Survival Study (4-S) (2) had only a 26% 6-year risk of MI.

Hypertension is very common in patients with carotid stenosis. In the North American Symptomatic Carotid Artery Surgery Trial (NASCET), only 20% of patients were reported as having blood pressure at entry above 160 mmHg systolic or 90 mmHg diastolic, but many had controlled pressures because they were on treatment. Overall, 61% of patients in NASCET were identified as having a history of hypertension. In the major asymptomatic trials, 64% of patients in the Asymptomatic Carotid Atherosclerosis Study (ACAS) were hypertensive and 65% of the Asymptomatic Carotid Surgery Trial (ACST) participants were diagnosed with hypertension. Among patients with carotid stenosis >50% in the Stroke Prevention Clinic of JDS, 75.5% had a history of hypertension or were on antihypertensive medications at the time of referral.

Hypertension is perhaps the most important stroke risk factor in that it is powerful, graded (3,4), and treatable. It is important to understand that hypertension is a much stronger risk factor for stroke than for CAD: After correction for this "regression dilution" bias, prolonged differences in usual diastolic blood pressure (DBP) of 5, 7.5, and 10 mmHg were respectively associated with at least 34, 46, and 56% less stroke and at least 21, 29, and 37% less CHD (4).

In order to understand this difference it is necessary to understand that hypertension contributes differently to atherosclerosis vs. hypertensive small vessel disease (5). Strokes due to high blood pressure per se are of two types: lacunar infarction and intracerebral hemorrhage; they occur in a particular distribution: the basal ganglia, thalamus, internal capsule, brainstem, and cerebellum. This distribution has been called by Hachinski the "vascular centrencephalon". In the ancient part of the brain, short straight arteries with few branches deliver systemic blood pressure directly to resistance vessels, which are damaged, reacting by hyaline degeneration or fibrinoid necrosis. When they occlude, the result is lacunar infarction; when they rupture, the result is intracerebral hemorrhage.

Control of blood pressure virtually eliminates this type of stroke. In London, Ontario we observed an experiment of nature that resulted from the coincidence of the arrival of the first CT scanner (which made it possible to distinguish stroke subtypes) the year before the opening of a new hypertension clinic, and the institution of a major study by the Department of Family Medicine aimed at increasing blood pressure detection and control. In 1978 we were seeing 500 strokes per year, of which half were due to hypertensive small vessel disease; nearly one patient with hypertensive intracerebral hemorrhage per day was admitted to our hospital. By 1984, strokes were down to 250 per year, and only 7% were due to hypertension. Strokes due to carotid atherosclerosis were unchanged.

Lawlor et al. documented a similar trend from autopsy data in England and Wales, from 1932 to 1999: The ratio of cerebral infarct to cerebral hemorrhage increased 4-fold from 0.5 in the 1930s to 2.0 by the 1990s; trends in estimated cerebral infarct mortality closely matched those for coronary heart disease mortality (6).

In the NASCET trial, strenuous efforts were made to control blood pressure. Investigators received pointed reminder letters whenever antihypertensive medication was not increased at follow-up visits at which a patient had blood pressures above 140 systolic or 90 diastolic. The result of this effort was that only 0.5% of strokes in the 5-year follow-up were due to hypertensive intracerebral hemorrhage or subarachnoid hemorrhage (7).

It is therefore clear that good blood pressure control is very important in the management of patients with carotid stenosis. How, though, can it be achieved?

1. DOES THE TYPE OF MEDICATION MATTER?

The way in which the blood pressure is lowered may make a difference. This issue has recently been debated (8–10). The PROGRESS trial (11) showed that among patients with previous stroke or transient ischemic attack (TIA), those randomized to perindopril and indapamide had significantly better outcomes than those randomized to placebo. This, taken with the stroke prevention results of the HOPE trial (12), suggested that perhaps treatment with angiotensin-converting enzyme inhibitors (ACEi) may be more effective than other treatments. The possibility that blockade of the rennin–angiotensin system may be the mechanism was supported by the findings of the LIFE trial, which showed that patients randomized to losartan had significantly better outcomes, with about a 25% relative risk reduction for stroke, compared with patients randomized to atenolol, despite identical blood pressure control (13). The Study on Cognition and Prognosis in the Elderly (SCOPE) also showed a significant reduction of non-fatal stroke with candesartan vs. alternative therapies (14). However, the ALL-HAT trial reported superior results in patients randomized to diuretic (15). It is very important to recognize that these results were driven by a major reduction of stroke in African-American participants, who represented 35% of patients in ALLHAT; the opposite result was obtained in the Second Australian National Blood Pressure Study (ANBP2) (16), in which only 0.55% of patients were of African origin. This difference in results of treatment with diuretics vs. other classes of antihypertensive therapy raises the issue of low-renin hypertension.

2. TREATING THE UNDERLYING CAUSE OF HYPERTENSION

In patients with difficult hypertension, it is necessary to identify the physiologic drivers of the hypertension in order to achieve control. A simple approach to this problem is to use renin/aldosterone profiling, which is very helpful in the management of resistant hypertension (17). The most neglected subset of hypertensives are those with low-renin hypertension. Table 1 summarizes causes of low-renin hypertension. Spence found that ∼20% of patients with resistant hypertension had renovascular hypertension, but 10% had adrenocortical hypertension, which was almost always due to bilateral adrenocortical hyperplasia; patients of African origin were approximately 10-fold more likely to have this problem (17). Among patients with carotid stenosis and resistant hypertension, 25% have renovascular hypertension, which would not be surprising given that atherosclerotic renal artery stenosis is more common among patients with severe atherosclerosis; what is surprising is that 8% had adrenocortical hyperplasia, a condition unknown to many "experts" in hypertension (18). Using renin/aldosterone profiling, Gallay et al. (19) found that 17% of patients referred

Table 1 Causes of Low-Renin Hypertension

Conn's syndrome
Primary adrenocortical hyperplasia
Adrenal enzyme deficiencies (11-OH, 17-OH)
Dexamethasone-suppressible hypertension
    Lifton's syndrome
    Laidlaw's syndrome: high 18-OH-DOC
Gordon's syndrome: treat with salt restriction
Renal tubular abnormality; Liddle's syndrome
    Na channel mutation: 5% of HT in blacks
    Low aldo and renin; treat with amiloride
GIP-dependent cortisol excess with nodular hyperplasia

---

for resistant hypertension had adrenocortical hypertension. Recently a new cause of hypertension was described, accounting for 5% of hypertension in patients of African descent, with low renin and low aldosterone levels. Baker et al. described a new sodium channel mutation (20), probably related to Liddle's syndrome (21), and treatable specifically with amiloride. Thus, particularly in patients of African origin, it is important to determine the rennin–aldosterone ratio. This physiological profiling permits selection of effective therapy. Among patients with primary hyperaldosteronism, with low renin and high aldosterone, the primary treatment is spironolactone in women, or eplerenone in either sex (in countries where eplerenone is not yet available, amiloride is probably preferable for men, because of gynecomastia from spironolactone). Among patients with abnormalities of sodium channels in the renal tubules, retention of salt and water suppresses both renin and aldosterone; the primary treatment is amiloride. Among patients with high renin and aldosterone levels (secondary hyperaldosteronism), a renal cause such as renovascular hypertension, obstruction, renal tumor, etc., must be investigated, and the primary treatment is angiotensin receptor blockers. (ACEi work mainly by raising levels of bradykinin; circulating levels of angiotensin II return to normal within weeks of initiating ACEi.) Table 2 summarizes these principles of therapy. Patients with renovascular hypertension, which is particularly common among patients with carotid stenosis, may require revascularization for control. This problem has recently been reviewed (22).

3. IS IT SAFE TO TREAT HYPERTENSION IN PATIENTS WITH SEVERE STENOSIS?

Despite the results of several trials now showing that antihypertensive therapy improves outcomes after stroke, some physicians remain concerned that lowering of blood pressure may be risky in patients with carotid

Table 2 Physiological Tailoring of Antihypertensive Therapy

	Primary Hyperaldosteronism	Liddle's, Na Channel Mutation	Renal/ Renovascular Hypertension
Renin	Low	Low	High
Aldosterone	High	Low	High
Primary treatment	Spironolactone for women, or eplerenone for either sex (amiloride where eplerenone not available)	Amiloride	Angiotensin receptor antagonists

stenosis. To address this issue, we analyzed data from NASCET (7), the European Carotid Surgery Trial (ECST) (23), and the UK-TIA trial (24). In all three studies, the risk of subsequent stroke increased as blood pressure increased, and this was true both for patients with stenosis above and below 70% (25). There was one very small group of patients, amounting to only 3% of the cases, with severe bilateral stenosis or severe stenosis and contralateral occlusion, in which there appeared to be protection from hypertension. In these patients, stroke risk declined as blood pressure increased (Fig. 1), but this protection was abolished by endarterectomy. Since patients with carotid stenosis represent only 20% of patients with stroke, and this group represented only 3% of the cases in these studies, such patients probably represent <1% of patients with TIA or stroke. Thus it is clear that the vast majority will benefit from antihypertensive therapy, including most patients with carotid stenosis.

4. CONCLUSIONS

Patients with carotid stenosis are at a high risk not only of stroke, but also of myocardial infarction. Effective treatment of hypertension substantially reduces the risk of recurrent stroke, and virtually eliminates stroke due to hypertensive small vessel disease. Even normotensive patients who have experienced stroke or TIA will benefit from treatment with ACE inhibitors or angiotensin receptor blockers, but in hypertensive patients, the choice of therapy is most effective when it is aimed at the underlying physiologic mechanism that is driving the hypertension. Among those with resistant hypertension, a high proportion have renovascular hypertension or adrenocortical hypertension. To achieve control in difficult cases it is very helpful to measure plasma renin and aldosterone.

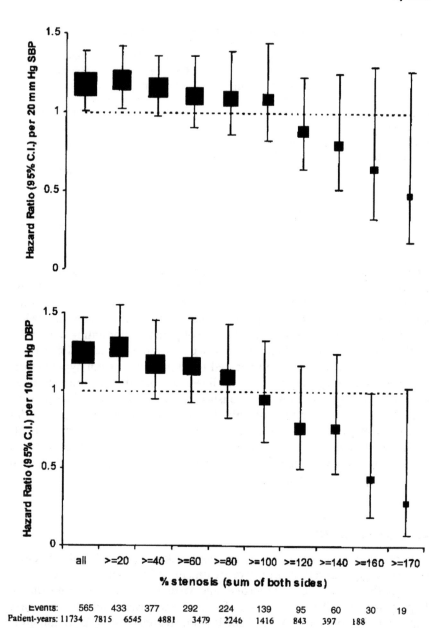

| Events: | 565 | 433 | 377 | 292 | 224 | 139 | 95 | 60 | 30 | 19 |
| Patient-years: | 11734 | 7815 | 6545 | 4881 | 3479 | 2246 | 1416 | 843 | 397 | 188 |

Figure 1 Hazard ratios for the change in stroke risk per increase in usual DBP (10 mmHg) and SBP (20 mmHg) in stenosis groups defined with different cut-off points based on the sum of the degrees of stenosis of both carotid arteries. In patients with bilateral severe carotid stenosis, elevated blood pressures are not associated with increased risk of stroke. This apparent protection of the brain from high pressure is lost following endarterectomy.

REFERENCES

1. Chimowitz MI, Weiss DG, Cohen SL, Starling MR, Hobson RW. (Veteran's Affairs Cooperative study group 167). Cardiac prognosis of patients with carotid stenosis and no history of coronary artery disease. Stroke 1994; 25: 759–765.
2. Scandinavian Simvastatin Survival Study Group. Randomized trial of cholesterol lowering in 4444 patients with coronary heart disease: the Scandinavian Simvastatin Survival Study (4S). Lancet 1994; 344:1383–1389.
3. Collins R, Peto R, MacMahon S, Hebert P, Fiebach NH, Eberlein KA, Godwin J, Qizilbash N, Taylor JO, Hennekens CH. Blood pressure, stroke, and coronary heart disease. Part 2. Short-term reductions in blood pressure: overview of randomised drug trials in their epidemiological context. Lancet 1990; 335(8693):827–838.
4. MacMahon S, Peto R, Cutler J, Collins R, Sorlie P, Neaton J, Abbott R, Godwin J, Dyer A, Stamler J. Blood pressure, stroke, and coronary heart disease. Part 1. Prolonged differences in blood pressure: prospective observational studies corrected for the regression dilution bias. Lancet 1990; 335(8692):765–774.
5. Spence JD. Cerebral consequences of hypertension. In: Laragh JH, Brenner B, eds. Hypertension: Pathophysiology, Diagnosis, and Management. New York: Raven Press, 1995:741–753.
6. Lawlor DA, Smith GD, Leon DA, Sterne JA, Ebrahim S. Secular trends in mortality by stroke subtype in the 20th century: a retrospective analysis. Lancet 2002; 360(9348):1818–1823.
7. Barnett HJ, Taylor DW, Eliasziw M, Fox AJ, Ferguson GG, Haynes RB, Rankin RN, Clagett GP, Hachinski VC, Sackett DL, Thorpe KE, Meldrum HE, Spence JD. Benefit of carotid endarterectomy in patients with symptomatic moderate or severe stenosis. North American Symptomatic Carotid Endarterectomy Trial Collaborators [see comments]. N Engl J Med 1998; 339(20): 1415–1425.
8. Anderson C. Blood pressure lowering for secondary prevention of stroke: ACE inhibition is the key. Stroke 2003; 34:1333–1334.
9. Bath P. Blood-pressure lowering for secondary prevention of stroke: ACE inhibition is not the key. Stroke 2003; 34:1334–1335.
10. Davis SM, Donnan GA. Blood pressure reduction and ACE inhibition in secondary stroke prevention: mechanism uncertain. Stroke 2003; 34(1335):1336.
11. PROGRESS Collaborative Group. Randomised trial of a perindopril-based blood pressure-lowering regimen among 6105 individuals with previous stroke or transient ischemic attack. Lancet 2001; 358:1033–1041.
12. Bosch J, Yusuf S, Pogue J, Sleight P, Lonn E, Rangoonwala B, Davies R, Ostergren J, Probstfield J. Use of ramipril in preventing stroke: double blind randomised trial. Br Med J 2002; 324(7339):699–702.
13. Dahlof B, Devereux RB, Kjeldsen SE, Julius S, Beevers G, Faire U, et al. Cardiovascular morbidity and mortality in the Losartan Intervention For End-point reduction in hypertension study (LIFE): a randomised trial against atenolol. Lancet 2002; 359(9311):995–1003.
14. Lithella H, Hansson L, Skoog I, Elmfeldt D, Hofmand A, Olofsson B, Trenkwalder P, Zanchetti A. The Study on Cognition and Prognosis in the

Elderly (SCOPE): principal results of a randomized double-blind intervention trial. J Hypertens 2003; 21:875–886.

15. The ALLHAT Officers and Coordinators for the ALLHAT Collaborative Research Group. Major outcomes in high-risk hypertensive patients randomized to angiotensin-converting enzyme inhibitor or calcium channel blocker vs diuretic: The Antihypertensive and Lipid-Lowering Treatment to Prevent Heart Attack Trial (ALLHAT). JAMA 2002; 288(23):2981–2997.

16. Wing LM, Reid CM, Ryan P, Beilin LJ, Brown MA, Jennings GL, Johnston CI, McNeil JJ, Marley JE, Morgan TO, Shaw J, Steven ID, West MJ. Second Australian National Blood Pressure Study (ANBP2). Australian Comparative Outcome Trial of ACE inhibitor- and diuretic-based treatment of hypertension in the elderly. Management Committee on behalf of the High Blood Pressure Research Council of Australia. Clin Exp Hypertens 1997; 19(5–6):779–791.

17. Spence JD. Physiologic tailoring of therapy for resistant hypertension: 20 year' experience with stimulated renin profiling. Am J Hypertens 1999; 12:1077–1083.

18. Spence JD. Management of resistant hypertension in patients with carotid stenosis: High prevalence of renovascular hypertension. Cerebrovasc Dis 2000; 10:249–254.

19. Gallay BJ, Ahmad S, Xu L, Toivola B, Davidson RC. Screening for primary aldosteronism without discontinuing hypertensive medications: plasma aldosterone-renin ratio. Am J Kidney Dis 2001; 37(4):699–705.

20. Baker EH, Duggal A, Dong Y, Ireson NJ, Wood M, Markandu ND, MacGregor GA. Amiloride, a specific drug for hypertension in black people with T594M variant? Hypertension 2002; 40:13–17.

21. Warnock DG. Liddle syndrome: genetics and mechanisms of Na+ channel defects. Am J Med Sci 2001; 322(6):302–307.

22. Spence JD. Treatment options for renovascular hypertension. Exp Opin Pharmacother 2002; 3:411–416.

23. European Carotid Surgery Trialists' Collaborative Group. Randomised trial of endarterectomy for recently symptomatic carotid stenosis: final results of the MRC European Carotid Surgery Trial (ECST). Lancet 1998; 351:1379–1387.

24. UK-TIA Study group. The United Kingdom transient ischaemic attack (UK-TIA) aspirin trial: final results. J Neurol Neurosurg Psychiatr 1991; 54:1044–1054.

25. Rothwell PM, Howard SC, Spence D. Relationship between blood pressure and stroke risk in patients with symptomatic carotid occlusive disease. Stroke 2003; 34:2583–90.

9

Hyperhomocyst(e)inemia and Carotid Atherosclerosis

Houta S. Sabet and L. Creed Pettigrew

Stroke Program of the Sanders-Brown Center on Aging and the Department of Neurology, University of Kentucky College of Medicine, Lexington, Kentucky, U.S.A.

1. INTRODUCTION

Homocyst(e)ine refers to a family of sulfated amino acids associated with premature, systemic atherosclerosis and prothrombotic disorders. In 1962, the first observation of elevated homocyst(e)ine associated with cerebrovascular disease was reported in children and young adults with homozygous homocystinuria secondary to deficiency of cystathionine synthase (1,2). In 1969, McCully suggested that moderate levels of homocyst(e)ine could be associated with atherosclerosis (3). Boers and co-workers reported in 1985 that homocyst(e)ine levels of 14 μmol/L or higher were present in approximately 30% of patients with symptomatic peripheral and cerebrovascular disease, but not coronary artery disease (4). This observation was corroborated by Clarke et al. who noted that about 30% of patients with premature atherosclerosis have plasma homocyst(e)ine levels >14 μmol/L (5). Several observational studies have shown that elevated homocyst(e)ine is associated with a high risk of ischemic stroke (6–11). Plasma homocyst(e)ine >10.2 μmol/L doubles the vascular risk of patients with lower levels (12). If plasma homocyst(e)ine rises above 20 μmol/L, then vascular risk increases 8-fold compared to levels below 9 μmol/L (13).

In this chapter, we will consider the relationship between hyperhomocyst(e)inemia and carotid atherosclerosis, a common cause of ischemic stroke. The metabolism of homocyst(e)ine will be reviewed with emphasis on the contribution of vitamin co-factors needed for the enzymatic conversion of the base molecule into inactive species. The role of homocyst(e)ine in the pathogenesis of atherosclerosis and prothrombotic conditions will then be considered. A survey of investigations reporting an association between hyperhomocyst(e)inemia and carotid atherosclerosis will be presented. The chapter will conclude with a discussion of clinical trials that have been performed to date for attempted treatments of hyperhomocyst(e)inemia with comments on the implications for the management of carotid atherosclerosis.

2. METABOLISM OF HOMOCYST(E)INE

Homocyst(e)ine encompasses the total of free and protein-bound sulfated amino acids that include homocysteine, homocystine, and mixed disulfides (14,15), as shown in Fig. 1. The regulation of homocyst(e)ine has been reviewed extensively elsewhere (16–18), requiring only a brief summary in this chapter for the convenience of the reader. Homocyst(e)ine is derived in humans from the methylation of dietary methionine that is abundant in animal protein. Once formed, homocyst(e)ine is metabolized by either the remethylation cycle or the transulfuration pathway (Fig. 2). In the remethylation cycle, ∼50% of homocyst(e)ine is converted back to methionine from methylene-tetrahydrofolate (MTHF) precursors by folate-dependent MTHF reductase (MTHFR) and cobalamin-dependent methionine synthase. The methyl group of methionine is activated by conversion to S-adenosyl methionine (SAM), an important methyl group donor. The product of SAM methylation is S-adenosyl homocysteine (SAH) which is in turn hydrolyzed to form homocyst(e)ine in a reversible reaction. In the transulfuration pathway, the remaining 50% of homocyst(e)ine is converted to cystathionine by

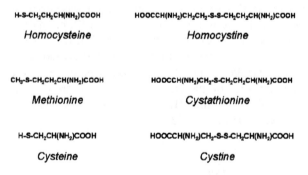

Figure 1 Structural formulas of molecules participating in homocyst(e)ine metabolism.

Remethylation Cycle

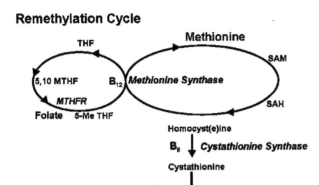

Trans-sulfuration Pathway

Figure 2 Simplified diagram of the methionine–homocysteine remethylation cycle and the transulfuration pathway for conversion of homocysteine to cystathionine. The enzymes methionine synthase, cystathionine synthase, and MTHFR (see italic typeface) are shown with their essential co-factor vitamins. SAM = S-adenyl-methionine; SAH = S-adensylhomocysteine; THF = tetrahydrofolate; 5,10-MTHF= 5,10-methylenetetrahydrofolate; 5-Me THF=5-methyltetrahydrofolate; MTHFR= methylenetetrahydrofolate reductase.

pyridoxine-dependent cystathionine synthase. Cystathionine is then metabolized further to form the end product of the pathway, cysteine.

The cofactor dependency of the three key enzymes in homocyst(e)ine metabolism, methionine synthase, MTHFR, and cystathionine synthase, forms the basis of megavitamin therapy to lower plasma homocyst(e)ine levels. The intake of large quantities of pyridoxine will augment the catabolism of homocyst(e)ine to cysteine by cystathionine synthase. Remethylation of homocyst(e)ine to form methionine will be accelerated if folic acid, the cofactor of MTFHR, and cobalamin, the cofactor of methionine synthase, are consumed in abundance (14). In most tissues within the human body, homocyst(e)ine is remethylated and detoxified by methionine synthase. However, hepatocytes in the liver, the most important organ for the metabolism of homocyst(e)ine (19), also contain MTFHR functioning within the alternate "loop" of the remethylation cycle to detoxify homocyst(e)ine through the formation of methionine.

The interaction between the remethylation cycle and the transulfuration pathway is complex. If SAM concentrations are low, then homocyst(e)ine is directed primarily by methionine synthase through the remethylation cycle to form methionine. If SAM concentrations are high, the transulfuration pathway is favored and more homocyst(e)ine is condensed irreversibly with serine to form cystathione and cysteine by two pyridoxine-dependent reactions, the first of which, shown in Fig. 2, is governed by cystathionine synthase. Cysteine is a metabolic precursor of glutathione, a major protector of cells against oxidative stress and other types of damage. Approximately half of the intracellular glutathione pool in the human liver was recently shown to be derived from homocyst(e)ine (20). The transulfuration pathway also directs homocyst(e)ine to degradation and its ultimate removal as sulfate.

3. HOMOCYST(E)INE AND THE PATHOGENESIS OF ATHEROTHROMBOSIS

Elevated levels of homocyst(e)ine may initiate arterial thrombosis and prevent natural thrombolysis by inhibiting thrombomodulin or the expression of heparin sulfate in the plasma membrane of endothelial cells constituting the vascular intima (21–26). Hydrogen peroxide released as a byproduct of homocyst(e)ine metabolism may exert oxidative stress to cause secondary injury of vascular endothelia (27–32). In vitro and animal model studies confirm that elevated levels of homocyst(e)ine promote cellular oxidative damage and may threaten endothelia, neurons, and other cell populations constituting, or dependent upon, the integrity of the intimal surface in the extracranial vessels and in the vasculature of the brain. These putative actions of homocyst(e)ine include the inhibition of nitric oxide (NO) in endothelial cells, direct cellular toxicity due to inadequate catabolism through impaired remethylation, and interactions with N-methyl-D-aspartate receptors to affect neuronal calcium conductance. As an important contributor to the pathogenesis of systemic atherosclerosis, homocyst(e)ine at peak levels may cause toxic injury to endothelial cells (33), activate platelets (34), induce procoagulant activity (35), enhance smooth muscle cell proliferation (36–38), and promote intravascular synthesis of collagen (39,40). Rats with hyperhomocyst(e)inemia that are fed a lipogenic diet become even more susceptible to intima-media hyperplasia (41). Durand et al. (42) showed that hyperhomocyst(e)inemic rats have enhanced thromboxane biosynthesis and accelerated platelet aggregation. Morita et al. (43) found excessive neo-intima formation in the wall of the carotid artery after induced endothelial injury in hyperhomocyst(e)inemic rats. In correlation with these in vitro and animal model experiments, observational studies in humans demonstrate a strong association between elevated homocyst(e)ine levels and enhanced lipid peroxidation (44) as well as increased total serum cholesterol levels (45). Hyperhomocyst(e)inemia may promote increased oxidation of LDL and cause unfavorable alterations in the level of lipoprotein (a) (46).

4. HYPERHOMOCYST(E)INEMIA AND THE RISK OF CAROTID ATHEROSCLEROSIS

Table 1 provides a summary of observational studies that have identified the correlative relationship between plasma homocyst(e)ine level and carotid atherosclerosis as measured by duplex ultrasonography. The most common technique used for the measurement of carotid atherosclerosis has been quantification of intima-media thickness (IMT), usually defined as the distance between the characteristic echoes from the lumen–intima and media–adventitia interfaces (47). The IMT is well accepted as a reproducible, non-invasive measure of peripheral atherosclerosis, although its correlation with coronary artery disease is less convincing (48). Although the studies described in Table 1 are heterogeneous in experimental design, inclusion criteria, and population (ranging from Northern Europeans to Japanese), they document that homocyst(e)ine as a continuous analytical variable will correlate with increasing severity of carotid atherosclerosis. With the exception of one study published by Voutilainen et al. (44) that observed this effect only in men, the robust association between the severity of carotid atherosclerosis and homocyst(e)ine has no gender preference. Other notable exceptions among the studies listed in Table 1 are those conducted by Taylor et al. (49) and Fagerberg et al. (50), both of which found no relationship between homocyst(e)ine level and measurements of carotid atherosclerosis (49,50). In the former report, 169 patients with symptomatic peripheral arterial disease (claudication, rest pain, digital gangrene, or amputation) and/or cerebrovascular disease (ischemic stroke or transient ischemic attack) were dichotomized into two groups with "elevated" or normal levels of homocyst(e)ine and were evaluated by serial ultrasonography. There was no difference between the groups in progression of carotid atherosclerosis as defined by conversion of a patent to an occluded vessel or by advancement to a more severe compromise of the arterial lumen. However, worsening of the ankle-brachial index measuring arterial perfusion in the leg was observed selectively in the "elevated" homocyst(e)ine group. In the second study by Fagerberg et al. (50), 800 men with insulin sensitivity and of the same age (58 years) showed no association between measurements of common carotid artery IMT and plasma homocyst(e)ine levels that were controlled appropriately for vitamin B_{12} and folic acid levels.

5. RECOMMENDATIONS FOR THERAPEUTIC MANAGEMENT OR REFINEMENT OF DIAGNOSIS

As of this writing, the first clinical trial of vitamin therapy to reduce elevated homocyst(e)ine and prevent recurrent stroke or symptomatic coronary artery disease (CAD), Vitamins in Stroke Prevention (VISP), has been terminated because of futility. Sponsored by the National Institutes of

Table 1 Representative Studies Predicting Risk of Carotid Atherosclerosis Associated with Elevated Homocyst(e)ine Levels

Ref.	Study Population	Sample Size	Experimental Design	Outcome Measure	Method of Carotid Atherosclerosis Measurement
(49)	Symptomatic cases of PAD or CVD examined by serial duplex (range of follow-up after initial study 3–36 months)	169 cases with serial duplex	Case control	No difference in progression of carotid stenosis between elevated (mean 14.4 μmol/L) and normal (mean 9.8–10.1 μmol/L) H(e)	Frequency/wave form analysis defining stenosis in six bands (0–100%)
(52)	Healthy adults aged 45–64 years	287 paired cases [defined by thickened IMT exceeding 90% threshold in ARIC[a] cohort] and controls	Case control sample derived from ARIC[a] study	Increase in H(e) of 1 SD (3.2 μmol/L) associated with 35% increase in OR for case designation	IMT of CCA and ICA
(53)	Men and women (67–96 years)	1041 (418 men; 623 women)	Cross-sectional cohort of prospective Framingham study	OR = 2.00 for stenosis ≥25% with H(e) ≥14.4 μmol/L	IMT of CCA and ICA
(54)	Men and women (60–99 years)	400 (121 men; 279 women)	Prospective	H(e) > 17 μmol/L in 40% of patients with stenosis ≥40%	Peak systolic flow velocity defining stenosis ≥40%
(55)	Men and women (60.1%) 55+ years	630	Random sample of population-based Rotterdam Study	Mean IMT 0.04 mm greater in subjects aged 55–74 years with H(e) ≥18.6 μmol/L	CCA-IMT

(56)	Healthy adults aged 22–75 years	75	Cross-sectional	H(e) level associated with IMT ($P < 0.001$) after adjustment for age, BMI, and LDL cholesterol	CCA-IMT
(57)	Japanese men aged 60–74 years with or without hypertension	474	Cross-sectional	OR = 5.8 for increased IMT (> 1.0 mm in CCA) in non-hypertensive subjects with H(e) level ≥ 10.4 μmol/L	IMT in CCA and ICA
(58)	Australian men and women aged 27–77 years	1111	Randomly selected, cross-sectional sample	OR = 2.6 for increased IMT (> 0.8 mm in CCA) associated with increased H(e) in men (≥ 14.4 μmol/L) and women (≥ 12.8 μmol/L)	CCA-IMT
(50)	Men with insulin sensitivity aged 58 years with mean H(e) 13 μmol/L	103	Population-based	No correlation between H(e) and mean IMT	Mean of linear measurements of IMT in both CCAs
(59)	Subjects aged 25+ years recruited from Framingham, Utah Family Tree Study, and ARIC[a]	1216/200	Population-based	Mean IMT significantly greater ($P < 0.02$) in subjects of 55+ years with H(e) ≥ 9.36 μmol/L	Mean IMT from six sites in CCA, carotid bifurcation, and ICA
(60)	Patients with ESRD on dialysis; not taking vitamin or folate supplements	55	Baseline analysis of ESRD patients in prospective follow-up study	Regression analysis showing IMT correlated with H(e) levels ($F = 4.63$, $P < 0.01$)	CCA-IMT

(Continued)

Table 1 Representative Studies Predicting Risk of Carotid Atherosclerosis Associated with Elevated Homocyst(e)ine Levels (*Continued*)

Ref.	Study Population	Sample Size	Experimental Design	Outcome Measure	Method of Carotid Atherosclerosis Measurement
(61)	Native Japanese in the 40–94 age range	1111	Single-center, population-based	Regression analysis showing mean IMT correlated with H(e) levels ($P < 0.05$ for trend)	CCA-IMT

[a]ARIC: Atherosclerosis Risk in Community Study; BMI: body mass index; CCA: common carotid artery; CVD: cerebrovascular disease; ESRD: end-stage renal disease; H(e): homocyst(e)ine; ICA: internal carotid artery; IMT: intima-media thickness; LDL: low-density lipoprotein; OR: odds ratio; PAD: peripheral arterial disease.

Health, VISP was a double-masked, randomized, prospective comparison of high- vs. low-dose vitamin therapy with the primary outcome of recurrent stroke and secondary outcomes of symptomatic CAD or death (51). Eligible subjects were at least 35 years of age who had a non-disabling ischemic stroke within 120 days prior to randomization and whose plasma homocyst(e)ine level at entry exceeded the 25th percentile for the US population (62). The trial was conducted at 56 centers in the United States, Canada, and Scotland, enrolling 3680 patients between August 1997 and December 2001. Each VISP patient was randomized to take a high-dose multi-vitamin containing supplemented levels of folic acid (2.5 mg), B_6 (25 mg), and B_{12} (400 μg) or a low-dose formulation containing quantities of these three essential co-factors that did not exceed the Recommended Daily Allowance (RDA) promulgated by the federal government. Both the high-and low-dose multi-vitamins contained uniform quantities of vitamins A, D, E, C, B_1, B_2, and K, biotin, niacinamide, and pantothenic acid in RDA quantities. The trial was terminated prematurely at the end of 1 year of follow-up after enrollment of the last subject. The unadjusted risk ratio for stroke, coronary heart disease event, or death was 1.0. For ischemic stroke alone, the 2 year risk was 9.2% for the high-dose and low-dose groups, respectively (risk ratio 1.0). There was an association, however, between lower total homocysteine levels and vascular events within the individual groups. A 3 umol/L lower total homocyst(e)ine level was associated with a 10% ($P = 0.05$) and 2% lower risk for stroke in the low-and high-dose groups.

In VISP, information regarding stroke subtype was not systematically collected. Therefore, it is unclear if there was a different treatment effect in patients with a large vessel atherosclerosis stroke subtype.

Similarly, the VISP study did not include systematic measurement of IMT or any other indicator of carotid plaque deposition, so that the impact of high-dose vitamin therapy on atherosclerosis cannot be determined. The high or therapeutic dose of vitamins evaluated in VISP was successful in accomplishing a rapid, sustained reduction of ~2 μmol/L from baseline homocyst(e)ine levels. Because measurements of carotid duplex studies were not performed, the hypothesis that the progression of peripheral atherosclerosis may be slowed by vitamin therapy that is effective in reducing homocyst(e)ine shall remain untested. Until future clinical trials confirm or refute this hypothesis, the management of hyperhomocyst(e)inemia in association with carotid stenosis must remain speculative.

The ongoing VITAmins TO Prevent Stroke (VITATOPS) trial has a larger sample size and broader inclusion criteria than VISP. VITATOPS aims to recruit 8000 patients with stroke of any type or TIA from 70 centers in 19 countries (63). Patients receive either multivitamins or placebo and are allowed in the study if they have had an event within 7 months of study enrollment. Patients receive folic acid 2.0 mg, cobalamin 0.5 mg, and pyridoxine 25 mg. Follow-up is for a median of 4 years and the study is testing a more modest hypothesis of a 15% risk reduction for the outcome of stroke, MI, or vascular death.

It is unlikely that VITATOPS will be able to provide information on patients with stroke due to carotid stenosis. Therefore, until future clinical trials confirm or refute this hypothesis, the management of hyperhomocyst(e)inemia in association with carotid stenosis must remain speculative, although meta-analyses are available (64,65).

Another study which will provide useful information on the value of treating elevated homocysteine is the Study of the Effectiveness of Additional Reductions in Cholesterol and Homocysteine (SEARCH). This study has recruited 12,000 patients with previous MI, and the results on risks of recurrent stroke and MI are expected in 2005 (66).

To assist with the characterization of vascular risk factors in a patient with symptomatic carotid stenosis, a fasting plasma homocyst(e)ine level should be obtained no earlier than 72 h after transient ischemic attack, angina, atherothrombotic cerebral infarction, or myocardial infarction. Renal failure as a cause of hyperhomocyst(e)inemia should be excluded by an assay of serum creatinine and urea nitrogen or by calculation of creatinine clearance. All patients with carotid stenosis and elevated plasma levels of homocyst(e)ine should be tested for cobalamin deficiency with vitamin B_{12} levels. A careful review of medication history should identify recent exposure to phenytoin, colestipol plus niacin, nitrous oxide, or other medications that are known to increase plasma levels of homocyst(e)ine. Although most patients with symptomatic carotid atherosclerosis will not present with hyperhomocyst(e)inemia that is genetic in origin, family history suggestive of recurrent atherothrombotic infarction in brain and heart that is not associated with other risk factors should prompt screening for MTHFR deficiency that may occur in an intermediate form without homocystinuria.

ACKNOWLEDGMENTS

Support for this work was provided through K30 HL004163, P20 RR015592, and M01RR002602 awarded to Dr. Sabet and from the General Clinical Research Center of the University of Kentucky Hospital M01RR002602. We thank Sherry Chandler Williams, MA, ELS for editorial assistance and preparation of the illustrations.

REFERENCES

1. Carson NAJ, Neill DW. Metabolic abnormalities detected in a survey of mentally backward individuals in Northern Ireland. Arch Dis Child 1962; 37:503–513.

2. Gerritsen T, Vaughn JG, Waisman HA. The identification of homocystine in the urine. Biochem Biophys Res Commun 1962; 9:493–496.
3. McCully KS. Vascular pathology of homocysteinemia: implications for the pathogenesis of arteriosclerosis. Am J Pathol 1969; 56:111–128.
4. Boers GH, Smals AG, Trijbels FJ, Fowler B, Bakkeren JA, Schoonderwaldt HC, Kleijer WJ, Kloppenborg PW. Heterozygosity for homocystinuria in premature peripheral and cerebral occlusive arterial disease. N Engl J Med 1985; 313:709–715.
5. Clarke R, Daly L, Robinson K, Naughten E, Cahalane S, Fowler B, Graham I. Hyperhomocysteinemia: an independent risk factor for vascular disease. N Engl J Med 1991; 324:1149–1155.
6. Brattstrom LE, Hardebo JE, Hultberg BL. Moderate homocysteinemia—a possible risk factor for arteriosclerotic cerebrovascular disease. Stroke 1984; 15:1012–1016.
7. Brattstrom L, Lindgren A, Israelsson B, Malinow MR, Norrving B, Upson B, Hamfelt A. Hyperhomocysteinaemia in stroke: prevalence, cause, and relationships to type of stroke and stroke risk factors. Eur J Clin Invest 1992; 22:214–221.
8. Coull BM, Malinow MR, Beamer N, Sexton G, Nordt F, de Garmo P. Elevated plasma homocyst(e)ine concentration as a possible independent risk factor for stroke. Stroke 1990; 21:572–576.
9. Perry IJ, Refsum H, Morris RW, Ebrahim SB, Ueland PM, Shaper AG. Prospective study of serum total homocysteine concentration and risk of stroke in middle-aged British men. Lancet 1995; 346:1395–1398.
10. Verhoef P, Hennekens CH, Malinow MR, Kok FJ, Willett WC, Stampfer MJ. A prospective study of plasma homocyst(e)ine and risk of ischemic stroke. Stroke 1994; 25:1924–1930.
11. Yoo JH, Chung CS, Kang SS. Relation of plasma homocyst(e)ine to cerebral infarction and cerebral atherosclerosis. Stroke 1998; 29:2478–2483.
12. Graham IM, Daly LE, Refsum HM, Robinson K, Brattstrom LE, Ueland PM, Palma-Reis RJ, Boers GH, Sheahan RG, Israelsson B, Uiterwaal CS, Meleady R, McMaster D, Verhoef P, Witteman J, Rubba P, Bellet H, Wautrecht JC, de Valk HW, Sales Luis AC, Parrot-Rouland FM, Tan KS, Higgins I, Garcon D, Medrano MJ, Candito M, Evans AE, Andria G. Plasma homocysteine as a risk factor for vascular disease. The European Concerted Action Project. JAMA 1997; 277:1775–1781.
13. Nygård O, Nordrehaug JE, Refsum H, Ueland PM, Farstad M, Vollset SE. Plasma homocysteine levels and mortality in patients with coronary artery disease. N Engl J Med 1997; 337:230–236.
14. Mudd SH, Levy HL. Plasma homocysteine or homocysteine? N Engl J Med 1995; 333:325.
15. Mudd SH, Finkelstein JD, Refsum H, Ueland PM, Malinow MR, Lentz SR, Jacobsen DW, Brattstrom L, Wilcken B, Wilcken DE, Blom HJ, Stabler SP, Allen RH, Selhub J, Rosenberg IH. Homocysteine and its disulfide derivatives: a suggested consensus terminology. Arterioscler Thromb Vasc Biol 2000; 20:1704–1706.

16. Finkelstein JD. Pathways and regulation of homocysteine metabolism in mammals. Semin Thromb Hemost 2000; 26:219–225.

17. Kruger WD. Vitamins and homocysteine metabolism. Vitam Horm 2000; 60:333–352.

18. Selhub J. Homocysteine metabolism. Annu Rev Nutr 1999; 19:217–246.

19. Blom HJ. Consequences of homocysteine export and oxidation in the vascular system. Semin Thromb Hemost 2000; 26:227–232.

20. Mosharov E, Cranford MR, Banerjee R. The quantitatively important relationship between homocysteine metabolism and glutathione synthesis by the transsulfuration pathway and its regulation by redox changes. Biochemistry 2000; 39:13005–13011.

21. den Heijer M, Koster T, Blom HJ, Bos GM, Briet E, Reitsma PH, Vandenbroucke JP, Rosendaal FR. Hyperhomocysteinemia as a risk factor for deepvein thrombosis. N Engl J Med 1996; 334:759–762.

22. Lentz SR, Sadler JE. Inhibition of thrombomodulin surface expression and protein C activation by the thrombogenic agent homocysteine. J Clin Invest 1991; 88:1906–1914.

23. Macko R, Kittner S, Refsum H, Cox D, Epstein A, Sparks M, al. e. Effect of vitamin therapy on plasma homocysteine, endogenous fibrinolysis, and markers of endothelial injury in stroke patients: a placebo-controlled trial [abstract]. Stroke 1998; 29:286.

24. Nishinaga M, Ozawa T, Shimada K. Homocysteine, a thrombogenic agent, suppresses anticoagulant heparan sulfate expression in cultured porcine aortic endothelial cells. J Clin Invest 1993; 92:1381–1386.

25. Nishinaga M, Shimada K. Heparan sulfate proteoglycan of endothelial cells: homocysteine suppresses anticoagulant active heparan sulfate in cultured endothelial cells. Rinsho Byori 1994; 42:340–345.

26. Simioni P. The molecular genetics of familial venous thrombosis. Baillieres Best Pract Res Clin Haematol 1999; 12:479–503.

27. Chambers JC, McGregor A, Jean Marie J, Kooner JS. Acute hyperhomocysteinaemia and endothelial dysfunction. Lancet 1998; 351:36–37.

28. Chambers JC, McGregor A, Jean-Marie J, Obeid OA, Kooner JS. Demonstration of rapid onset vascular endothelial dysfunction after hyperhomocysteinemia: an effect reversible with vitamin C therapy. Circulation 1999; 99:1156–1160.

29. Stamler JS, Osborne JA, Jaraki O, Rabbani LE, Mullins M, Singel D, Loscalzo J. Adverse vascular effects of homocysteine are modulated by endothelium-derived relaxing factor and related oxides of nitrogen. J Clin Invest 1993; 91:308–318.

30. Stamler JS, Slivka A. Biological chemistry of thiols in the vasculature and in vascular-related disease. Nutr Rev 1996; 54:1–30.

31. van den Berg M, Franken DG, Boers GH, Blom HJ, Jakobs C, Stehouwer CD, Rauwerda JA. Combined vitamin B_6 plus folic acid therapy in young patients with arteriosclerosis and hyperhomocysteinemia. J Vasc Surg 1994; 20:933–940.

32. van den Berg M, Boers GH, Franken DG, Blom HJ, van Kamp GJ, Jakobs C, Rauwerda JA, Kluft C, Stehouwert CD. Hyperhomocysteinaemia and endothelial dysfunction in young patients with peripheral arterial occlusive disease. Eur J Clin Invest 1995; 25:176–181.

33. Blundell G, Jones BG, Rose FA, Tudball N. Homocysteine mediated endothelial cell toxicity and its amelioration. Atherosclerosis 1996; 122:163–172.

34. Di Minno G, Davi G, Margaglione M, Cirillo F, Grandone E, Ciabattoni G, Catalano I, Strisciuglio P, Andria G, Patrono C, Mancini M. Abnormally high thromboxane biosynthesis in homozygous homocystinuria. Evidence for platelet involvement and probucol-sensitive mechanism. J Clin Invest 1993; 92:1400–1406.

35. Khajuria A, Houston DS. Induction of monocyte tissue factor expression by homocysteine: a possible mechanism for thrombosis. Blood 2000; 96:966–972.

36. Chen C, Halkos ME, Surowiec SM, Conklin BS, Lin PH, Lumsden AB. Effects of homocysteine on smooth muscle cell proliferation in both cell culture and artery perfusion culture models. J Surg Res 2000; 88:26–33.

37. Tsai JC, Perrella MA, Yoshizumi M, Hsieh CM, Haber E, Schlegel R, Lee ME. Promotion of vascular smooth muscle cell growth by homocysteine: a link to atherosclerosis. Proc Natl Acad Sci USA 1994; 91:6369–6373.

38. Woo DK, Dudrick SJ, Sumpio BE. Homocysteine stimulates MAP kinase in bovine aortic smooth muscle cells. Surgery 2000; 128:59–66.

39. Tyagi SC. Homocysteine redox receptor and regulation of extracellular matrix components in vascular cells. Am J Physiol 1998; 274:C396–C405.

40. Tyagi SC, Smiley LM, Mujumdar VS, Clonts B, Parker JL. Reduction-oxidation (Redox) and vascular tissue level of homocyst(e)ine in human coronary atherosclerotic lesions and role in extracellular matrix remodeling and vascular tone. Mol Cell Biochem 1998; 181:107–116.

41. Southern FN, Cruz N, Fink LM, Cooney CA, Barone GW, Eidt JF, Moursi MM. Hyperhomocysteinemia increases intimal hyperplasia in a rat carotid endarterectomy model. J Vasc Surg 1998; 28:909–918.

42. Durand P, Lussier-Cacan S, Blache D. Acute methionine load-induced hyperhomocysteinemia enhances platelet aggregation, thromboxane biosynthesis, and macrophage-derived tissue factor activity in rats. Faseb J 1997; 11:1157–1168.

43. Morita H, Kurihara H, Yoshida S, Saito Y, Shindo T, Oh-Hashi Y, Kurihara Y, Yazaki Y, Nagai R. Diet-induced hyperhomocysteinemia exacerbates neointima formation in rat carotid arteries after balloon injury. Circulation 2001; 103:133–139.

44. Voutilainen S, Morrow JD, Roberts LJ 2nd, Alfthan G, Alho H, Nyyssonen K, Salonen JT. Enhanced in vivo lipid peroxidation at elevated plasma total homocysteine levels. Arterioscler Thromb Vasc Biol 1999; 19:1263–1266.

45. Nygård O, Vollset SE, Refsum H, Stensvold I, Tverdal A, Nordrehaug JE, Ueland M, Kvale G. Total plasma homocysteine and cardiovascular risk profile. The Hordaland Homocysteine Study. JAMA 1995; 274:1526–1533.

46. Leerink CB, van Ham AD, Heeres A, Duif PF, Bouma BN, van Rijn HJ. Sulfhydryl compounds influence immunoreactivity, structure and functional aspects of lipoprotein(a). Thromb Res 1994; 74:219–232.

47. Pignoli P, Tremoli E, Poli A, Oreste P, Paoletti R. Intimal plus medial thickness of the arterial wall: a direct measurement with ultrasound imaging. Circulation 1986; 74:1399–1406.

48. Adams MR, Nakagomi A, Keech A, Robinson J, McCredie R, Bailey BP, Freedman SB, Celermajer DS. Carotid intima-media thickness is only weakly correlated with the extent and severity of coronary artery disease. Circulation 1995; 92:2127–2134.

49. Taylor LM Jr, DeFrang RD, Harris EJ Jr, Porter JM. The association of elevated plasma homocyst(e)ine with progression of symptomatic peripheral arterial disease. J Vasc Surg 1991; 13:128–136.

50. Fagerberg B, Wallenfeldt K, Alenhag EL, Bokemark L, Wikstrand J. High-normal serum homocysteine concentrations are associated with an increased risk of early atherosclerotic carotid artery wall lesions. J Hypertens 2000; 18:1523–1525.

51. Spence JD, Malinow MR, Barnett PA, Marian AJ, Freeman D, Hegele RA. Plasma homocyst(e)ine concentration, but not MTHFR genotype, is associated with variation in carotid plaque area. Stroke 1999; 30:969–973.

52. Malinow MR, Nieto FJ, Szklo M, Chambless LE, Bond G. Carotid artery intimal-medial wall thickening and plasma homocyst(e)ine in asymptomatic adults. The Atherosclerosis Risk in Communities Study. Circulation 1993; 87:1107–1113.

53. Selhub J, Jacques PF, Bostom AG, D'Agostino RB, Wilson PW, Belanger AJ, O'Leary DH, Wolf PA, Schaefer EJ, Rosenberg IH. Association between plasma homocysteine concentrations and extracranial carotid-artery stenosis. N Engl J Med 1995; 332:286–291.

54. Aronow WS, Ahn C, Schoenfeld MR. Association between plasma homocysteine and extracranial carotid arterial disease in older persons. Am J Cardiol 1997; 79:1432–1433.

55. Bots ML, Launer LJ, Lindemans J, Hofman A, Grobbee DE. Homocysteine, atherosclerosis and prevalent cardiovascular disease in the elderly: The Rotterdam Study. J Intern Med 1997; 242:339–347.

56. Willinek WA, Ludwig M, Lennarz M, Holler T, Stumpe KO. High-normal serum homocysteine concentrations are associated with an increased risk of early atherosclerotic carotid artery wall lesions in healthy subjects. J Hypertens 2000; 18:425–430.

57. Okamura T, Kitamura A, Moriyama Y, Imano H, Sato S, Terao A, Naito Y, Nakagawa Y, Kiyama M, Tamura Y, Iida M, Suzuki H, Komachi Y. Plasma level of homocysteine is correlated to extracranial carotid-artery atherosclerosis in non-hypertensive Japanese. J Cardiovasc Risk 1999; 6:371–377.

58. McQuillan BM, Beilby JP, Nidorf M, Thompson PL, Hung J. Hyperhomocysteinemia but not the C677T mutation of methylenetetrahydrofolate reductase is an independent risk determinant of carotid wall thickening. The Perth Carotid Ultrasound Disease Assessment Study (CUDAS). Circulation 1999; 99:2383–2388.

59. Tsai MY, Arnett DK, Eckfeldt JH, Williams RR, Ellison RC. Plasma homocysteine and its association with carotid intimal-medial wall thickness and prevalent coronary heart disease: NHLBI Family Heart Study. Atherosclerosis 2000; 151:519–524.

60. Haraki T, Takegoshi T, Kitoh C, Kajinami K, Wakasugi T, Hirai J, Shimada T, Kawashiri M, Inazu A, Koizumi J, Mabuchi H. Hyperhomocysteinemia, diabetes mellitus, and carotid atherosclerosis independently increase athero-

sclerotic vascular disease outcome in Japanese patients with end-stage renal disease. Clin Nephrol 2001; 56:132–139.

61. Adachi H, Hirai Y, Fujiura Y, Matsuoka H, Satoh A, Imaizumi T. Plasma homocysteine levels and atherosclerosis in Japan: epidemiological study by use of carotid ultrasonography. Stroke 2002; 33:2177–2181.

62. Toole JF, Malinow MR, Chambless LE, Spence JD, Pettigrew LC, Howard VJ, Sides EG, Wang CH, Stampfer M. Lowering homocysteine in patients with ischemic stroke to prevent recurrent stroke, myocardial infarction, and death: the Vitamin Intervention for Stroke Prevention (VISP) randomized control trial. JAMA 2004; 291:565–575.

63. Hankey GJ, Eikelboom JW. Folic acid-based multivitamin therapy to prevent stroke. Stroke 2004; 35:1995–1998.

64. Danesh J, Lewington S. Plasma homocysteine and coronary heart disease: systematic review of published epidemiological studies. J Cardiovasc Risk 1998; 5:229–232.

65. Homocysteine Lowering Trialists' Collaboration. Lowering blood homocysteine with folic acid based supplements: meta-analysis of randomized trials. Br Med J 1998; 316:894–898.

66. Clarke R, Collins R. Can dietary supplements with folic acid or vitamin B6 reduce cardiovascular risk? Design of clinical trials to test the homocysteine hypothesis of vascular disease. J Cardiovasc Risk 1998; 5:249–255.

10

Diet in the Management of Patients with Carotid Stenosis

J. David Spence

Stroke Prevention and Atherosclerosis Research Centre, Robarts Research Institute, London, Ontario, Canada

In the era of powerful lipid-lowering drugs, a common and mistaken assumption is that diet is unimportant, because the drugs are so much more effective in lowering fasting lipids. On average, a low-fat diet only reduces fasting LDL by about 9%, whereas statin drugs reduce it by 50–60%. However, this approach ignores the importance of post-prandial fat. I have commented recently (1) on the conceptual error of focusing only on fasting lipids; they can be thought of as a baseline, on top of which post-prandial fats are superimposed. Since post-prandial fat is what affects the endothelium for about 18 hours of the day, diet is much more important than is appreciated when it is seen only thoursough the lens of fasting lipids. Indeed, a number of studies show that post-prandial fat is probably more important than fasting lipids (2,3).

A high-fat meal impairs endothelial function for about 4 hours (4). It is likely that this effect is via oxidative stress, since antioxidant vitamins (C and E) partly prevent the impairment of endothelial function (5). A Mediterranean diet, which is not only low in harmful fats, but also high in vitamins and antioxidants, improves endothelial function compared to a usual North American diet.

A Mediterranean diet has been shown to improve endothelial function in hyperlipidemic men (6), perhaps in part because it has a higher content of

175

antioxidants, and significantly lower indices of plasma lipid peroxidation
(7). Vogel et al. studied the effect of components of the Mediterranean diet
on endothelial function and found that the beneficial components appeared
to be antioxidant-rich foods, including vegetables, fruits, balsamic vinegar,
and omega-3 rich fish and canola oil (8).

Carluccio et al. (9) found that oleic acid had a direct anti-atherosclerotic effect in endothelial cells. Tsimikas et al. (10) showed monocyte adhesion
and chemotaxis induced by LDL from subjects consuming an American
diet, which did not occur with LDL from subjects on a normal Greek diet.
This effect was reversed by oleic acid supplementation to the American diet.

The focus on fasting lipids has led us to mistakenly underestimate the
importance of diet. It may be true that this morning's egg only raises fasting
LDL cholesterol by a moderate (though statistically significant) amount
($\sim$10%); but we need to pay more attention to what it does for a few hours
after breakfast (see below). Similarly, the focus on "red meat" is based on
the effect of saturated fat on liver metabolism and next morning's fasting
lipids, and ignores the fact that the cholesterol is in the cell membrane of
every muscle cell. Chicken with the skin off and fish have less saturated
fat than beef, but just as much cholesterol.

Dietary cholesterol intake *is* important. Ginsberg et al. (11) showed a
dose–response relationship between increases in plasma cholesterol and dietary cholesterol, in a study using eggs. Even though egg consumption
increases fasting LDL by only about 10% (12), egg consumption increases
oxidized LDL levels by 34% (13). An analysis from the Health Professionals
study showed a doubling of coronary risk among diabetics who consumed
one egg per day vs. less than one per week. Even the Step 2 diet recommends
a daily intake of cholesterol < 200 mg per day, and a single egg contains
275 mg of cholesterol. Eggs, therefore, are not appropriate food for patients
with vascular disease.

The Dean Ornish regression diet, together with smoking cessation and
exercise, has been shown to regress coronary disease without drugs (14).
However, it is very difficult for patients to persist with it. Among more than
15,000 patients with vascular disease that I have followed, only two were
able to persist with the Ornish diet. A more palatable and acceptable diet
is a Mediterranean diet, which though not low in fat, is low in harmful
fat, high in beneficial oils, and high in vitamins and antioxidants.

Two important studies have shown that a Mediterranean diet significantly reduced vascular events compared to a usual Western diet.

In the Lyon Diet Heart Study, 423 survivors of myocardial infarction
(MI) were randomized to a prudent Western diet amounting to a Step I
NCEP diet, or to a Mediterranean diet from Crete. This diet was low in cholesterol, low in animal fat, high in olive oil, canola oil, fruits, and vegetables;
canola margarine was substituted for butter. The proportion of calories
from fat was the same ($\sim$30%) in the two diets, but the Mediterranean diet

provided a significant reduction in dietary cholesterol, and a significant increase of beneficial oils such as α-linolenic acid, as opposed to the animal fats of the "prudent Western diet". The patients assigned to the Mediterranean diet (15) had a 60% reduction in cardiac death and myocardial infarction over 4 years ($P = 0.0001$) compared with those to the prudent Western diet, which amounted to a Step I diet. Importantly, there was no difference in alcohol consumption between the two diets.

This reduction in MI and death was twice that achieved by simvastatin in the 4-S trial (a reduction of coronary risk by 40% over 6 years) (16). Importantly, this benefit was achieved without any difference in fasting lipids between the two groups. It seems very likely that the benefit was due to reduction of postprandial fat and oxidative stress.

Recently, these results have been replicated in a study in India, among 1000 coronary patients. Despite a vegetarian diet in 60% of the patients, a Mediterranean diet high in α-linolenic acid reduced coronary events by more than half, in 2 years. This was achieved by consuming less cholesterol, and more fruits, vegetables, walnuts, almonds, whole grains, and mustard or soybean oil, compared to the control diet, which was an Indian version of an NCEP Step II diet (17).

Patients with carotid stenosis have a systemic process that affects all arteries. They have a higher risk of myocardial infarction than do patients with a history of coronary disease. Chimowitz et al. reported (18) that among patients with asymptomatic carotid stenosis, the 4-year risk of coronary events was 33% with no history of coronary artery disease, and 40% with a previous history. In contrast, the patients in the 4-S trial had a 6-year risk of coronary events of only 26% (16). Among patients with carotid stenosis followed in endarterectomy trials, 25% of those with resistant hypertension had renovascular hypertension (19).

Because patients with carotid stenosis have a high risk of vascular events, they need intensive treatment of all the risk factors for atherosclerosis. In addition to optimal treatment of blood pressure, antiplatelet agents, and drugs to reduce fasting lipids, it is very important for them to follow an anti-atherosclerotic diet. Furthermore, because many are hypertensive, the diet should also be low in salt. The DASH salt diet study showed that a low-salt diet that was low in saturated fats, high in fruits and vegetables, and had low-fat dairy products reduced blood pressure by 11.5 mmHg, as much as an antihypertensive drug.

Salt restriction is not as difficult as many patients think it will be. Adding salt to food causes downregulation of salt receptors on the tongue, so that more salt is needed to appreciate its presence. Salt restriction leads to upregulation of salt receptors, so that after about 3 weeks, the patient can taste the salt that is already in the food, and does not miss it as much as expected. In the meantime, the patient can learn to flavor food with anything but salt: pepper, spices, herbs, garlic, ginger, green peppers, onions, paprika, curry powder, hot peppers, and balsamic vinegar are a few examples to suggest. Patients who salt their food before tasting on average consume ~20 g a day of salt; those who taste first consume ~10 g; the body needs only half a gram! To get down to a target of 2 to 3 g per day requires no added salt, and avoidance of salty foods such as pickles, potato chips (crisps), cured meats, and some canned goods. If something tastes salty, it should be avoided.

Weight loss is an important issue for overweight patients, particularly if they are diabetic or pre-diabetic. A waistline bigger than the hips, or high triglycerides with a low HDL-cholesterol level, are predictors of insulin resistance, a precursor of Type II diabetes. Patients with such attributes need to exercise to a level equivalent to 30 minutes/day of brisk walking (2 miles or 3 km). They should not delude themselves that this will make much difference to their weight: running a 6-minutes mile burns only 100 calories, the equivalent of 4 soda crackers.

One pound of fat represents 3500 stored calories. This means that to lose a pound, the patient needs to reduce caloric intake by 500 calories per day for 7 days. To lose 50 pounds requires 50 weeks at that reduced caloric intake; to keep the weight off requires permanent reduction in caloric intake.

For most patients the richest source of calorie reduction will be fat, because fat contains 9 calories/g, compared to 4 calories for carbohydrates or protein. A serving of meat, pie, cake, or ice cream will each be about 400 calories. Because of the oils in nuts, they are also high in calories: 100 calories represents 7 cashews or 15 peanuts. In addition to avoiding nuts, cake, pie, ice cream, and the like, overweight patients need to reduce their intake of meat, and avoid fried foods. A large baked potato is about 200 calories, but when it is converted to French fries it absorbs 400 calories of bad fat. (Oils heated for a long time break down into trans fats.) A potato chip is so thin that it has a huge surface area; 1 calorie of potato chip can soak up 9 calories of bad fat.

Carbohydrates represent another opportunity for caloric restriction. One piece of bread, 4 crackers, half a bagel, a glass of juice or a serving of fruit each contains 100 calories.

Most overweight people cannot lose weight eating the number of calories recommended for normal people. They need to reduce their intake of animal flesh to about 4 oz every other day, and keep the carbohydrates that are not on the plate to about 5 or 6 servings per day. In order to do so, they need to try a lot of recipes for low-fat vegetarian meals in order to have enough variety to make their new way of eating enjoyable.

Low-fat vegetarian pasta dishes, curries, chili, grilled vegetables, omelettes, or frittata made with egg substitutes are some examples of meatless alternatives. In order to obtain complete protein (i.e., a combination of all the essential amino acids), it is necessary to combine grains and legumes.

Table 1 Dietary Recommendations for Patients with Carotid Stenosis

---

No egg yolks: use egg whites or egg substitutes such as Egg Beaters®
Keep the intake of the flesh of *any* animal[a] to 4 oz every *other* day
Use non-hydrogenated canola margarine instead of butter
Olive oil and canola oil are preferable to other oils
Skim milk; low-fat cheese
Avoid fried foods and foods containing hydrogenated vegetable oils
Make low-fat vegetarian meals delicious not with salt, cheese, and butter, but with
 spices, herbs, onion, garlic, ginger, green peppers, lime juice, balsamic vinegar, etc.
Favor whole grain bread and pasta, and brown rice

---

[a]An animal is anything that walks, swims, flies, or crawls; anything with eyes, a face, or a mother.

Options include beans, lentils, peas, chickpeas, tofu, etc., with rice, pasta, couscous, barley, etc. Doing so makes vegetarian meals more satisfying.

For patients with carotid stenosis, a prudent diet would be as described in Table 1: No egg yolks; use of non-hydrogenated canola margarine in place of butter; one serving of animal flesh of any kind every other day; use of skim milk and low-fat cheeses (the latter in small quantities), with frequent low-fat vegetarian meals.

Physicians often think they are not knowledgeable about nutrition. However, they know a lot about the digestive system, the metabolism of carbohydrates, proteins, fats, vitamins, and so on. What many do not know is cooking. It is important to understand that when the doctor says to the patient "You need to go on a diet, so I will send you to the dietitian", the message received is: "Diet is not important enough for the doctor to spend time on." It is important for the physician to at least begin the discussion of the importance of diet. In order to be effective at this, the physician needs to learn to cook.

REFERENCES

1. Spence JD. Fasting lipids: the carrot in the snowman. Can J Cardiol. 2003; 19:890–892.
2. Steiner G. Triglyceride-rich lipoproteins and atherosclerosis, from fast to feast. Annal Med 1993; 25:431–435.
3. Gronholdt ML, Nordestgaard BG, Nielsen TG, Sillesen H. Echolucent carotid artery plaques are associated with elevated levels of fasting and postprandial triglyceride-rich lipoproteins. Stroke 1996; 27:2166–2172.
4. Vogel RA, Corretti MC, Plotnick GD. Effect of a single high-fat meal on endothelial function in healthy subjects. Am J Cardiol 1997; 79(3):350–354.
5. Plotnick GD, Corretti MC, Vogel RA. Effect of antioxidant vitamins on the transient impairment of endothelium-dependent brachial artery vasoactivity following a single high-fat meal [see comments]. JAMA 1997; 278(20):1682–1686.

6. Fuentes F, Lopez-Miranda J, Sanchez E, Sanchez F, Paez J, Paz-Rojas E, Marin C, Gomez P, Jimenez-Pereperez J, Ordovas JM, Perez-Jimenez F. Mediterranean and low-fat diets improve endothelial function in hypercholesterolemic men. Ann Intern Med 2001; 134:1115–1119.

7. Mancini M, Parfitt VJ, Rubba P. Antioxidants in the Mediterranean diet. Can J Cardiol 1995; 11(suppl G):105G–109G.

8. Vogel RA, Corretti MC, Plotnick GD. The postprandial effect of components of the Mediterranean diet on endothelial function. J Am Coll Cardiol 2000; 36:1455–1460.

9. Carluccio MA, Massaro M, Bonfrate C, Siculella L, Maffia M, Nicolardi G, Distante A, Storelli C, De Caterina R. Oleic acid inhibits endothelial activation: a direct vascular antiatherogenic mechanism of a nutritional component in the Mediterranean diet. Arterioscler Thoursomb Vasc Biol 1999; 19:220–228.

10. Tsimikas S, Philis-Tsimikas A, Alexopoulos S, Sigari F, Lee C, Reaven PD. LDL isolated from Greek subjects on a typical diet or from American subjects on an oleate-supplemented diet induces less monocyte chemotaxis and adhesion when exposed to oxidative stress. Arterioscler Thoursomb Vasc Biol 1999; 19(122):130.

11. Ginsberg HN, Karmally W, Siddiqui M, Holleran S, Tall AR, Rumsey SC, Deckelbaum RJ, Blaner WS, Ramakrishnan R. A dose-response study of the effects of dietary cholesterol on fasting and postprandial lipid and lipoprotein metabolism in healthy young men. Arterioscler Thoursomb 1994; 14(4):576–586.

12. Schnohours P, Thomsen OO, Riis HP, Boberg-Ans G, Lawaetz H, Weeke T. Egg consumption and high-density-lipoprotein cholesterol. J Intern Med 1994; 235(3):249–251.

13. Levy Y, Maor I, Presser D, Aviram M. Consumption of eggs with meals increases the susceptibility of human plasma and low-density lipoprotein to lipid peroxidation. Ann Nutr Metab 1996; 40(5):243–251.

14. Ornish D, Schwerwitz LW, Billings JH, Brown SE, Gould KL, Merritt TA, Sparler S, Armstrong WT, Ports TA, Kirkeeide RL, Hogeboom C, Brand RJ. Intensive lifestyle changes for reversal of coronary heart disease. JAMA 1998; 280:2001–2007.

15. de Lorgeril M, Salen P, Martin JL, Monjaud I, Delaye J, Mamelle N. Mediterranean diet, traditional risk factors, and the rate of cardiovascular complications after myocardial infarction: final report of the Lyon Diet Heart Study [see comments]. Circulation 1999; 99(6):779–785.

16. Scandinavian Simvastatin Survival Study Group. Randomized trial of cholesterol lowering in 4444 patients with coronary heart disease: the Scandinavian Simvastatin Survival Study (4S). Lancet 1994; 344:1383–1389.

17. Singh RB, Dubnov G, Niaz MA, Gosh S, Singh R, Rastogi SS, Manor O, Pella D, Berry EM. Effect of an Indo-Mediterranean diet on progression of coronary artery disease in high-risk patients (Indo-Mediterranean Diet Heart Study): a randomized single-blind trial. Lancet 2002; 360:1455–1461.

18. Chimowitz MI, Weiss DG, Cohen SL, Starling MR, Hobson RW. (Veteran's Affairs Cooperative study group 167). Cardiac prognosis of patients with carotid stenosis and no history of coronary artery disease. Stroke 1994; 25:759–765.

19. Spence JD. Management of resistant hypertension in patients with carotid stenosis: high prevalence of renovascular hypertension. Cerebrovasc Dis 2000; 10:249–254.

11

Angiogenesis and Angiogenic Growth Factors as Future Therapies for Cerebrovascular Disease

Brian H. Annex and Christopher D. Kontos
Division of Cardiology, Department of Medicine, Duke University School of Medicine, Durham, North Carolina, U.S.A.

1. INTRODUCTION

Angiogenesis is defined as the growth and proliferation of blood vessels from existing vascular structures (1,2). Since blood vessels sub-serve the critical biological function of delivering oxygen and removing toxins from target organs, this part of the circulatory system plays a critical role in normal body homeostasis. Therefore, evolutionary pressures have put a great deal of emphasis on the development of a complex circulatory system in larger animals, and the growth of new blood vessels in the adult is tightly regulated to prevent disruption of the delicate homeostatic balance. In a number of physiologic and pathologic states, however, metabolic changes in a target organ may result in the need to modulate the delivery of oxygen and the removal of waste products, which may best be achieved by an increased vascular supply to that organ. This chapter will: (i) review some basic concepts of blood vessel growth and development (i.e., angiogenesis); (ii) describe some of the growth factors and receptors that mediate angiogenesis; (iii) discuss examples of the signal transduction pathways that appear to be critical for this process; (iv) highlight potential targets for therapeutic angiogenesis agents that have been studied in different human disease states with basic fibroblast growth factor

(FGF-2) as the focus; (v) discuss FGF-2 in studies of cerebrovascular disease; and (vi) discuss the potential toxicities of therapeutic angiogenesis agents and the potential evolution of these factors that may eventually lead to novel approaches to treat ischemic cerebrovascular disease.

2. VASCULOGENESIS AND ANGIOGENESIS

In contrast to angiogenesis, vasculogenesis is defined as the formation of blood vessels de novo. Over the past two decades, a great deal of information has been learned about the basic mechanisms of blood vessel growth and development (1–3). One critical factor that is now understood as a central observation is that the delivery of oxygen to tissues is limited by passive diffusion to a distance of approximately 100 µm and that all cells must be relatively close to a capillary network (4). Even in post-natal development, tissue hypoxia is considered a driving force for the generation of a new vascular supply. However, in contrast to tissues like skeletal muscle, the brain is intolerant to episodic bouts of ischemia. During embryonic vascular development, the initial step in this process is *vasculogenesis*, or the differentiation of endothelial cells from their embryonic precursors, the angioblasts (5). Once endothelial cells have developed, they begin to assemble into a primitive vascular network, called the primary capillary plexus. This process requires the interplay and effects of a number of cytokine growth factors, including vascular endothelial growth factor (VEGF), basic fibroblast growth factors (bFGF), and their receptors in order to permit the differentiation of the endothelium and vascular cells that will comprise mature blood vessels (6). While vascularization of the endocardium of the heart and the dorsal aorta occurs by vasculogenesis, the brain is vascularized by *angiogenesis*, which is defined as the sprouting of new blood vessels from a pre-existing vascular network (7).

The same process, i.e., angiogenesis, is largely recapitulated and appears to serve as the primary mechanism for most new blood vessel growth in the adult, whether it is due to physiologic or pathologic stimuli (2). A number of molecular mechanisms that mediate normal embryonic vascular development are known to play a similar role in pathologic angiogenesis. Angiogenesis can be divided into several distinct phases based upon the characteristic responses of endothelial cells to an angiogenic stimulus, including (i) protease production, (ii) migration or chemotaxis, (iii) proliferation, (iv) capillary morphogenesis, and (v) vascular maturation or stabilization. The initiating factor in this process is the secretion of angiogenic growth factors, such as VEGF and bFGF, into the extracellular matrix in response to tissue hypoxia. Endothelial cells in nearby vessels respond to these angiogenic factors by producing proteases in order to degrade the basement membrane and allow endothelial cell migration (8). Endothelial cells then migrate out from the original vessel toward the source of the angiogenic stimulus, producing nascent vascular sprouts. Endothelial cells in these sprouts proliferate (i.e., undergo mitosis) and then form tubular structures in a process called capillary morphogenesis (9). The primitive blood vessels are still leaky but subsequently undergo a multifaceted and still poorly understood process known as vascular maturation or stabilization (10).

Although vascular maturation is a critical step in all tissues, this is perhaps even more so in the cerebral vasculature, where it contributes to formation of the blood–brain barrier. Vascular maturation involves the formation of endothelial cell–cell junctions and the recruitment of surrounding pericytes and smooth muscle cells. These changes are largely responsible for the development of organ-specific endothelial characteristics that define the blood–tissue barrier in organs such as the brain and the glomerular endothelium in the kidney (10,11). A key aspect of this phase of vascular development is that endothelial cells stop proliferating, or become quiescent. In contrast to many epithelial tissues, which are replaced over hours to days, the mature endothelium is characterized by a long survival and slow turnover, both on the order of years, while it continues to regulate a number of critical homeostatic processes.

Finally, even the "simple" process of angiogenesis has its complexities. In adult tissues, new blood vessel growth was previously thought to occur only by angiogenesis. However, in some situations the growth of blood vessels appears to exceed the rate of endothelial cell proliferation. As a result, it has been hypothesized that circulating endothelial progenitor cells contribute to vascular formation in states of rapid blood vessel growth (12). Interestingly, some factors that are known to promote angiogenesis, such as VEGF, may also enhance the migration or localization of these circulating progenitor cells to the newly forming blood vessels. An understanding of all of these processes within the context-dependent tissue considerations imparted by the brain and the blood–brain barrier will be necessary in order to translate the advances made in the area of therapeutic angiogenesis in other vascular beds to the cerebral vasculature.

3. ANGIOGENIC GROWTH FACTORS AND THE CORRESPONDING RECEPTORS

A host of factors have been shown to stimulate endothelial cell proliferation in vitro and/or to modulate angiogenesis in vivo. The most biologically and physiologically important are the polypeptide growth factors, including VEGF, acidic and basic fibroblast growth factors (aFGF, bFGF), placental growth factor (PlGF), hepatocyte growth factor (HGF), the angiopoietins, the ephrins, and others (11,13,14). These growth factors, or ligands, mediate their actions upon binding to specific cell surface receptor tyrosine kinases (RTKs) expressed on endothelial cells. Whereas some receptors, such as those for FGF, are expressed on a variety of different cell types, the receptors for VEGF and the Tie family of receptors are expressed almost exclusively on endothelial cells, and as a result the ligands for these receptors have effects that are more specific to the endothelium.

Receptor tyrosine kinases transduce their signals to the vasculature through mechanisms that include receptor dimerization and phosphorylation of specific tyrosine residues (15). Receptor tyrosine phosphorylation serves to recruit certain signaling proteins to each receptor at the plasma membrane, thereby activating downstream signal transduction pathways. These signaling cascades translate into the cellular responses required for angiogenesis, such as chemotaxis and proliferation. The specificity of function of each ligand–receptor pair is due, at least in part, to the particular subset of signaling proteins that bind each receptor. However, some additional level of organ and tissue specificity must exist with regard to the presence, function, and sequelae of receptor–ligand signaling during angiogenesis.

Angiogenesis is a multi-stage process, and particular angiogenic growth factors may exert their effects at one or more stages of the process while others may be more restricted. For example, VEGF has been shown to be required for most of the early steps of angiogenesis, including vasculogenesis, hematopoietic cell differentiation, endothelial cell protease production, chemotaxis, and proliferation (16). In related situations, VEGF has been shown to be a potent mediator of endothelial cell survival (17), a process that may be required during the early stages of angiogenesis as well as in the maintenance of the adult endothelium. In contrast, the functions of the angiopoietins appear to be more restricted to vascular maturation. Ang1 and Tie2 play key roles in directing complex vascular branching (vascular morphogenesis) and apparently in recruitment of pericytes and smooth muscle cells that support mature veins and arteries (18,19). Tie1 appears to play a key role in vascular integrity, as mice that lack functional Tie1 receptors die late in gestation from diffuse edema and hemorrhage (18,20). Although the ligand for Tie1 has not yet been identified, both Tie1 and Tie2 appear to promote endothelial cell survival (21–23), which is likely an important aspect of vascular maturation and stabilization of the adult endothelium.

Finally it must be appreciated that the endothelium is not uniform throughout the vascular tree, and an understanding of the complexity of the endothelium is beginning to be appreciated (11,13). For example, while some receptors like Tie2 are expressed throughout the vasculature, a member of the Eph receptor family, Eph-B4, is expressed only on venous endothelial cells while its corresponding cell surface-bound ligand, ephrin-B2, is present on arterial endothelium (24). This differential expression pattern allows a molecular distinction between developing arteries and veins, which join at the capillary plexus. Similarly, in atherosclerosis, a difference in expression patterns of CD31 and von Willebrand factor, two known endothelial cell markers, has been noted (25). This complexity of the endothelium allows for distinct receptor–ligand interactions that may be important during both physiologic and pathologic angiogenesis, and this may be further compounded by tissue vascular bed specificity.

4. EXAMPLES OF SIGNAL TRANSDUCTION PATHWAYS USED DURING ANGIOGENESIS

Angiogenic growth factors serve as ligands that bind to and thereby activate their corresponding receptors, and this in turn leads to the activation of downstream signal transduction pathways. Interestingly, and most relevant for the potential "other" effects of angiogenic growth factors that will be discussed later, some of the signal transduction pathways are unique to a receptor while others have common downstream effects and functions. For example, most RTKs expressed on endothelial cells, including VEGFR-2 (Flk-1), HGFR, and both of the Tie receptors, are capable of activating at least one common pathway, the phosphatidylinositol (PI) 3-kinase/Akt pathway (17,23,26,27). Following growth factor binding and receptor activation, PI 3-kinase is recruited to the plasma membrane where it is activated in part through phosphorylation by RTKs. This serves to localize PI 3-kinase in close proximity to its substrates, the plasma membrane-bound phosphoinositides, particularly PI (4,5) *bis*-phosphate. Pi 3-kinase transfers a phosphate group to the d-3 position of the inositol ring of these lipid substrates. This leads to the recruitment of a number of other proteins to the cell surface, including the serine/threonine kinases pdk1 and Akt, or protein kinase B. Signaling through other intermediate effector proteins, PI 3-kinase also plays a role in cell proliferation and chemotaxis (16,28,29), both of which are important for VEGF-mediated angiogenesis.

As noted, both VEGF and Ang1 promote endothelial cell survival, which is a key component of vascular maturation and maintenance. Cell survival mediated by these and other factors has been linked to the activation of PI 3-kinase and Akt (17,21–23). Activation of Akt following growth factor binding induces a potent anti-apoptotic effect in a variety of cell types (28). Interestingly, although the Tie receptors can activate PI 3-kinase/Akt to inhibit apoptosis, they are not mitogenic, demonstrating a degree of specificity in these receptors' signaling pathways. However, the precise mechanisms by which PI 3-kinase and Akt promote endothelial cell survival or distinguish between survival and proliferation are unknown. Some of the potential downstream signaling molecules that may play a role in these distinctive processes include BAD, caspase-9, Ras, ERK, and endothelial nitric oxide synthase (28–30).

5. BALANCING PRO-ANGIOGENESIS AND ANTI-ANGIOGENESIS

A final potential site of regulation of vascular growth is at the level of endogenous inhibition of angiogenesis, and this importance is underscored by the low rate of endothelial proliferation in the mature endothelium of the adult, such as in the cerebrovascular tree. Two known endogenous inhibitors of angiogenesis are angiostatin and endostatin (31,32). These proteins were identified based upon their ability to inhibit tumor neovascularization and were subsequently identified as cleavage products of other known proteins; angiostatin from plasminogen and endostatin from collagen XVIII. These proteins inhibit endothelial proliferation and they induce endothelial cell apoptosis (33,34). Angiostatin binds and inhibits ATP synthase on the endothelial cell surface, thereby shutting off the cell's energy supply (35). Another factor that may play an inhibitory role in angiogenesis is Angiopoietin-2, Ang2 (36). Ang1 activates the Tie2 receptor while Ang2 appears to be a context-dependent inhibitor of Tie2. Ang1 is a potent endothelial cell survival factor that helps stabilize the adult vasculature (21,23). In contrast, Ang2 is thought to facilitate VEGF-mediated angiogenesis by inhibiting the stabilizing actions of Ang1 while in the absence of an appropriate angiogenic stimulus like VEGF, Ang2 may promote endothelial cell apoptosis by blocking the protective effects of Ang1 (23). Thus, from these and other studies, it is clear that a number of factors play important roles in regulating the complex balance that is required to change vascular density and/or to stabilize the vascular tree.

6. THERAPEUTIC ANGIOGENESIS

While angiogenesis is the growth and proliferation of new vessels from existing vascular structures, *therapeutic angiogenesis* seeks to treat disorders of inadequate tissue perfusion through the growth and proliferation of new blood vessels or through the modulation of endothelial cell function (37). A number of pre-clinical studies using models of hindlimb and myocardial ischemia have demonstrated the feasibility of this approach, and early reports in humans were quite exciting (38–42). A number of angiogenic growth factors have been or are currently being tested as sole agents for therapeutic angiogenesis. However, the complexity of this process offers multiple targets for modulation, and the opportunity exists for multiple different pharmacological agents, and perhaps mechanical approaches, to act together at the same target or synergistically at multiple targets. Ultimately, these approaches could benefit hundreds of thousands of patients with advanced coronary artery and peripheral vascular disease. The following section will focus on basic fibroblast growth factor; the clinical testing of bFGF in patients with cerebrovascular disease actually preceded its testing as an agent to promote perfusion in states of myocardial and peripheral arterial disease.

7. BASIC FIBROBLAST GROWTH FACTOR AND THERAPEUTIC ANGIOGENESIS

The two major clinical targets for therapeutic angiogenesis in humans at present are cardiac and peripheral skeletal muscle. Chronic myocardial ischemia is almost universally caused by atherosclerotic coronary artery disease (CAD) and may manifest as "angina pectoris", an exertional chest discomfort that is relieved by rest. In more severe cases myocardial ischemia may manifest as angina with minimal exertion or even at rest, life-threatening ischemic dysrhythmia, and/or reversible ischemic myocardial dysfunction. Finally, small-vessel disease or microvascular dysfunction may also cause chronic myocardial ischemia. Importantly, while increases in myocardial perfusion would be expected to attenuate the adverse impact of an acute myocardial infarction, the biological time-scale for angiogenesis probably exceeds the time required to salvage myocardium, but BFGF could be considered as an agent that can block apoptosis and thereby have a beneficial effect on the long-term outcome of this disease.

Just as atherosclerotic vascular disease causes obstruction of (epicardial) coronary arteries, the same process in the lower (and rarely) upper extremities causes peripheral artery obstructive disease with inducible or persistent skeletal muscle ischemia. Though originally considered to be relatively rare compared with coronary artery disease, it is now well recognized that an estimated 15% of North American adults over the age of 55 have detectable hemodynamic impairments attributed to peripheral artery disease (43).

Intermittent claudication (IC), muscular leg discomfort provoked by exercise and relieved by rest, is the leg equivalent of angina pectoris and the most common manifestation of peripheral artery disease (43). Even patients with "atypical" leg discomfort have a marked functional impairment with otherwise "subclinical" intermittent claudication (44). Patients with IC are limited in walking distance, speed, functional status, and other measures of life quality. As opposed to coronary artery disease, in which patients will change their clinical status frequently, the annual incidence of progression to critical limb ischemia from intermittent claudication is as low as 1% per year in selected populations such non-smokers and non-diabetics (45). Intermittent claudication is an attractive clinical target for the study of therapeutic angiogenesis because the functional impairment (decreased ability to walk) is directly attributable to the pathophysiology (impaired lower extremity blood flow) and can be measured easily in the majority of patients (46). Moreover, the affected organ is accessible for direct observation and measurement. In contrast, functional measures of myocardial ischemia are potentially confounded by non-myocardial phenomena, including pulmonary and skeletal muscle abnormalities.

Critical limb ischemia (CLI) is the most profound manifestation of peripheral arterial disease (PAD) and is characterized by a constellation of syndromes: rest pain, ulcers that fail to heal, or frank gangrene (47). These patients are at a very high risk for limb loss without revascularization. Patients with CLI frequently have a large number of co-morbid diseases and high rates of cardiovascular events and mortality. Clearly, strategies to improve perfusion, even on a temporary basis, and permit wound healing would be of enormous clinical benefit.

8. CLINICAL TRIALS TESTING THE SAFETY AND EFFICACY OF FGF-2

8.1. Early Experience

The first human studies of parenteral FGF-2 were conducted at the National Institutes of Health (47,48). Unger et al. (47) treated patients with angina and observed sustained hypotension following bolus therapy with 30 or 100 µg/kg, but there was little evidence of clinical efficacy in this small trial. Lazarous et al.(48) treated patients with IC with FGF-2 and found no significant toxicity. This group was the first to report a "therapeutic effect", with plethysmographic evidence of improved lower extremity blood flow. Doses up to 30 µg/kg on two consecutive days were well tolerated, and there were no blood pressure problems even at the highest dose. Laham et al. (49) performed a dose-escalating (0.33–48 µg/kg), open-label, uncontrolled, phase I trial of FGF-2 in 52 patients with CAD who were not amenable to revascularization. This trial again confirmed the safety of this approach, and the investigators noted the efficacy in a sub-study that used thallium perfusion imaging.

8.2. The FIRST Trial

The FGF-2 Initiating Revascularization Trial, or FIRST trial, randomized 337 patients with CAD in a 1:1:1:1 ratio to placebo, 0.3, 3, or 30 µg/kg of FGF-2 administered via a 10 minutes intra-coronary infusion (50). The primary end-point of this study showed no significant difference in the change in exercise treadmill time or myocardial thallium perfusion imaging in patients treated with FGF-2 compared to placebo. Importantly, a post-hoc analysis suggested that the most symptomatic patients who were treated with FGF-2 did have improvements in a number of quality-of-life measures. Notably, the differences between the open-label and the randomized trials are numerous. Overall, the patients in FIRST were not as symptomatic as those in the earlier trials. A sizeable fraction of the patients in FIRST stopped their exercise tests both initially and at follow-up due to non-cardiovascular symptoms. Over time, trials tend to alter the types of patients they select with regard to their potential options for revascularization. Finally, the 3 μg/kg dose of FGF-2 was actually superior to the 30 μg/kg dose, suggesting the possibility that dose optimization might have resulted in better efficacy and that simple dose responses may not be present with these biological agents.

8.3. Surgical Delivery of Sustained-Release FGF-2

One approach to achieving therapeutic angiogenesis in the myocardium also deserves mention with regard to the applicability of FGF-2 treatment. An interesting double-blind, placebo-controlled, randomized clinical trial tested the safety and efficacy of a sustained-release FGF-2 formulation (heparin alginate microspheres) delivered at the time of coronary artery bypass surgery to regions of "viable" myocardium where the coronary artery vessels were too small for arterial bypass grafting. A small number of patients were assigned in a 1:1:1 ratio to receive placebo, or 10 or 100 μg of FGF-2 pellets. The study focused on nuclear perfusion imaging, and patients treated with 100 μg of FGF-2 reportedly had less angina and a significant reduction in stress perfusion defects (19 vs. 9.1%, $P < 0.01$) at 3 months compared to the other groups (51). The long-term effects of FGF-2 persisted through 32.2 ± 6.8 months of follow-up (52). While this specific approach of pharmacologic administration is not well suited for large-scale clinical trials that will be necessary for approval of the drug by regulatory agencies, these findings support the concept of therapeutic angiogenesis in a placebo-controlled trial and the findings highlight the potential utility of prolonged exposure of a growth factor.

8.4. Basic Fibroblast Growth Factor for PAD: The TRAFFIC Study

The Therapeutic Angiogenesis with FGF-2 for Intermittent Claudication trial (TRAFFIC) was a randomized, double-blind, placebo-controlled, phase II clinical trial testing the efficacy and safety of FGF-2 in patients with moderate-to-severe intermittent claudication (53). In total, 190 patients were randomized 1:1:1 to receive bilateral intra-arterial infusions of placebo and placebo, FGF-2 and placebo, or FGF-2 and FGF-2 on day 1 and day 30, respectively. The primary end-point in TRAFFIC was the change in peak walking time (PWT) from baseline to 90 days. Patients treated with FGF-2 (single or double) had a slightly greater than 1 minutes increase in PWT compared with placebo, and there was a corresponding improvement in the ankle-brachial systolic blood pressure index (ABI), supporting the proposed mechanism of action of improved lower extremity blood flow following FGF-2 treatment. Interestingly, the time to onset of claudication did not show important improvement with treatment. Overall, TRAFFIC showed that a single infusion of FGF-2 (30 μg/kg) improved treadmill performance, but a second infusion after 30 days did not provide incremental benefit. These data again suggest that the biological properties of FGF-2 may not follow the classic dose–response parameters.

9. BASIC FIBROBLAST GROWTH FACTOR IN STUDIES OF CEREBROVASCULAR DISEASE

Before FGF-2 investigation began in humans with coronary artery and lower extremity peripheral arterial disease, studies of FGF-2 and other forms of FGF were being explored to treat cerebrovascular disease. Basic fibroblast growth factor is involved in the normal development of multiple cell types in the brain, and interestingly FGF-2 expression was shown to increase following experimental cerebrovascular injury and in the recovery period (54). In its normal state, the blood–brain barrier prevents systemic FGF-2 from entering the brain, but studies showed that systemic (i.e., intravenous) administration of FGF-2 led to significant reductions in cerebral infarct size in experimental models, an effect that is likely due to the breakdown of the blood–brain barrier that occurs during injury (55,56). Although the mechanisms responsible for the beneficial effects of FGF-2 in stroke are not completely understood, they appear to include neuronal protection from cell death and promotion of neuronal plasticity as a form of remodeling (57,58). Although it has not been studied in models of cerebrovascular injury, VEGF has also been shown to have beneficial effects on cell survival, and it has been shown to bind to the neuropilin receptor; this receptor plays a role in axonal development and targeting (2,59).

The largest placebo-controlled trial of FGF-2 in patients with stroke included a total of 286 patients who were randomized to placebo, 5 mg, or 10 mg FGF-2 intravenously over 24 h (60). Patients who presented within 6 h of onset of a stroke and had a moderate-to-large clinical event were included in the trial, and the end-points of the study were the magnitude of the neurological defect and mortality. The results of FGF-2 treatment were modest at best. When compared to the control group, the 5 mg group showed a small but not statistically significant advantage in neurological function with no difference in mortality, while the 10 mg group showed a slightly worse neurological outcome and an increase in mortality, although neither effect was statistically significant. Somewhat in contrast to the pre-clinical models, patients treated later following the onset of symptoms may have done better than those treated earlier, and the authors suggested that this finding correlates with a potential effect on neuronal plasticity and remodeling. Finally, although the target of the outcome of therapy was different from the outcomes sought in patients with ischemic heart or lower extremity peripheral arterial disease, a recurrent theme appears to be that higher doses of FGF-2 are no better, or even worse, than lower doses.

10. POTENTIAL TOXICITY OF FGF-2 AS AN EXAMPLE OF AN ANGIOGENIC GROWTH FACTOR

Potential non-target organ toxicities of FGF-2 include neoangiogenesis, acceleration of atherosclerosis, and spread of malignancy (61,62). Neoangiogenesis in the retina is causally linked to macular degeneration and diabetic proliferative retinopathy, but studies reviewed in the sections above have failed to show an increase in either of these conditions.

Neoangiogenesis may also contribute to nephropathy in diabetes mellitus and other conditions, and FGF-2 has been linked to transient, clinically insignificant, proteinuria (60). Basic fibroblast growth factor and other angiogenic growth factors may promote favorable or deleterious neointimal formation after therapeutic vascular injury (angioplasty and stenting) or may accelerate underlying atherosclerosis progression (63), although this has not been demonstrated in human trials. Angiogenic growth factors were first characterized by their ability to promote tumor blood supply, and growth or metastasis of subclinical malignancy or angioma is a theoretical concern (1,2). To date, six human trials of FGF-2 have not demonstrated any evidence of non-target organ neoangiogenesis, and only low rates of proteinuria and spontaneously resolving episodes of hypotension.

11. FUTURE STEPS WITH FGF-2 AND OTHER ANGIOGENIC GROWTH FACTORS

The preceding sections reviewed the data on FGF-2 as an example of an angiogenic growth factor that has been through several stages of development, and fibroblast growth factor remains a subject of ongoing investigation (64). The mechanisms involved in the formation of functional vascular networks are complex and involve multiple factors and pathways. Evidence for synergy between VEGF and FGF-2 can be found in in-vitro and in-vivo studies (65,66). However, understanding and capitalizing on this synergy for therapeutic purposes is not likely to be easy. Cao et al. (67) showed that FGF-2 and platelet-derived growth factor-BB synergistically promote the formation of new blood vessel networks, but there was no synergy between VEGF and platelet-derived growth factor-BB. Finally, studies have also suggested that there is a "systemic" component to all angiogenic responses, and circulating and/or bone marrow-derived progenitor cell populations contribute to new vessel formation (12); therefore, approaches utilizing angiogenic growth factors to treat aspects of cerebrovascular disease will also need to consider recent advances in this area.

12. SUMMARY

Angiogenesis, the growth and proliferation of blood vessels from existing vascular structures, is a tightly regulated process in adult tissues, and abnormalities in angiogenesis are associated with a number of pathologic states. Strategies designed to promote angiogenesis to treat disorders of inadequate tissue perfusion, such as occurs in coronary artery and peripheral vascular disease, have led to the area of therapeutic angiogenesis. In addition to promoting the growth of blood vessels, angiogenic growth factors have the potential to influence important biological processes such as the response to injury and cell survival. This chapter reviewed some of the basic concepts of vascular development and the mechanisms involved in angiogenesis. Discussion focused on fibroblast growth factors and receptors that are known to mediate angiogenesis. The potential use of these agents as targets within the cerebrovascular system was discussed.

REFERENCES

1. Folkman J. Angiogenesis—retrospect and outlook. In: Steiner R, Weisz PB, Langer R, eds. Angiogenesis: Key Principles-Science-Technology-Medicine. Switzerland: Birkhauser Verlag Basel, 1992:4–13.
2. Folkman J. Clinical applications of research on angiogenesis. N Engl J Med 1995; 333:1757–1763.
3. Risau W. Mechanisms of angiogenesis. Nature 1997; 386:671–674.
4. Gimbrone MA, Gullino PM. Angiogenic capacity of preneoplastic lesions of the murine mammary gland as a marker of neoplastic transformation. J Cancer Res 1976; 36:2611–2620.
5. Risau W, Flamme I. Vasculogenesis. Annu Rev Cell Dev Biol 1995; 11:73–91.
6. Shalaby F, Rossant J, Yamaguchi TP, Gertsenstein M, Wu X-F, Breitman ML, Schuh AC. Failure of blood-island formation and vasculogenesis in Flk-1-deficient mice. Nature 1995; 376:62–66.
7. Folkman J, Shing Y. Angiogenesis. J Biol Chem 1992; 267:10931–10934.
8. Kalebic T, Garbish S, Glaser B, Liotta LA. Basement membrane collagen: degradation by migrating endothelial cells. Science 1983; 221:281–283.
9. Burger PC, Chandler DB, Klintworth GK. Corneal neovascularization as studied by scanning electron microscopy of vascular casts. Lab Invest 1983; 48:169–180.
10. Garlanda C, Dejana E. Heterogeneity of endothelial cells. specific markers. Arterioscler Thromb Vasc Biol 1997; 17:1193–1202.
11. Pepper MS. Manipulating angiogenesis. From basic science to the bedside. Arterioscler Thromb Vasc Biol 1997; 17:605–619.
12. Asahara T, Murohara T, Sullivan A, Silver M, van der Zee R, Li T, Witzenbichler B, Schatteman G, Isner JM. Isolation of putative progenitor endothelial cells for angiogenesis. Science 1997; 275:964–967.
13. Yancopoulos GD, Klagsbrun M, Folkman J. Vasculogenesis, angiogenesis, and growth factors: ephrins enter the fray at the border. Cell 1998; 93:661–664.
14. Folkman J, D'Amore PA. Blood vessel formation: what is its molecular basis? Cell 1996; 87:1153–1155.
15. Schlessinger J. Cell signaling by receptor tyrosine kinases. Cell 2000; 103: 211–225.

16. Ferrara N, Davis-Smyth T. The biology of vascular endothelial growth factor. Endocrine Rev 1997; 18:4–25.

17. Gerber H-P, McMurtrey A, Kowalski J, Yan M, Keyt BA, Dixit V, Ferrara N. Vascular endothelial growth factor regulates endothelial cell survival through the phosphatidylinositol 3'-kinase/Akt signal transduction pathway. J Biol Chem 1998; 273:30336–30343.

18. Sato TN, Tozawa Y, Deutsch U, Wolburg-Bucholz K, Fujiwara Y, Gendron-Maguire M, Gridley T, Wolburg H, Risau W, Qin Y. Distinct roles of the receptor tyrosine kinases Tie-1 and Tie-2 in blood vessel formation. Nature 1995; 376:70–74.

19. Suri C, Jones PF, Patan S, Bartunkova S, Maisonpierre PC, Davis S, Sato TN, Yancopoulos GD. Requisite role of angiopoietin-1, a ligand for the Tie-2 receptor, during embryonic angiogenesis. Cell 1996; 87:1171–1180.

20. Puri MC, Rossant J, Alitalo K, Bernstein A, Partanen J. The receptor tyrosine kinase Tie is required for integrity and survival of vascular endothelial cells. Embo J 1995; 14:5884–5891.

21. Holash J, Maisonpierre PC, Compton D, Boland P, Alexander CR, Zagzag D, Yancopoulos GD, Wiegand SJ. Vessel cooption, regression, and growth in tumors mediated by angiopoietins and VEGF. Science 1999; 284:1994–1998.

22. Papapetropoulos A, Garcia-Cardena G, Dengler TJ, Maisonpierre PC, Yancopoulos GD, Sessa WC. Direct actions of angiopoietin-1 on human endothelium: evidence for network stabilization, cell survival, and interaction with other angiogenic growth factors. Lab Invest 1999; 79:213–223.

23. Kontos CD, Annex BH. Angiogenesis. Curr Atheroscler Rep 1999; 1:165–171.

24. Wang HU, Chen Z-F, Anderson DJ. Molecular distinction and angiogenic interaction between embryonic arteries and veins revealed by ephrin-B2 and its receptor Eph-B4. Cell 1998; 93:741–753.

25. Tenaglia AN, Peters KP, Sketch MH, Annex BH. Neovascularization in atherectomy specimens from patients with unstable angina: implications for pathogenesis of unstable angina. Am Heart J 1998; 135:10–14.

26. Kontos C, Stauffer T, Yang W-P, York J, Huang L, Blanar M, Meyer T, Peters K. Tyrosine 1101 of Tie2 is the major site of association of p85 and is required for activation of phosphatidylinositol 3-kinase and Akt. Mol Cell Biol 1998; 18:4131–4140.

27. Thakker GD, Hajjar DP, Muller WA, Rosengart TK. The role of phosphatidylinositol 3-kinase in vascular endothelial growth factor signaling. J Biol Chem 1999; 274:10002–10007.

28. Rousseau S, Houle F, Landry J, Huot J. p38 Map kinase activation by vascular endothelial growth factor mediates actin reorganization and cell migration in human endothelial cells. Oncogene 1997; 15:2169–2177.

29. Murohara T, Asahara T, Silver M, Bauters C, Masuda H, Kalka C, Kearney M, Chen D, Symes JF, Fishman MC, Huang PL, Isner JM. Nitric oxide synthase modulates angiogenesis in response to tissue ischemia. J Clin Invest 1998; 101:2567–2578.

30. Fulton D, Gratton JP, McCabe TJ, Fontana J, Fujio Y, Walsh K, Franke TF, Papapetropoulos A, Sessa WC. Regulation of endothelium-derived nitric oxide production by the protein kinase Akt. Nature 1999; 399:597–601.

31. O'Reilly MS, Boehm T, Shing Y, Fukai N, Vasios G, Lane WS, Flynn E, Birkhead JR, Olsen BR, Folkman J. Endostatin: an endogenous inhibitor of angiogenesis and tumor growth. Cell 1997; 88:277–285.

32. O'Reilly MS, Holmgren L, Shing Y, Chen C, Rosenthal RA, Moses M, Lane WS, Cao Y, Sage EH, Folkman J. Angiostatin: a novel angiogenesis inhibitor that mediates the suppression of metastases by a Lewis lung carcinoma. Cell 1994; 79:315–328.

33. Dhanabal M, Ramchandran R, Waterman MJ, Lu H, Knebelmann B, Segal M, Sukhatme VP. Endostatin induces endothelial cell apoptosis. J Biol Chem 1999; 274:11721–11726.

34. Claesson-Welsh L, Welsh M, Ito N, Anand-Apte B, Soker S, Zetter B, O'Reilly M, Folkman J. Angiostatin induces endothelial cell apoptosis and activation of focal adhesion kinase independently of the integrin-binding motif RGD. Proc Natl Acad Sci USA 1998; 95:5579–5583.

35. Moser TL, Stack MS, Asplin I, Enghild JJ, Hojrup P, Everitt L, Hubchak S, Schnaper HW, Pizzo SV. Angiostatin binds ATP synthase on the surface of human endothelial cells. Proc Natl Acad Sci USA 1999; 96:2811–2816.

36. Maisonpierre PC, Suri C, Jones PF, Bartunkova S, Wiegand SJ, Radziejewski C, Compton D, McClain J, Aldrich TH, Papadopoulos N, Daly TJ, Davis S, Sato TN, Yancopoulos GD. Angiopoietin-2, a natural antagonist for Tie2 that disrupts in vivo angiogenesis. Science 1997; 277:55–60.

37. Engler DA. Use of vascular endothelial growth factor for therapeutic angiogenesis. Circulation 1996; 94:1496–1498.

38. Lopez JJ, Laham RJ, Stamler A, Pearlman JD, Bunting S, Kaplan A, Carrozza JP, Sellke FW, Simons M. VEGF administration in chronic myocardial ischemia in pigs. Cardiovasc Res 1998; 40:272–281.

39. Takeshita S, Zheng LP, Brogi E, Kearney M, Pu LQ, Bunting S, Ferrara N, Symes JF, Isner JM. Therapeutic angiogenesis: a single intra-arterial bolus of vascular endothelial growth factor augments revascularization in a rabbit ischemic hind limb model. J Clin Invest 1994; 93:662–670.

40. Losordo DW, Vale PR, Symes JF, Dunnington CH, Esakof DD, Maysky M, Ashare AB, Lathi K, Isner JM. Gene therapy for myocardial angiogenesis: initial clinical results with direct myocardial injection of PHVEGF165 as sole therapy for myocardial ischemia. Circulation 1998; 98:2800–2804.

41. Schumacher B, Pecher P, von Specht BU, Stegmann T. Induction of neoangiogenesis in ischemic myocardium by human growth factors: first clinical results of a new treatment of coronary heart disease. Circulation 1998; 97:645–650.

42. Isner JM, Pieczek A, Schainfeld R, Blair R, Haley L, Asahara T, Rosenfield K, Razvi S, Walsh K, Symes JF. Clinical evidence of angiogenesis after arterial gene transfer of PHVEGF165 in patient with ischaemic limb. Lancet 1996; 348:370–374.

43. Criqui, MH. Peripheral arterial disease—epidemiological aspects. Vasc Med 2001; 6:3–7.

44. McDermott MM, Greenland P, Liu K, Guralnik JM, Criqui MH, Dolan NC, Chan C, Celic L, Pearce WH, Schneider JR, Sharma L, Clark E, Gibson D, Martin GJ. Leg symptoms in peripheral arterial disease: associated clinical characteristics and functional impairment. JAMA 2001; 286:1599–1606.

45. Hiatt WR, Hirsch AT, Regensteiner JG, Brass EP. Clinical trials for claudication. assessment of exercise performance, functional status, and clinical end-points. Circulation 1995; 92:614–621.
46. Isner JM, Asahara T. Angiogenesis and vasculogenesis as therapeutic strategies for postnatal neovascularization. J Clin Invest 1999; 103:1231–1236.
47. Unger EF, Goncalves L, Epstein SE, Chew EY, Trapnell CB, Cannon RO 3rd, Quyyumi, AA. Effects of a single intracoronary injection of basic fibroblast growth factor in stable angina pectoris. Am J Cardiol 2000; 85:1414–1419.
48. Lazarous DF, Unger EF, Epstein SE, Stine A, Arevalo JL, Chew EY, Quyyumi AA. Basic fibroblast growth factor in patients with intermittent claudication: results of a phase I trial. J Am Coll Cardiol 2000; 36:1239–1244.
49. Laham RJ, Chronos NA, Pike M, Leimbach ME, Udelson JE, Pearlman JD, Pettigrew RI, Whitehouse MJ, Yoshizawa C, Simons M. Intracoronary basic fibroblast growth factor (FGF-2) in patients with severe ischemic heart disease: results of a phase I open-label dose escalation study. J Am Coll Cardiol 2000; 36:2132–2139.
50. Simons M, Annex BH, Laham RJ, Kleiman N, Henry T, Dauerman H, Udelson JE, Gervino EV, Pike M, Whitehouse MJ, Moon T, Chronos NA. Pharmacological treatment of coronary artery disease with recombinant fibroblast growth factor-2: double-blind, randomized, controlled clinical trial. Circulation 2002; 105:788–793.
51. Laham RJ, Sellke FW, Edelman ER, Pearlman JD, Ware JA, Brown DL, Gold JP, Simons M. Local perivascular delivery of basic fibroblast growth factor in patients undergoing coronary bypass surgery: results of a phase I randomized, double-blind, placebo-controlled trial. Circulation 1999; 100: 1865–1871.
52. Ruel M, Laham RJ, Parker JA, Post MJ, Ware JA, Simons M, Sellke FW. Long-term effects of surgical angiogenic therapy with fibroblast growth factor 2 protein. J Thorac Cardiovasc Surg 2002; 124:28–34.
53. Lederman RJ, Mendelsohn FO, Anderson RD, Saucedo JF, Tenaglia AN, Hermiller JB, Hillegass WB, Rocha-Singh K, Moon TE, Whitehouse MJ, Annex BH. Therapeutic angiogenesis with recombinant fibroblast growth factor-2 for intermittent claudication (the traffic study): a randomised trial. Lancet 2002; 359:2053–2058.
54. Lin DA, Finkelstein SP. Basic fibroblast growth factor: a new treatment for stroke? Neuroscientist 1997; 3:247–250.
55. Fisher M, Meadows ME, Do T, Charette M, Finklestein SP. Delayed treatment with intravenous basic fibroblast growth factor reduces infarct size following permanent focal cerebral ischemia in rats. J Cereb Blood Flow Metab 1995; 15:953–959.
56. Jing N, Finklestein SP, Do T, Caday CG, Charette M, Chopp M. Delayed intravenous administration of basic fibroblast growth factor (BFGF) reduces infarct volume in a model of focal cerebral ischemia/reperfusion in the rat. J Neurol Sci 1996; 139:173–179.
57. Kawamata T, Dietrich WD, Schallert T, Gotts JE, Cocke RR, Benowitz LI, Finklestein SP. Intracisternal basic fibroblast growth factor enhances functional recovery and up-regulates the expression of a molecular marker of neuronal

sprouting following focal cerebral infarction. Proc Natl Acad Sci (USA) 1997; 94:8179–8184.

58. Kawamata T, Ren JM, Cha JH, Finklestein SP. Intracisternal antisense oligonucleotides to growth associated protein-43 blocks the recovery-promoting effects of basic fibroblast growth factor after acute stroke. Exp Neurol 1999; 158:89–96.

59. Ailatolo Veikkola T, Karkkainen M, Claesson-Welsh L, Alitalo K. Regulation of angiogensis via vascular endothelial growth factor receptors. Cancer Res 2000; 60:203–212.

60. Bougousslavsky J, Victor SJ, Salinas EO, Pallay A, Donnan GA, Fieschi C, Kaste M, Orgogozo JM, Chamorro A, Desmet A. (for the European-Australian Fiblast (Trafermin) in acute stroke group: Fiblast (Trafermin) in acute stroke. Results of the European-Australian Phase II/III Safety and efficacy trial. Cerebrovasc Dis 2002; 14:239–251.

61. Mazue G, Bertolero F, Jacob C, Sarmientos P, Roncucci R. Preclinical and clinical studies with recombinant human basic fibroblast growth factor. Ann NY acad Sci 1991; 638:329–340.

62. Post MJ, Laham R, Sellke FW, Simons M. Therapeutic angiogenesis in cardiology using protein formulations. Cardiovasc Res 2001; 49:522–531.

63. Moulton KS, Heller E, Konerding MA, Flynn E, Palinski W, Folkman J. Angiogenesis inhibitors endostatin or TNP-470 reduce intimal neovascularization and plaque growth in apolipoprotein e-deficient mice. Circulation 1999; 99:1726–1732.

64. Comerota AJ, Throm RC, Miller KA, Henry T, Chronos N, Laird J, Sequeira R, Kent CK, Bacchetta M, Goldman C, Salenius JP, Schmieder FA, Pilsudski R. Naked plasmid DNA encoding fibroblast growth factor type 1 for the treatment of end-stage unreconstructible lower extremity ischemia: preliminary results of a phase I trial. J Vasc Surg 2002; 35:930–936.

65. Goto F, Goto K, Weindel K, Folkman J. Synergistic effects of vascular endothelial growth factor and basic fibroblast growth factor on the proliferation and cord formation of bovine capillary endothelial cells within collagen gels. Lab Invest 1993; 69:508–517.

66. Asahara T, Bauters C, Zheng LP, Takeshita S, Bunting S, Ferrara N, Symes JF, Isner JM. Synergistic effect of vascular endothelial growth factor and basic fibroblast growth factor on angiogenesis in vivo. Circulation 1995; 92(II):365–371.

67. Cao R, Brakenhielm E, Pawliuk R, Wariaro D, Post MJ, Wahlberg E, Leboulch P, Cao Y. Angiogenic synergism, vascular stability and improvement of hind-limb ischemia by a combination of PDGF-BB and FGF-2. Nat Med 2003; 9:604–613.

12

What Are the Current Operative Risks of Carotid Endarterectomy?

Peter M. Rothwell

*Stroke Prevention Research Unit, University Department of Neurology,
University of Oxford, Radcliffe Infirmary, Oxford, U.K.*

Carotid endarterectomy (CEA) reduces the risk of stroke in patients with recently symptomatic severe carotid stenosis and to a lesser extent in patients with recently symptomatic moderate stenosis or severe asymptomatic stenosis (1–4). However, the procedure has a relatively high rate of complications, which limit the benefit of surgery in patients at low and moderate risk of stroke on medical treatment alone. Reliable data on the risk of CEA in relation to clinical indication are necessary to target surgery more effectively, to properly inform patients, to adjust risks for case-mix, and to understand the mechanisms of operative stroke. This chapter will briefly consider what we know about the overall operative risk of CEA and how the risk is related to the clinical indication, the characteristics of the patient, and the timing of surgery. Other important issues, such as surgical technique (e.g., patching, shunting, monitoring, etc.) (5–7), surgical workload, and experience, and type of anesthetic (8) are covered in other chapters.

1. WHAT IS THE RISK OF CEA FOR SYMPTOMATIC STENOSIS?

In the European Carotid Surgery Trial (ECST), 1729 patients underwent trial surgery. There were 17 deaths (1.0%, 95% CI $= 0.5$–1.6) and 105 non-fatal strokes with symptoms lasting longer than 7 days (6.1%, 5.0–7.2) within 30 days of surgery (9). The operative risk of stroke or death was

7.1% (5.8–8.4). The risk of disabling or fatal stroke was 3.0% (2.1–3.8). There were also 19 (1.1%, 0.7–1.7) transient ischemic attacks (TIAs) and 15 (0.9%, 0.5–1.4) minor strokes (symptoms < 7 days). In addition to four deaths due to myocardial infarction (MI), there were four non-fatal myocardial infarctions and four episodes of unstable angina. The most common minor complications were cranial nerve palsy (6.4%, 5.3–7.7) and neck hematoma requiring re-operation (3.1%, 2.3–4.0). Of the 111 cranial nerve palsies, only nine patients (0.5%, 0.2–1.0) had a deficit still present at the 4-month follow-up (10).

Among the 3157 patients who underwent trial surgery in the pooled analysis of the three major randomized trials of CEA for symptomatic stenosis, there were 222 operative strokes or deaths (7.0%, 6.2–8.0) (2). This risk and the other complication rates reported in the ECST and NASCET are consistent with those from published case series in which post-operative outcome was also assessed by a neurologist (11). However, some surgeons now argue that the surgical data from trials such as the ECST and NASCET are out of date because refinements in surgical technique have reduced operative risks, and that the indications for CEA should therefore be broadened beyond those determined in the trials. Yet, routinely collected data suggest that operative mortality is still higher than in the trials (12–15).

A systematic review of all studies published between 1980 and 2001 inclusive that reported the risks of stroke and death due to CEA for symptomatic carotid stenosis found no evidence of a reduction over the last decade in operative risks, current risks still being comparable to those reported in ECST and NASCET (16). Of 383 studies published during 1994–2001, only 45 reported operative risks for patients with symptomatic stenosis separately. Comparison of these studies with 47 similar studies published prior

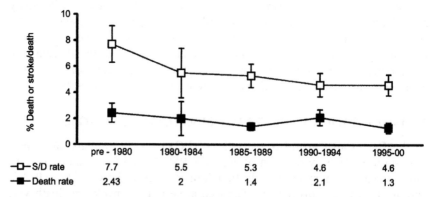

Figure 1 Time trends in operative mortality and risk of stroke and death due to carotid endarterectomy for symptomatic stenosis in published case series from 1980 to 2001 (16).

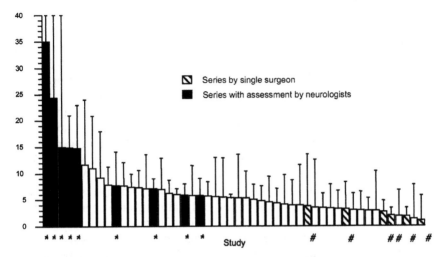

Figure 2 Risks (95% CI) of stroke and death due to carotid endarterectomy for symptomatic carotid stenosis in studies published by single surgeons (#), studies that involved post-operative assessment by neurologists (*), and studies published by multiple surgeons without involvement of neurologists (unmarked) (17).

to 1995 (11) showed no evidence of a reduction in risks of death or stroke or death due to CEA for symptomatic stenosis between 1980 and 2001 (Fig. 1) (16). Interestingly, in keeping with the reports of routinely collected mortality data (12–15), operative mortality in case series published between 1994 and 2001 was significantly higher than that in ECST and NASCET (16).

The reported operative risks of stroke due to CEA are very dependent on the specialty of the authors reporting them. For example, in a review of studies published prior to 1995 (11,17) the operative risk of stroke and death was 7.7% (5.0–10.0) in studies that involved neurologists vs. 2.3% (1.8–2.7) in studies in which single surgeons reported their own data (Fig. 2) (17). The importance of involvement of a neurologist or stroke physician was highlighted again in the more recent review, in which the pooled operative risk of stroke and death reported in studies published by surgeons only was 4.2% (2.9–5.5, 34 studies) whereas that reported in studies that involved neurologists was 6.5% (4.3–8.7, 11 studies) (16).

2. WHAT IS THE RISK OF CEA FOR ASYMPTOMATIC STENOSIS?

Several studies have shown that the operative risk for patients with asymptomatic stenosis is less than that for patients with symptomatic stenosis (18). A recent systematic review of all studies published from 1980 to 2001 inclusive that reported the risk of stroke and death due to CEA identified 59 studies that reported the operative risk separately for patients with symptomatic stenosis and patients with asymptomatic stenosis (19). The operative risk of stroke and death for symptomatic stenosis was about 60% higher than for asymptomatic stenosis (OR = 1.62, 95% CI = 1.45–1.81, $P < 0.00001$). This difference was highly consistent across all studies (heterogeneity: $P = 0.94$). Taking all studies together (irrespective of assessment by neurologists), the pooled operative risk of stroke and death for asymptomatic stenosis was 3.4% (2.5–4.4) in 29 studies published prior to 1995 and 3.0% (2.5–3.5) in 28 studies published since 1995. The corresponding risks for patients with symptomatic stenosis were 5.0% (4.4–5.5) and 5.1 (4.7–5.6), respectively. The operative risk of stroke and death due to CEA in the eight published case series in which post-operative outcome was assessed by a neurologist was 4.3% (3.5–5.2) (20). Importantly, although the operative risk of stroke is lower, there is no consistent evidence of a lower operative mortality due to CEA for asymptomatic stenosis than symptomatic stenosis. Among 46 published case series, the operative mortality for asymptomatic carotid stenosis was 1.1% (0.9–1.3) (20). This risk is similar to that reported for symptomatic stenosis and is considerably greater than the 0.14% (0–0.40) risk reported in the ACAS trial (3).

3. DOES THE TYPE OF PRESENTING SYMPTOM MATTER?

There is good evidence that operative risk for patients with symptomatic stenosis differs depending on the type of symptomatic event (19,21). A systematic review of all surgical case series published from 1980 to 2001 inclusive that reported the risk of stroke and death due to CEA identified 103 studies that stratified risk by indication (19). Operative risk was the same for CEA for stroke and cerebral TIA (OR = 1.16, 0.99–1.35, $P = 0.08$, 23 studies), but was higher for cerebral TIA than for ocular events only (OR = 2.31, 1.72–3.12, $P < 0.00001$, 19 studies), and the risk of CEA for re-stenosis was higher than for primary surgery (OR = 1.95, 1.21–3.16, $P = 0.018$, six studies). Interestingly, the operative risk in patients with only ocular events only tended to be even lower than for asymptomatic stenosis (OR = 0.75, 0.50–1.14, 15 studies). Thus, the risk of stroke and death due to CEA is highly dependent on the clinical indication. Audits of risk should be stratified accordingly, and patients should be informed of the risk that relates to their presenting event.

4. IS OPERATIVE RISK RELATED TO SEX?

Reliable data on the risk of CEA in relation to other clinical characteristics of the patient are also useful in order to target surgery effectively, to properly inform patients, and to adjust risks for case-mix. In the ECST, several baseline characteristics predicted the operative risk of stroke and death in univariate analyses, but apart from the type of presenting event, only three were independent risk factors in a multiple regression analysis: female sex (HR = 2.04, 95% CI = 1.37–3.06, P = 0.001), systolic hypertension (HR = 1.01 per 10 mmHg, 1.00–1.02, P = 0.034), and peripheral vascular disease (HR = 2.17, 1.17–2.89, P = 0.001) (9).

A recent analysis of pooled data from ECST and NASCET showed that benefit from CEA is decreased in women, partly to a higher operative risk than in men (22). A recent systematic review of all publications reporting data on the association between sex and perioperative risk of stroke and/or death following CEA from 1980 to 2003 showed that the higher operative risk in women is also seen in routine clinical practice (23). Among 21 studies that reported data on sex and perioperative risk, the rate of operative stroke and death was nearly 50% higher in women than in men (1.45, 95% CI = 1.2–1.6, P < 0.001).

It is uncertain why operative risk of stroke should be increased in women. Some surgeons are more likely to use a patch graft in women, but this seems to be associated with a reduced operative risk in randomized trials of patching vs. no-patching (5). Sex differences in anatomy may play a part. Women have smaller-diameter blood vessels which may make them more difficult to operate upon or more likely to acutely thrombose. However, women also tend to have longer necks and many surgeons find them easier to operate upon than men (7). A further possibility is referral bias. Women are less likely than men to be selected for both cardiac and peripheral vascular surgery (24), and recent studies have found that women are also less likely to receive carotid endarterectomy or angioplasty than men in the same situation (25) possibly because of a relative disinclination to have surgery amongst women. It is possible, therefore, that those women who choose to have surgery are at higher risk of complications than those who do not.

The systematic review did not find a consistent increase in operative mortality in women (23). Nor do the large number of studies of routinely collected mortality data following CEA suggest a sex difference in operative mortality (12–15). It would seem therefore that the increased operative risk in women is due to an excess of non-fatal strokes. Unfortunately, there are few data on the severity of operative stroke by sex, although there was no evidence in the ECST of any sex difference in the case-fatality or disability scores at 6 months after operative strokes (unpublished data).

5. DOES AGE MATTER?

The average age of patients undergoing CEA has increased progressively over the last 20 years (16). Although chronological age is not always proportional to the degree of ill health, concern has been expressed that the perioperative risk of CEA for "old" patients may be too high to allow them any benefit. Yet, the pooled individual patient data from the randomized trials of endarterectomy for symptomatic carotid stenosis showed that benefit was increased in patients aged over 75 years, due to a high risk of stroke without surgery but no increase in operative risk (22). However, these trials had specific inclusion and exclusion criteria, and trial recruitment tends to be particularly selective in the elderly (26). It does not follow therefore that a major increase in operative risk in the elderly could not still be found in routine clinical practice. In fact, the trial observations do appear to be generalizable. A systematic review of case series reporting operative risk by age showed that whilst operative mortality was increased in patients aged ≥75 years (17 studies, 1.36, 1.1–1.7, $P = 0.02$) and ≥80 years (10 studies, 1.6, 1.1–2.3, $P < 0.001$), there was no major increase in the rate of stroke and death: ≥75 years (20 studies, 1.18, 0.94–1.44, $P = 0.06$); ≥80 years (10 studies, 1.09, 0.8–1.4, $P = 0.59$) (23).

Thus, although there probably is an increased risk of perioperative death in older patients undergoing CEA, there is no increase in risk of operative stroke and hence only a minimal increase in risk of stroke and death combined. Provided patients are selected carefully, age should not therefore be a barrier to undergoing CEA. It has also been shown that about 75% of patients aged ≥80 years will survive for at least 4 years after successful CEA (27) and will therefore benefit from the prevention of stroke.

6. DOES TIMING MATTER?

Early studies showed that CEA carries a high risk, particularly of intracranial hemorrhage, if performed within hours or days after a large cerebral infarction (28,29). Such patients rarely undergo CEA today, but many surgeons still delay CEA for 4–6 weeks after non-disabling stroke. Yet data from NASCET suggested that operative risk was not increased in patients operated within 30 days of a non-disabling stroke (30) and a recent systematic review of surgical case series has confirmed this (19). Urgent CEA for evolving symptoms had a much higher risk (19.2%, 10.7–27.8) than CEA for stable symptoms (OR = 3.9, 2.7–5.7, $P < 0.001$, 13 studies), but there was no difference between early (< 3–6 weeks) and late (>3–6 weeks) CEA for stroke in stable patients (OR = 1.13, 0.79–1.62, $P = 0.62$, 11 studies) (19). In pooled data from ECST and NASCET, there was no evidence of an increased operative risk either in patients with TIA or non-disabling stroke operated within 1 week of presenting symptoms (31).

If early CEA is not associated with an increased operative risk after non-disabling stroke, any delay is likely to lead to reduced benefit because of the risk of stroke on medical treatment prior to surgery. As has recently become clear (32,33), the risk of stroke after a TIA or non-disabling ischemic stroke is highest in the first few days and weeks after the presenting event, particularly in patients with carotid stenosis (34). Although current clinical guidelines in North America and Europe simply state that surgery should be performed within 6 months of last symptoms (35,36), recent subgroup analyses of the pooled individual patient data from the ECST and NASCET showed that the absolute reduction in risk of ipsilateral ischemic stroke with CEA fell rapidly with increasing time from last symptomatic event to randomization (22), particularly in women (31). For patients with ≥50% stenosis, the number of patients needed to undergo surgery (NNT) to prevent one ipsilateral stroke in 5 years was 5 for patients randomized within 2 weeks after their last ischemic event vs. 125 for patients randomized > 12 weeks. Thus, in neurologically stable patients with TIA or non-disabling stroke, CEA should be performed within a few days of the presenting event.

7. SUMMARY

The overall operative risk of stroke and death due to CEA is ~7% for symptomatic carotid stenosis and ~3–5% for asymptomatic stenosis, and there is no evidence that risks are falling. However, the risk in patients with symptomatic carotid stenosis does vary in relation to the clinical indication and the characteristics of the patient. Early surgery in neurologically stable patients with a recent TIA or non-disabling stroke is not associated with a significant increase in operative risk.

REFERENCES

1. North American Symptomatic Carotid Endarterectomy Trialists' Collaborative Group. The final results of the NASCET trial. N Engl J Med 1998; 339: 1415–1425.
2. Rothwell PM, Eliasziw M, Gutnikov SA, Fox AJ, Taylor W, Mayberg MR, Warlow CP, Barnett HJM. Analysis of pooled data from the randomized controlled trials of endarterectomy for symptomatic carotid stenosis. Lancet 2003; 361:107–116.
3. Executive Committee for the Asymptomatic Carotid Atherosclerosis Study. Endarterectomy for asymptomatic carotid artery stenosis. JAMA 1995; 273:1421–1428.
4. Halliday A, Mansfield A, Marro J, Peto C, Peto R, Potter J, Thomas D. Prevention of disabling and fatal strokes by successful carotid endarterectomy in patients without recent neurological symptoms: randomised controlled trial. Lancet 2004; 363:1491–1502.
5. Bond R, Warlow CP, Naylor R, Rothwell PM. Variation in surgical and anaesthetic technique and associations with operative risk in the European Carotid Surgery Trial: implications for trials of ancillary techniques. Eur J Vasc Endovasc Surg 2002; 23:117–126.
6. Bond R, Rerkasem K, Rothwell PM. Routine or selective carotid artery shunting for carotid endarterectomy. Cochrane Database Syst Rev 2002; 2: CD000190.

7. Bond R, Rerkasem K, Shearman CP, Rothwell PM. Patch angioplasty versus primary closure for carotid endarterectomy. Cochrane Database Syst Rev 2004; 2:CD000160.

8. Rerkasem K, Bond R, Rothwell PM. Local versus general anaesthetic for carotid endarterectomy. Cochrane Database Syst Rev 2004; 2:CD000126.

9. Bond R, Narayan S, Rothwell PM, Warlow CP. Clinical and radiological risk factors for operative stroke and death in the European Carotid Surgery Trial. Eur J Vasc Endovasc Surg 2002; 23:108–116.

10. Cunningham EJ, Bond R, Mayberg MR, Warlow CP, Rothwell PM (for the European Carotid Surgery Trialists' Collaborative Group). Risk of persistent cranial nerve injury after carotid endarterectomy. J Neurosurg 2004; 101; 455–458.

11. Rothwell PM, Slattery J, Warlow CP. A systematic review of the risks of stroke and death due to carotid endarterectomy for symptomatic stenosis. Stroke 1996; 27:260–265.

12. Huber TS, Wheeler KG, Cuddeback JK, Dame DA, Flynn TC, Seeger JM. Effect of the Asymptomatic Carotid Atherosclerosis Study on carotid endarterectomy in Florida. Stroke 1998; 29:1099–1105.

13. Hannan EL, Popp AJ, Tranmer B, Fuestel P, Waldman J, Shah D. Relationship between provider volume and mortality for carotid endarterectomies in New York state. Stroke 1998; 29:2292–2297.

14. O'Neill L, Lanska DJ, Hartz A. Surgeon characteristics associated with mortality and morbidity following carotid endarterectomy. Neurology 2000; 55: 773–781.

15. Wennberg DE, Lucas FL, Birkmeyer JD, Bredenberg CE, Fisher ES. Variation in carotid endarterectomy mortality in the Medicare population: trial hospitals, volume, and patient characteristics. JAMA 1998; 279:1278–1281.

16. Bond R, Rerkasem K, Shearman CP, Rothwell PM. Time trends in the published risks of stroke and death due to endarterectomy for symptomatic carotid stenosis. Cerebrovasc Dis 2004; 18:37–46.

17. Rothwell PM, Warlow CP. Is self-audit reliable? Lancet 1995; 346:1623.

18. Rothwell PM, Slattery J, Warlow CP. A systematic comparison of the risks of stroke and death due to carotid endarterectomy for symptomatic and asymptomatic stenosis. Stroke 1996; 27:266–269.

19. Bond R, Rerkasem K, Rothwell PM. A systematic review of the risks of carotid endarterectomy in relation to the clinical indication and the timing of surgery. Stroke 2003; 34:2290–2301.

20. Rothwell PM, Goldstein LB. Carotid endarterectomy for asymptomatic stenosis: Asymptomatic Carotid Surgery Trial. Stroke 2004; 35:2425–2427.

21. Rothwell PM, Slattery J, Warlow CP. A systematic review of clinical and angiographic predictors of stroke and death due to carotid endarterectomy. Br Med J 1997; 315:1571–1577.

22. Rothwell PM, Eliasziw M, Gutnikov SA, Warlow CP, Barnett HJM (for the Carotid Endarterectomy Trialists Collaboration). Effect of endarterectomy for symptomatic carotid stenosis in relation to clinical subgroups and to the timing of surgery. Lancet 2004; 363:915–924.

23. Bond R, Rerkasem K, Rothwell PM. A systematic review of the associations between age and sex and the operative risk of carotid endarterectomy. Cerebrovasc Dis In press.
24. Feinglass J, McDermott MM, Foroohar M, Pearce WH. Gender differences in interventional management of peripheral vascular disease: evidence from a blood flow laboratory population. Ann Vasc Surg 1994; 8:343–349.
25. Ramani S, Byrne-Logan S, Freund KM, Ash A, Yu W, Moskowitz MA. Gender differences in the treatment of cerebrovascular disease. J Am Geriatr Soc 2000; 48:741–745.
26. Bungeja G, Kumar A, Banerjee AK. Exclusion of elderly people from clinical research: a descriptive study of published reports. Br Med J 1997; 315:1059.
27. Schneider JR, Droste JS, Schindler N, Golan JF. Carotid endarterectomy in octogenarians: comparison with patient characteristics and outcomes in younger patients. J Vasc Surg 2000; 31:927–935.
28. Bruteman ME, Fields WS, Crawford ES, Debakey ME. Cerebral haemorrhage in carotid artery surgery. Arch Neurol 1963; 9:458–467.
29. Blaisdell WF, Clauss RH, Galbraith JG, Imparato AM, Wylie EJ. Joint Study of Extracranial Arterial Occlusion, IV: a review of surgical considerations. JAMA 1969; 209:1889–1895.
30. Gasecki AP, Ferguson GG, Eliasziw M, Clagett GP, Fox AJ, Hachinski V, Barnett HJM. Early endarterectomy for severe carotid artery stenosis after a non-disabling stroke: results from the North American Symptomatic Carotid Endarterectomy Trial. J Vasc Surg 1994; 20:288–295.
31. Rothwell PM, Gutnikov SA, Eliasziw M, Warlow CP, Barnett HJM. Sex difference in effect of time from symptoms to surgery on benefit from endarterectomy for transient ischaemic attack and non-disabling stroke. Stroke 2004; 35: 2855–2861.
32. Lovett J, Dennis M, Sandercock PAG, Bamford J, Warlow CP, Rothwell PM. The very early risk of stroke after a first transient ischaemic attack. Stroke 2003; 34:e138–e140.
33. Coull A, Lovett JK, Rothwell PM (on behalf of the Oxford Vascular Study). Early risk of stroke after a TIA or minor stroke in a population-based incidence study. Br Med J 2004; 328:326–328.
34. Lovett JK, Coull A, Rothwell PM (on behalf of the Oxford Vascular Study). Early risk of recurrent stroke by aetiological subtype: implications for stroke prevention. Neurology 2004; 62:569–574.
35. The Intercollegiate Working Party for Stroke. National Clinical Guidelines for Stroke. London: Royal College of Physicians, 2000.
36. Biller J, Feinberg WM, Castaldo JE, Whittemore AD, Harbaugh RE, Dempsey RJ, Caplan LR, Kresowik TF, Matchar DB, Toole JF, Easton JD, Adams HP, Brass LM, Hobson RW, Brott G, Sternau L. Guidelines for carotid endarterectomy: a statement for healthcare professionals from a special writing group of the Stroke Council, American Heart Association. Circulation 1998; 97: 501–509.

13

Benefits of Endarterectomy for Recently Symptomatic Carotid Stenosis

Peter M. Rothwell

Stroke Prevention Research Unit, University Department of Neurology, University of Oxford, Radcliffe Infirmary, Oxford, U.K.

Most of the strokes that occur within the first few years after a transient ischemic attack (TIA) or minor stroke in patients with carotid stenosis are ischemic and occur in the territory of the symptomatic artery. All patients with recently symptomatic carotid stenosis require treatment to reduce their risk of stroke and other vascular events. Medical treatment has been discussed in the preceding chapters. This chapter will concentrate on the selection of patients for carotid surgery based on data from relevant randomized controlled trials and based on the risk of stroke on medical treatment alone.

1. WHICH RANGE OF STENOSIS?

To target carotid endarterectomy appropriately, it is first necessary to determine as precisely as possible the overall effect of surgery and how it relates to the degree of carotid stenosis. There have been five randomized controlled trails (RCTs) of endarterectomy for symptomatic carotid stenosis (1–7). The first two were small and no longer reflect current practice (3,4). The larger VA trial [VA#309] 5 reported a non-significant trend in favor of surgery, but was stopped early when the two largest trials, ECST (1) and NASCET(2), reported their initial results. The analyses of these trials were stratified by the severity of stenosis of the symptomatic carotid artery, but different methods of measurement of the degree of stenosis on pre-randomization angiograms were used (Fig. 1), the NASCET method under-estimating stenosis as compared with the ECST method. Stenoses reported to be 70–99% in the NASCET were equivalent to 82–99% by the ECST method, and stenoses reported to be 70–99% by the ECST were 55–99% in the NASCET method (8).

In 1998, the ECST showed that there was no benefit from surgery in patients with [ECST]30–49% stenosis or [ECST]50–69% stenosis, but that there was a major benefit in patients with [ECST]70–99% stenosis (6). When the results of the ECST were stratified by decile of stenosis, endarterectomy was only beneficial in patients with [ECST]80–99% stenosis. The 11.6% absolute reduction in the risk of major stroke or death at 3 years was consistent with the 10.1% reduction in major stroke or death at 2 years reported in the NASCET in patients with [NASCET]70–99% stenosis (7). However, in contrast

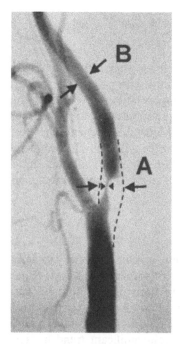

Figure 1 A selective arterial angiogram of the carotid bifurcation showing a 90% stenosis. To calculate the degree of stenosis, the lumen diameter at the point of maximum stenosis (A) was measured as the numerator in both the ECST and NASCET. However, the NASCET used the lumen diameter of the distal ICA (B) as the denominator, whereas the ECST used the estimated normal lumen diameter (dotted lines) at the point of maximum stenosis.

to the ECST, the NASCET reported a 6.9% ($P = 0.03$) absolute reduction in the risk of disabling stroke or death in patients with [NASCET]50–69% stenosis ([ECST]65–82% stenosis) (7).

Given this apparent disparity between the results of the trials, the ECST group re-analyzed their results such that they were comparable with the results of the NASCET (9). This required that the original ECST angiograms be re-measured by the method used in the NASCET and that outcome events be re-defined. Re-analysis of the ECST showed that endarterectomy had reduced the 5-year risk of *any stroke* or *surgical death* by 5.7% (95% CI: 0–11.6), in patients with [NASCET]50–69% stenosis ($n = 646$, $P = 0.05$) and by 21.2% (95% CI: 12.9–29.4) in patients with [NASCET]70–99% stenosis without 'near-occlusion' ($n = 429$, $P < 0.0001$) (9). Surgery was harmful in patients with <30% stenosis ($n = 1321$, $P = 0.007$) and of no benefit in patients with 30–49% stenosis ($n = 478$, $P = 0.6$). Thus, the results of the two trials were therefore consistent when analyzed in the same way. This allowed a pooled analysis of data from the ECST, NASCET, and VA#309 trials, which included over 95% of patients with symptomatic carotid stenosis ever randomized to endarterectomy vs. medical treatment (10).

The pooled analysis showed that there was no statistically significant heterogeneity between the trials in the effect of the randomized treatment allocation on the relative risks of any of the main outcomes in any of the stenosis groups. Data were therefore merged on 6092 patients with 35,000 patient-years of follow-up. The overall operative mortality was 1.1% (95% CI: 0.8–1.5), and the operative risk of stroke and death was 7.1% (95% CI: 6.3–8.1). The effect of surgery on the risks of the main trial outcomes is shown by the stenosis group in (Fig. 2). Endarterectomy reduced the 5-year absolute risk of *any stroke* or *death* in patients with [NASCET] 50–69% stenosis (ARR = 7.8%, 95% CI: 3.1–12.5) and was highly beneficial in patients with [NASCET] 70–99% stenosis (ARR = 15.3%, 95% CI: 9.8–20.7), but was of no benefit in patients with near-occlusion. The confidence intervals around the estimates of treatment effect in the near-occlusions were wide, but the difference in the effect of surgery between this group and patients with ≥70% stenosis without near-occlusion was highly significant statistically for each of the outcomes. Qualitatively similar results were seen for disabling stroke.

The results of these pooled analyses show that with the exception of near-occlusions, the degree of stenosis above which surgery is beneficial is [NASCET]50% (equivalent to about [ECST]65% stenosis). Given the confusion generated by the use of different methods of the measurement of stenosis in the original trials, it has been suggested that the NASCET method be adopted as the standard in future (10). There are several arguments in favor of the continued use of selective arterial angiography in the selection of patients for endarterectomy (11,12). However, if non-invasive techniques are used to select patients for surgery, then they must be properly validated

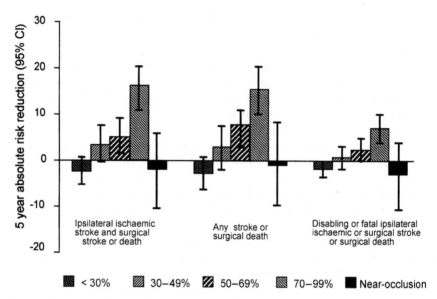

Figure 2 The effect of endarterectomy on the 5-year risks of each of the main trial outcomes in patients with <30% stenosis, 30–49% stenosis, 50–69% stenosis, ≥70% stenosis without near-occlusion, and in near-occlusions, in an analysis of pooled data from the ECST, NASCET, and VA#309 trials (10).

against catheter angiography within individual centers (13). More work is also required to assess the accuracy of non-invasive methods of carotid imaging in detecting near-occlusion (14,15).

2. WHAT ABOUT NEAR-OCCLUSIONS?

Near-occlusions were identified in the NASCET, because it is not possible to measure the degree of stenosis using the NASCET method in cases where the post-stenotic internal carotid artery (ICA) is narrowed or collapsed due to markedly reduced post-stenotic blood flow (16). Patients with 'abnormal post-stenotic narrowing' of the ICA were also identified in the ECST (17). In both trials, these patients had a paradoxically low risk of stroke on medical treatment (16,17). The low risk of stroke is most likely due to the presence of a good collateral circulation, which is visible on angiography in the vast majority of the patients with narrowing of the ICA distal to a severe stenosis (Fig. 3). The benefit from surgery in near-occlusions in the NASCET had been minimal,(16) and both the re-analysis of the ECST and the pooled analysis suggested no benefit at all in this group in terms of preventing stroke (9,10). Some patients with near-occlusion may still wish to undergo surgery, particularly if they experience recurrent TIAs. In the

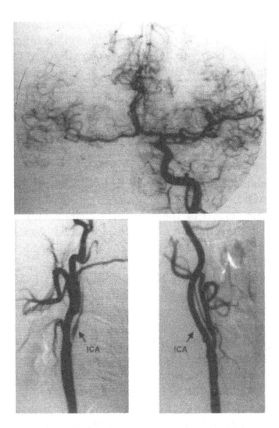

Figure 3 Selective arterial angiograms of both carotid circulations in a patient with a recently symptomatic carotid "near-occlusion" (left), and a mild stenosis at the contralateral carotid bifurcation (right). The near-occluded ICA is markedly narrowed, and flow of contrast into the distal ICA is delayed. After selective injection of contrast into the contralateral carotid artery, significant coilateral flow can be seen across the anterior communicating arteries with filling of the middle cerebral artery of the symptomatic hemisphere (top).

re-analysis of the ECST, endarterectomy did reduce the risk of recurrent TIA in patients with near-occlusion (absolute risk reduction 15%, $P = 0.007$) (9). However, patients should be informed that endarterectomy does not prevent stroke.

3. WHICH SUBGROUPS BENEFIT MOST?

The overall trial results are of only limited help to patients and clinicians in making decisions about surgery. Although endarterectomy reduces the relative risk of stroke by about 30% over the next 3 years in patients with a recently symptomatic severe stenosis, only 20% of such patients have a stroke on medical treatment alone. The operation is of no value in the other 80% of patients who, despite having a symptomatic stenosis, are destined to remain stroke-free without surgery and can only be harmed. It would, therefore, be useful to be able to identify in advance, and operate on, only those patients with a high risk of stroke on medical treatment alone, but a relatively low operative risk. The degree of stenosis is a major determinant of benefit from endarterectomy, but there are several other clinical and angiographic characteristics that might influence the risks and benefits of surgery, including the delay between symptoms and surgery (18).

The NASCET trial published 11 reports of different univariate subgroup analyses (Table 1) (16,19–28). Although interesting, the results are difficult to interpret because several of the subgroups contain only a few tens of patients, with some of the estimates of the effect of surgery based on only one or two outcome events in each treatment group, the 95% confidence intervals around the absolute risk reductions in each subgroup have generally not been given, and there have been no formal tests of the interaction between the subgroup variable and the treatment effect. It is, therefore, impossible to be certain whether differences in the effect of surgery between subgroups are real or due to chance.

Subgroup analyses of pooled data from ECST and NASCET have greater power to determine subgroup-treatment interactions reliably and several clinically important interactions were recently reported (29). Sex ($P=0.003$), age ($P=0.03$), and time from the last symptomatic event to randomization ($P=0.009$) modified the effectiveness of surgery (Fig. 4). Benefit from surgery was greatest in men, patients aged ≥ 75 years, and patients randomized within 2 weeks after their last ischemic event and fell rapidly with increasing delay. For patients with $\geq 50\%$ stenosis, the number of patients needed to undergo surgery (NNT) to prevent one ipsilateral stroke in 5 years was 9 for men vs. 36 for women, 5 for age ≥ 75 years vs. 18 for age <65 years, and 5 for patients randomized within 2 weeks after their last ischemic event vs 125 for patients randomized >12 weeks. These observations were consistent across the 50–69% and $\geq 70\%$ stenoses groups, and similar trends were present in both ECST and NASCET.

Women had a lower risk of ipsilateral ischemic stroke on medical treatment and a higher operative risk in comparison to men. For recently symptomatic carotid stenosis, surgery is very clearly beneficial in women with $\geq 70\%$ stenosis, but not in women with 50–69% stenosis (Fig. 4). In contrast, surgery reduced the 5-year absolute risk of stroke by 8.0% (3.4–12.5) in men with 50–69% stenosis. This sex difference was statistically significant even when the analysis of the interaction was confined to the 50–69% stenosis group. These same patterns were also shown in both of the large published trials of endarterectomy for asymptomatic carotid stenosis (30,31).

Table 1 The Univariate Subgroup Analyses of the Effect of Carotid Endarterectomy in Relation to Baseline Clinical Characteristics that have been published by NASCET

Subgroup	Patients (n) Medicine	Surgery	Follow-up (Years)	Treatment Effect ARR (95% CI)	Statistical Significance[a] Treatment Effect	Interaction
Clinical characteristics						
Age (19)			2			0.04
<65	143	160		9.7% (1.5–17.9)	<0.05	
65–74	144	141		15.1% (7.2–23.0)	<0.05	
75+	44	27		28.9% (12.9–44.9)	<0.05	
Ocular versus cerebral TIA (20)[b]			3			Not reported
Ocular TIA only	142	142		1.3% (not given)	Not reported	
Cerebral TIA	215	197		9.5% (not given)	Not reported	
Type of presenting event (21)			2			Not reported
Recent (for <6 months)	224	220		10.8% (not given)	0.02	
Recurrent (for >6 months)	74	90		30.4% (not given)	0.0003	
Type of presenting event (22)[b]			3			Not reported
Probable lacunar stroke	41	38		10% (not given)	0.53	
Possible lacunar stroke	57	69		8.5% (not given)	0.22	
Non-lacunar stroke	172	160		15.2% (not given)	0.002	
Leukoariosis on CT brain scan (23)[b]			3			Not reported
Widespread	36	36		11.6% (−9.6–32.8)	0.46	
Restricted	86	87		7.6% (−4.8–20.0)	0.39	
None	585	574		10.9% (6.7–15.1)	<0.001	
Angiographic characteristics						

(Continued)

Table 1 The Univariate Subgroup Analyses of the Effect of Carotid Endarterectomy in Relation to Baseline Clinical Characteristics that have been published by NASCET (*Continued*)

Subgroup	Patients (n) Medicine	Surgery	Follow-up (Years)	Treatment Effect ARR (95% CI)	Statistical Significance[a] Treatment Effect	Interaction
Ipsilateral plaque surface morphology (24)			2			
70–79% stenosis						Not reported
Ulcerated	Not given			19.4% (not given)	Not reported	
Not ulcerated	Not given			10.6% (not given)	Not reported	
80–89% stenosis						Not reported
Ulcerated	Not given			32.4% (not given)	Not reported	
Not ulcerated	Not given			10.7% (not given)	Not reported	
90–99% stenosis						Not reported
Ulcerated	Not given			54.0% (not given)	Not reported	
Not ulcerated	Not given			10.6% (not given)	Not reported	
Near-occlusion (16)			1			0.89
Yes	14		15	4.4% (not given)	Not reported	
String sign	44		33	9.2% (not given)	Not reported	
No string sign	141		130	8.2% (not given)	Not reported	
70–79%	110		127	9.8% (not given)	Not reported	
80–89%	22		23	26.4% (not given)	Not reported	
90–94%					Not reported	

Ipsilateral intracranial stenosis (25)	3					Not reported
70–84% stenosis						
Yes		Not given		22.7% (not given)	Not reported	
No		Not given		13.4% (not given)	Not reported	
85–89% stenosis						
Yes		Not given		37.1% (not given)	Not reported	
No		Not given		15.3% (not given)	Not reported	
Intracranial collateral blood flow towards the symptomatic hemisphere (26)	2					Not reported
Yes		111	136	5.4% (not given)	Not reported	
No		228	206	19.4% (not given)	Not reported	
Ipsilateral intracranial aneurysm (27)c	5					Not reported
Yes		23	25	12.7% (not given)	Not reported	
Contralateral ICA stenosis (28)	2					Not reported
Occlusion		22	21	57.3% (not given)	Not reported	
70–99% stenosis		32	25	20.0% (not given)	Not reported	
<70% stenosis		277	282	17.9% (not given)	Not reported	

aUnless otherwise stated, the outcome is the risk of ipsilateral ischemic stroke and operative stroke or death; analyses are by intention-to-treat; and analyses are confirmed to patients with 70–99% stenosis.
bAnalysis included 50–99% stenosis.
cAnalysis included all degress of stenosis.

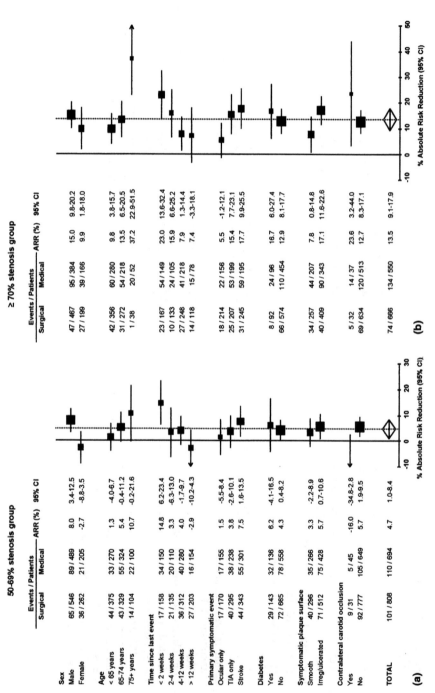

Figure 4 Absolute reduction with surgery in the 5-year risk of ipsilateral carotid territory ischemic stroke and any stroke or death within

Benefit from CEA increased with age in the pooled analysis of trials in patients with recently symptomatic stenosis, particularly in patients aged 75 years (Fig. 4). Although patients randomized in trials generally have a good prognosis (32), and there is some evidence of an increased operative mortality in elderly patients in routine clinical practice, particularly in those aged 85 years (33), a recent systematic review of all published surgical case-series reported no increase in the operative risk of stroke and death in older age groups (34). There is therefore no justification for withholding CEA in patients aged 75 years who are deemed to be medically fit to undergo surgery. The evidence suggests that benefit is likely to be greatest in this group because of their high risk of stroke on medical treatment. However, it is important to understand that it does take a year for overall benefit from surgery to accrue in patients with >70% stenosis and over 2 years in patients with 50–69% stenosis, and so elderly patients who are considered for surgery should ideally have a life expectancy that goes beyond these periods.

Benefit from surgery is probably also greatest in patients with stroke, intermediate in those with cerebral TIA, and lowest in those with retinal events (Fig. 4). There was also a trend in the trials towards greater benefit in patients with an irregular plaque than those with a smooth plaque.

4. HOW SOON SHOULD SURGERY BE PERFORMED?

The urgency with which endarterectomy should be performed has been much debated (35,36). The risk of stroke on medical treatment after a TIA or minor stroke is highest during the first few days and weeks (37,38), particularly in patients with carotid stenosis (39). However, the risk falls rapidly over the subsequent year (7,8), possibly because of the "healing" of the unstable atheromatous plaque or an increase in collateral blood flow to the symptomatic hemisphere, but there have been no reliable data on the extent to which the effectiveness of endarterectomy also falls with time. There has been concern that the operative risk may be increased if surgery is performed early, particularly in patients with major cerebral infarction or stroke-in-evolution (40,41). However, for neuroiogically stable patients, such as those enrolled into the trials, there was no evidence of any increase in operative risk in patients operated within 2 weeks of their last event (29). Moreover, in a systematic review of surgical case-series, early surgery in neurologically stable patients was not associated with an increased operative risk (42), although emergency surgery for stroke-in-evolution or crescendo TIA was associated with a markedly increased risk and is not advised.

Given the high early risk of stroke on medical treatment alone after a TIA or minor stroke in patients with carotid disease and the lack of an increased operative risk in neurologicaliy stable patients, early surgery is

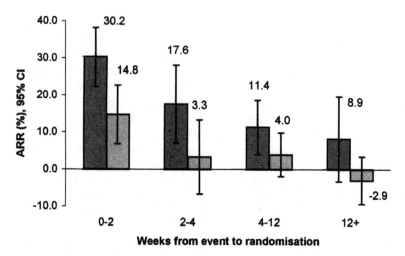

Figure 5 Absolute reduction with surgery in the 5-year risk of ipsilateral carotid territory ischemic stroke and any stroke or death within 30 days after trial surgery in
patients with 50–69% stenosis and 70% stenosis without near-occlusion stratified
by the time from last symptomatic event to randomization. The numbers above
the bars indicate the actual absolute risk reduction.

likely to be most effective. The pooled analysis of data from the trials
confirms this, showing that benefit from endarterectomy is greatest in
patients randomized within 2 weeks of their last event (Figs. 4 and 5). The
subgroup by treatment effect interaction with time from the last symptomatic event to randomization was highly significant ($P = 0.009$), and was
particularly important in patients with 50–69% stenosis, where the reduction
in the 5-year risk of stroke with surgery was considerable in those who were
randomized within 2 weeks of their last event (14.8%, 95% CI = 6.2–23.4),
but minimal in patients randomized later. Clinical guidelines currently state
that patients should be operated within 6 months of their presenting event
(43,44), and many patients wait for several months for surgery, but more
urgent intervention is clearly required.

5. WHICH INDIVIDUALS BENEFIT MOST?

There are some clinically useful subgroup observations in the pooled
analyses of the endarterectomy trials, but the results of univariate subgroup
analyses are often of only limited use in clinical practice. Individual patients
frequently have several important risk factors, each of which interacts in a
way that cannot be described using univariate subgroup analysis, and all
of which should be taken into account in order to determine the likely
balance of risk and benefit from surgery (18,29). For example, what would

be the likely benefit from surgery in a 78 year old (increased benefit) female (reduced benefit) with 70% stenosis who presented within 2 weeks (increased benefit) of an ocular ischemic event (reduced benefit) and was found to have an ulcerated carotid plaque (increased benefit)?

One way in which clinicians can weigh the often-conflicting effects of the important characteristics of an individual patient on the likely benefit from treatment is to base decisions on the predicted absolute risks of a poor outcome with each treatment option using prognostic models (18,45). Properly validated prognostic models are available to predict stroke risk in the general population (46), in patients with non-rheumatic atrial fibrillation (47,48), and in patients presenting with transient ischemic attacks (49,50). A model for predicting risk of stroke on medical treatment in patients with recently symptomatic carotid stenosis has been derived from the ECST (Table 2) (18,51). The model was validated using data from the NASCET and showed very good agreement between predicted and observed medical risk (Mantel-Haenszel $\chi^2_{Trend} = 41.3$, df= 1, $P < 0.0001$), reliably distinguishing between individuals with a 10% risk of ipsilateral ischemic stroke after 5 years follow-up and individuals with a risk of over 40% (Fig. 6) (51). Importantly, Fig. 6 also shows that the operative risk of stroke and death in patients who were randomized to surgery in NASCET was unrelated to the medical risk (Mantel-Haenszel $\chi^2_{Trend} = 0.98$, df = 1, $P = 0.32$). Thus, when the operative risk and the small additional residual risk of stroke following successful endarterectomy were taken into account, benefit from endarterectomy at 5 years varied significantly across the quintiles ($P=0.001$), with no benefit in patients in the lower three quintiles of predicted medical risk (ARR = 0 – 2%), moderate benefit in the fourth quintile (ARR = 10.8%, 95% CI = 1.0–20.6), and substantial benefit in the highest quintile (ARR = 32.0%, 95% CI = 21. 9–42.1).

Prediction of risk using models requires a computer, a pocket calculator with an *exponential* function, or internet access (the ECST model can be found at www.stroke.ox.ac.uk). As an alternative, a simplified risk score based on the hazard ratios derived from the relevant risk model can be derived. Table 2 shows a score for the 5-year risk of stroke on medical treatment in patients with recently symptomatic carotid stenosis derived from the ECST model. As is shown in the example, the total risk score is the product of the scores for each risk factor. Figure 7 shows a plot of the total risk score against the 5-year predicted risk of ipsilateral carotid territory ischemic stroke derived from the full model, and is used as a nomogram for the conversion of the score into a risk prediction.

Alternatively, risk tables allow a relatively small number of important variables to be considered and have the major advantage that they do not require the calculation of any score by the clinician or patient. Figure. 8 shows a risk table for the 5-year risk of ipsilateral ischemic stroke in patients with recently symptomatic carotid stenosis on medical treatment derived

Table 2 A Cox model for the 5-year risk of ipsilateral ischemic stroke on medical treatment in patients with recently symptomatic carotid stenosis derived from the ECST

Model				Scoring System[a]	
Risk Factor	HR (95% CI)	P-Value	Risk Factor	Score	Example
Stenosis (per 10%)	1.18 (1.10, 1.25)	<0.0001	Stenosis (%)		
			50–59	2.4	2.4
			60–69	2.8	
			70–79	3.3	
			80–89	3.9	
			90–99	4.6	
Near-occulusion	0.49 (0.19, 1.24)	0.1309	Near-occulusion	0.5	No
Male sex	1.19 (0.81, 1.75)	0.3687	Male sex	1.2	No
Algae (per 10 years)	1.12 (0.89, 1.39)	0.3343	Age (years)		
			31–40	1.1	
			41–50	1.2	
			51–60	1.3	
			61–70	1.5	1.5
			71–80	1.6	
			81–90	1.8	

	Hazard ratio (95% CI)	p-value		Score	Example
Time since last event (per 7 days)	0.96 (0.93, 0.99)	0.0039	Days since last event		8.7
			0–13	8.7	
			14–28	8.0	
			29–89	6.3	
			90–365	2.3	
Presenting event		0.0067	Presenting event		
Ocular	1.000		Ocular	1.0	
Single TIA	1.41 (0.75, 2.66)		Single TIA	1.4	
Multiple TIAs	2.05 (1.19, 3.60)		Multiple TIAs	2.0	
Minor stroke	1.82 (0.99, 3.34)		Minor stroke	1.8	
Major stroke	2.54 (1.48, 4.35)		Major stroke	2.5	2.5
Diabetes	1.35 (0.86, 2.11)	0.1881	Diabetes	1.4	1.4
Previous MI	1.57 (1.01, 2.45)	0.0471	Previous MI	1.6	No
PVD	1.18 (1.78, 1.77)	0.4368	PVD	1.2	No
Treated hypertension	1.24 (0.88, 1.75)	0.2137	Treated hypertension	1.2	1.2
Irregular/ulcerated plaque	2.03 (1.31, 3.14)	0.0015	Irregular/ulcerated plaque	2.0	2.0
			Total risk score		263
			Predicted risk using nomogram		37%

[a]Hazard ratios derived from the model are used for the scoring system. The score for the 5-year risk of stroke is the product of the individual scores for each of the risk factors present. The score is converted into a risk with the graphic in Fig. 7. An example is shown. Presenting event refers to the most "severe" event during the previous 6 months (stroke > TIA > ocular). Near-occlusions should be entered as 85% stenosis.

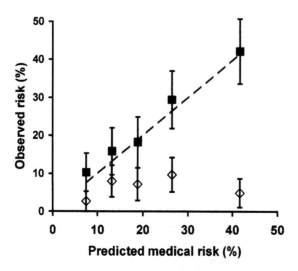

Figure 6 Validation of the ECST model (Table 2) for the 5-year risk of stroke on medical treatment in patients with 50–99% stenosis in NASCET (51). Predicted medical risk is plotted against observed risk of stroke in patients randomized to medical treatment in NASCET (squares) and against the observed operative risk of stroke and death in patients randomized to surgical treatment (diamonds). Groups are quintiles of predicted risk. Error bars represent 95% confidence intervals.

from the ECST model. The table is based on the five variables that were both significant predictors of risk in the ECST model (Table 2) and yielded clinically important subgroup–treatment effect interactions in the analysis of pooled data from the relevant trials (sex, age, time since last symptomatic event, type of presenting event(s), and carotid plaque surface morphology).

One potential problem with the ECST risk model is that it might over-estimate risk in current patients because of improvements in medical treatment, such as the increased use of statins. However, such improvements in treatment pose more problems for interpretation of the overall trial results than for the risk-modeling approach. For example, it would take only a relatively modest improvement in the effectiveness of medical treatment to erode the overall benefit of endarterectomy in patients with 50–69% stenosis. In contrast, very major improvements in medical treatment would be required in order to significantly reduce the benefit from surgery in patients in the high predicted-risk quintile in (Fig. 6). Thus, the likelihood that ancillary treatments have improved, and are likely to continue to improve, is an argument in favor of a risk-based approach to targeting treatment. However, it would be reasonable in a patient on treatment with a statin, for example, to reduce the risks derived from the risk model by 20% in relative terms.

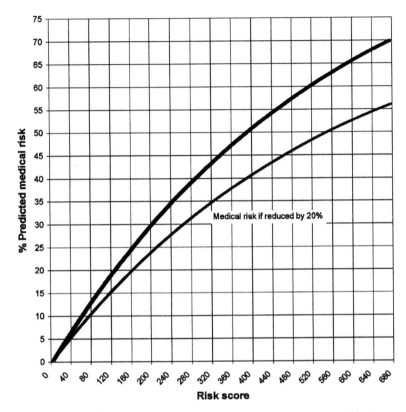

Figure 7 A plot of the total risk score derived from the table against the 5-year predicted risk of ipsilateral carotid territory ischemic stroke derived from the full model in the table in patients in the ECST (thick line). This should be used as a nomogram for the conversion of the score into a prediction of the percentage risk. The thin line represents a 20% reduction in risk as might be seen with more intensive medical treatment than was available in the ECST in the late 1980s and 1990s.

The risk model will also be useful in targeting angiopiasty and stenting, in which the main determinant of likely benefit in individuals is also the risk of stroke on medical treatment alone.

6. SUMMARY

We now have highly consistent, and reliable data on the degree of stenosis above which endarterectomy for symptomatic carotid stenosis is beneficial. There is a major benefit in patients with 70–99% stenosis, modest benefit in patients with 50–69% stenosis and, no evidence of benefit in patients with <50% stenosis or near-occlusion. However, benefit is also influenced by other factors, particularly age, sex, the timing of surgery, plaque surface

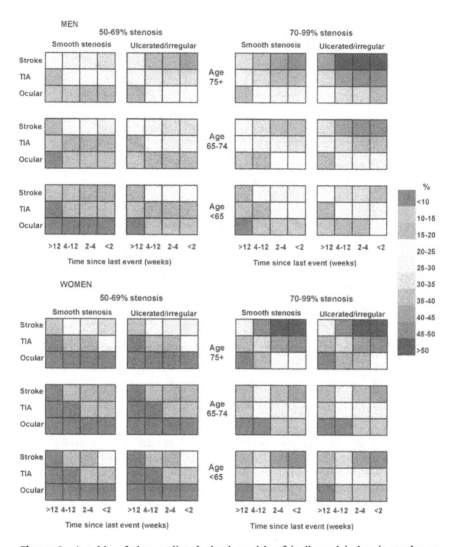

Figure 8 A table of the predicted absolute risk of ipsilateral ischemic stroke on medical treatment in ECST patients with recently symptomatic carotid stenosis derived from a Cox model based on six clinically important patient characteristics (51).

morphology, and the nature of the presenting symptomatic event. In order to take into account all of these different factors when considering the likely benefit from surgery in individual patients, it is necessary to use risk scores or prediction models.

REFERENCES

1. European Carotid Surgery Trialists' Collaborative Group. MRC European Carotid Surgery Trial. Interim results for symptomatic patients with severe (70–99%) or with mild (0–29%) carotid stenosis. Lancet 1991; 337:1235–1243.
2. North American Symptomatic Carotid Endarterectomy Trial Collaborators. Beneficial effect of carotid endarterectomy in symptomatic patients with high-grade carotid stenosis. N Engl J Med 1991; 325:445–453.
3. Fields WS, Maslenikov V, Meyer JS, Hass WK, Remington RD, MacDonald M. Joint study of extracranial arterial occlusion. V. Progress report on prognosis following surgery or non-surgical treatment for transient cerebral ischemic attacks and cervical carotid artery lesions. JAMA 1970; 211:1993–2003.
4. Shaw DA, Venables GS, Cartilidge NE, Bates D, Dickinson PH. Carotid endarterectomy in patients with transient cerebral ischaemia. J Neuroi Sci 1984; 64:45–53.
5. Mayberg MR, Wilson E, Yatsu F, Weiss DG, Messina L, Hershey LA, Colling C, Eskeridge J, Deykin D, Winn HR. Carotid endarterectomy and prevention of cerebral ischemia in symptomatic carotid stenosis. Veterans Affairs Cooperative Studies Program 309 Trialist Group. JAMA 1991; 266:3289–3294.
6. European Carotid Surgery Trialists' Collaborative Group: Randomised trial of endarterectomy for recently symptomatic carotid stenosis: final results of the MRC European Carotid Surgery Trial (ECST). Lancet 1998; 351:1379–1387.
7. North American Symptomatic Carotid Endarterectomy Trial Collaborators: Benefit of carotid endarterectomy in patients with symptomatic moderate or severe stenosis. N Engl J Med 1998; 339:1415–1425.
8. Rothwell PM, Gibson RJ, Slattery J, Sellar RJ, Warlow CP. Equivalence of measurements of carotid stenosis: a comparison of three methods on 1,001 angiograms. Stroke 1994; 25:2435–2439.
9. Rothwell PM, Gutnikov SA, Warlow CP. (for the ECST). Re-analysis of the final results of the European Carotid Surgery Trial. Stroke 2003; 34:514–523.
10. Rothwell PM, Eliasziw M, Gutnikov SA, Fox AJ, Taylor W, Mayberg MR, Warlow CP, Barnett HJ. (for the Carotid Endarterectomy Trialists' Collaboration). Pooled analysis of individual patient data from randomized controlled trials of endarterectomy for symptomatic carotid stenosis. Lancet 2003; 361:107–116.
11. Johnston DC, Goldstein LB. Clinical carotid endarterectomy decision making: non-invasive vascular imaging Vs. angiography. Neurology 2001; 56: 1009–1015.
12. Norris J, Rothwell PM. Noninvasive carotid imaging to select patients for endarterectomy: Is it really safer than conventional angiography? Neurology 2001; 56:990–991
13. Rothwell PM, Pendlebury ST, Wardlaw J, Warlow CP. Critical appraisal of the design and reporting of studies of imaging and measurement of carotid stenosis. Stroke 2000; 31:1444–1450.
14. Bermann SS, Devine JJ, Erdos LS, Hunter GC. Distinguishing carotid artery pseudo-occlusion with colour-flow Doppler. Stroke 1995; 26:434–438.

15. Ascher E, Markevich N, Hingorani A, Kallakuri S. Pseudo-occlusions of the internal carotid artery: a rationale for treatment on the basis of a modified duplex scan protocol. J Vase Surg 2002; 35:340–350.

16. Morgenstern LB, Fox AJ, Sharpe BL, Eliasziw M, Barnett HJ, Grotta JC (for the North American Symptomatic Carotid Endarterectomy Trial (NASCET) Group). The risks and benefits of carotid endarterectomy in patients with near-occlusion of the carotid artery. Neurology 1997; 48:911–915.

17. Rothwell PM, Warlow CP. (for the European Carotid Surgery Trialists' Collaborative Group). Low risk of ischemic stroke in patients with collapse of the internal carotid artery distal to severe carotid stenosis: Cerebral protection due to low post-stenotic flow? Stroke 2000; 31:622–630.

18. Rothweil PM, Warlow CP. (on behalf of the ECST Collaborators). Prediction of benefit from carotid endarterectomy in individual patients: A risk-modeling study. Lancet 1999; 353:2105–2110.

19. Alamowitch S, Eliasziw M, Algra A, Meldrum H, Barnett HJ. (for the North American Symptomatic Carotid Endarterectomy Trial (NASCET) Group). Risk, causes, and prevention of ischemic stroke in elderly patients with symptomatic internal carotid artery stenosis. Lancet 2001; 357;1154–1160.

20. Benavente O, Eliasziw M, Streifler JY, Fox AJ, Barnett HJ, Meldrum H (for the NASCET Collaborators). Prognosis after transient monocular blindness associated with carotid artery stenosis. N Engl J Med 2001; 345:1084–1090.

21. Paddock-Eliasziw LM, Eiiasziw M, Barr HW, Barnett HJ. (for the NASCET Group). Long-term prognosis and the effect of carotid endarterectomy in patients with recurrent ipsilateral ischemic events. Neurology 1996; 47:1158–1162.

22. Inzitari D, Eliasziw M, Shape BL, Fox AJ, Barnett HJ (for the NASCET Group). Risk factors and outcome of patients with carotid artery stenosis presenting with lacunar stroke. Neurology 2000; 54:660–666.

23. Streifler JY, Eliasziw M, Benavente OR, Alamowitch S, Fox AJ, Hachinski VC, Barnett HJ (for the NASCET Group). Prognostic importance of leukoaraiosis in patients with symptomatic internal carotid artery stenosis. Stroke 2002; 33:1651–1655.

24. Eliasziw M, Streifler JY, Fox AJ, Hachinski VC, Ferguson GG, Barnett HJ. Significance of plaque ulceration in symptomatic patients with high-grade carotid stenosis. North American Symptomatic Endarterectomy Trial. Stroke 1994; 25:304–308.

25. Kappelle LJ, Eliasziw M, Fox AJ, Sharpe BL, Barnett HJ (for the North American Symptomatic Carotid Endarterectomy Trial Group). Importance of intracranial atherosclerotic disease in patients with symptomatic stenosis of the internal carotid artery. Stroke 1999; 30:282–286.

26. Henderson RD, Eliasziw M, Fox AJ, Rothweil PM, Barnett HJ (for the NASCET Group). Angiographically defined collateral circulation and risk of stroke in patients with severe carotid artery stenosis. Stroke 2000; 31:128–132.

27. Kappelle LJ, Eliasziw M, Fox AJ, Barnett HJ (for the NASCET Group). Small, unruptured intracranial aneurysms and management of symptomatic carotid artery stenosis. Neurology 2000; 55:307–309.

28. Gasecki AP, Eliasziw M, Ferguson GG, Hachinski VC, Barnett HJ (for the NASCET Group). Long-term prognosis and effect of endarterectomy in

patients with symptomatic severe carotid stenosis and contralateral carotid stenosis or occlusion: Results from NASCET. J Neurosurg 1995; 83:778–782.

29. Rothweil PM, Eliasziw M, Gutnikov SA, Warlow CP, Barnett HJ (for the Carotid Endarterectomy Trialists' Collaboration). Endarterectomy for symptomatic carotid stenosis in relation to clinical subgroups and the timing of surgery Lancet 2004; 363:915–924.

30. Asymptomatic Carotid Atherosclerosis Study Group. Carotid endarterectomy for patients with asymptomatic internal carotid artery stenosis. JAMA 1995; 273:1421–1428.

31. Halliday A, Mansfield A, Marro J, Peto C, Peto R, Potter J, Thomas D MRC Asymptomatic Carotid Surgery Trial (ACST) Collaborative Group. Prevention of disabling and fatal strokes by successful carotid endarterectomy in patients without recent neurological symptoms: randomized controlled trial. Lancet 2004; 363:1491–1502.

32. Stiller CA. Centralised treatment, entry to trials and survival. Br J Cancer 1994; 70:352–362.

33. Wennberg DE, Lucas FL, Birkmeyer JD, Bredenberg CE, Fisher ES. Variation in carotid endarterectomy mortality in the Medicare population: trial hospitals, volume, and patient characteristics. JAMA 1998; 279:1278–1281.

34. Bond R, Rerkasem K, Rothweil PM. A systematic review of the associations between age and sex and the operative risks of carotid endarterectomy. Cerebrovascular Diseases. In press.

35. Pritz MB. Timing of carotid endarterectomy after stroke. Stroke 1997; 28: 2563–2567.

36. Golledge J, Cuming R, Beattie DK, Davies AH, Greenhalgh RM. Influence of patient-related variables on the outcome of carotid endarterectomy. J Vasc Surg 1996; 24:120–126.

37. Lovett J, Dennis M, Sandercock PAG, Bamford J, Wariow CP, Rothwell PM. The very early risk of stroke following a TIA. Stroke 2003; 34:e138–e140.

38. Coull A, Lovett JK, Rothwell PM (on behalf of the Oxford Vascular Study). Early risk of stroke after a TIA or minor stroke in a population-based incidence study. Br Med J 2004; 328:326–328.

39. Lovett JK, Coull A, Rothwell PM. Early risk of recurrent stroke by aetiological subtype: implications for stroke prevention. (on behalf of the Oxford Vascular Study). Neurology 2004; 62:569–574.

40. Blaisdell WF, Clauss RH, Galbraith JG, Imparato AM, Wylie EJ. Joint study of extracranial arterial occlusion, IV: a review of surgical considerations. JAMA 1969; 209:1889–1895.

41. Brandl R, Brauer RB, Maurer PC. Urgent carotid endarterectomy for stroke in evolution. Vasa 2001; 30:115–121.

42. Bond R, Rerkasem K, Rothwell PM. A systematic review of the risks of carotid endarterectomy in relation to the clinical indication and the timing of surgery. Stroke 2003; 34:2290–2301.

43. The Intercollegiate Working Party for Stroke. National Clinical Guidelines for Stroke. London: Royal College of Physicians, 2000.

44. Biller J, Feinberg WM, Castaldo JE, Whittemore AD, Harbaugh RE, Dempsey RJ, Caplan LR, Kresowik TF, Matchar DB, Toole JF, Easton JD, Adams HP,

Brass LM, Hobson RW, Brott G, Stemau L. Guidelines for carotid endarterectomy: a statement for healthcare professionals from a special writing group of the Stroke Council, American Heart Association. Circulaton 1998; 97:501–509.

45. Rothwell PM. Can overall results of clinical trials be applied to all patients? Lancet 1995; 345:1616–1619.

46. Nanchahal K, Duncan JR, Durrington PN, Jackson RT. Analysis of predicted coronary heart disease risk in England based on Framingham study risk appraisal models published in 1991 and 2000. Br Med J 2002; 325:194–195.

47. Laupacis A, Boysen G, Connolly S, et al. Risk factors for stroke and efficacy of antithrombotic therapy in atrial fibrillation. Analysis of pooled data from five randomized controlled trials. Arch Intern Med 1994; 154:1449–1457.

48. Pearce LA, Hart RG, Halpern JL. Assessment of three schemes for stratifying stroke risk in patients with non-valvular atrial fibrillation. Am J Med 2000; 109:45–51.

49. Hankey GJ, Slattery JM, Wariow CP. Transient ischemic attacks: which patients are at high (and low) risk of serious vascular events? J Neurol Neurosurg Psychiatry 1992; 55:640–652

50. Kernan WN, Viscoli CM, Brass LM, Makuch RW, Sarrel PM, Roberts RS, Gent M, Rothwell PM, Sacco R, Liu RC, Boden-Albala B, Horowitz Rl. The Stroke Prognosis Instrument II (SPIII): a clinical prediction instrument for patients with transient ischaemia and non-disabling ischemic stroke. Stroke 2000; 31:456–462.

51. Rothwell PM, Mehta Z, Howard SC, Gutnikov SA, Warlow CP. From subgroups to individuals: general principles and the example of carotid endartectomy. Lancet 2005; 365:256–265.

14

Management of Carotid Artery Disease: Carotid Endarterectomy for Asymptomatic Carotid Stenosis

Graeme J. Hankey

Stroke Unit, Department of Neurology, Royal Perth Hospital and School of Medicine and Pharmacology, University of Western Australia, Perth, Australia

Because up to 85% of all first-ever ischemic strokes are unheralded by "warning" transient ischemic attacks (TIAs), and about one-quarter of these are caused by carotid stenosis, it is likely that about one-fifth of all ischemic strokes can be attributed to carotid stenosis that was hitherto asymptomatic neurologically (1). If these asymptomatic carotid stenoses could be detected safely and cost-effectively *before* they become symptomatic, and removed safely and effectively by carotid endarterectomy or stenting, it is possible that many strokes could be prevented. But can we safely and cost-effectively identify neurologically asymptomatic carotid stenosis, quantify the risk of stroke that it affords, and balance the risks and benefits of screening for carotid stenosis and undertaking carotid endarterectomy to treat the carotid stenosis and reduce the risk of stroke?

1. DETECTING AND QUANTIFYING CAROTID ARTERY STENOSIS

Stenosis of the origin of the extracranial internal carotid artery (ICA) can be detected safely and non-invasively by duplex carotid ultrasound (U/S), computerized tomographic angiography (CTA), and magnetic resonance angiography (MRA) (2). The sensitivity and specificity of these techniques are not as optimal as invasive carotid artery imaging by catheter contrast angiography, but the latter carries up to a 1% risk of permanent disabling stroke (3). Furthermore, the methods of measuring the diameter of stenoses are also variable, and neither precise nor standardized throughout the world. Some investigators use the European Carotid Surgery Trial (ECST) method, others the North American Symptomatic Carotid Surgery Trial (NASCET) method, and others the common carotid artery method, as discussed in Chapter 10. Hence, measurements by different observers (and even the same observer) may vary considerably (4).

The circumstances under which carotid artery imaging studies are commonly performed in neurologically asymptomatic patients, and, hence, carotid stenosis is discovered, are:

- finding of a carotid bruit during general health checks;
- investigation (usually by carotid ultrasound or MRA) of patients with presumed symptoms of carotid territory brain or eye ischemia on the contralateral side;
- investigation (usually by angiography) of patients with symptoms of coronary heart disease and peripheral vascular disease;
- preoperative investigations (e.g., for vascular or general surgery).

2. PREVALENCE OF NEUROLOGICALLY ASYMPTOMATIC CAROTID STENOSIS

Atherosclerosis of the origin of the internal carotid artery, causing stenosis (narrowing) of the diameter of the lumen by 50% or more, is common, affecting about 0.5% of people in their sixth decade, to 3% in the seventh decade, 6% in the eighth decade, and 10% in people older than 80 years (5–7). In developed countries, this translates into 10% of men and 5–7% of women aged ≥65 years. In the Cardiovascular Health Study, carotid stenosis >50% was detected in 7% of men and 5% of women aged ≥65 years, and in the Framingham cohort, carotid stenosis ≥50% was detected in 9% of men and 7% of women aged 66–93 years (7,8).

3. PROGNOSIS OF ASYMPTOMATIC CAROTID STENOSIS

3.1. Prognosis for Stroke

Moderate-to-severe asymptomatic carotid stenosis (60–99% luminal obstruction) is associated with a low risk of *ipsilateral ischemic* stroke (which is what carotid endarterectomy can possibly prevent) of about 1–2% per year, and *any* stroke of about 2–3% per year, without carotid endarterectomy (9–13).

Mild-to-moderate asymptomatic carotid stenosis (<60% luminal obstruction) is associated with an even lower risk of *ipsilateral ischemic* stroke of about 0.5% per year (13).

The above annual risks of stroke in people with asymptomatic carotid stenosis remain stable during up to 15 years follow-up (13).

About half of the strokes among individuals with asymptomatic carotid stenosis are disabling. One-third of the strokes are due to intracranial small vessel disease (lacunar infarcts) or embolism from the heart, which are unlikely to be prevented by carotid endarterectomy (14,15).

3.2. Prognosis for Myocardial Infarction and Non-stroke Vascular Death

Individuals with asymptomatic carotid stenosis have a long-term risk of myocardial infarction and non-stroke vascular death of about 10% (95% CI: 4–16%) at 10 years, and 24% (95% CI: 14–34%) at 15 years (i.e., about 1–2% per year), which is at least as high, if not higher than, the risk of ipsilateral stroke (13).

4. PROGNOSTIC FACTORS

4.1. Stroke

It is difficult to predict the risk of stroke in patients with asymptomatic carotid stenosis. Baseline clinical characteristics have not been shown to predict the risk of stroke in long-term follow-up studies (13). There is some evidence that increasing degrees of asymptomatic carotid stenosis are associated with an increased risk of ipsilateral ischemic stroke, but this information is based on very small numbers of patients studied (13). Furthermore, there does not appear to be a relationship between plaque progression and risk of ipsilateral stroke (13).

The importance of carotid stenosis as a prognostic factor for stroke and other serious vascular events is clearly determined to some extent by other factors. One of these is whether the carotid stenosis has recently become unstable and active, causing focal neurological symptoms of a TIA or ischemic stroke. Symptomatic severe carotid stenosis (70–99%) has a risk of ipsilateral ischemic stroke of more than 7% per year (16,17). In addition to the severity of carotid stenosis and the presence or absence of neurological symptoms, other factors that have been associated with an increased risk of stroke, in the presence of carotid stenosis, include irregular plaque surface morphology, absence of angiographic collateral flow, impaired cerebral reactivity, a high frequency of transcranial Doppler-detected emboli to the brain, hypertension, and coronary heart disease (18–20). However, these associations need to be validated in other studies.

4.2. Myocardial Infarction and Non-stroke Vascular Death

In contrast to predicting stroke, there are several useful predictors of MI and non-stroke vascular death among individuals with neurologically asymptomatic carotid stenosis. The factors which each increase the risk of MI and non-stroke vascular death by at least 2-fold are increasing age (10 year increments), male sex, and diabetes mellitus, and asymptomatic carotid stenosis (13,17).

5. SURGICAL RISKS OF CAROTID ENDARTERECTOMY FOR ASYMPTOMATIC CAROTID STENOSIS

It is ironic that the precise purpose of carotid endarterectomy is to prevent stroke, and paradoxically its major potential complication is perioperative stroke. Other specific adverse effects of carotid endarterectomy, besides those inherent in any operation, include:

- lower cranial nerve palsy (about 5–9% of patients);
- peripheral nerve palsy (about 1% of patients);
- major neck hematoma requiring surgery or extended hospital stay (about 5–7% of patients); and
- wound infection (3%) (22).

5.1. Perioperative Stroke or Death

A systematic review of 57 studies, involving a total of 13,285 carotid endarterectomies, indicates that the perioperative risk of stroke and death varies widely from <1% to more than 30%, but is usually about 2–5%, and is on average 2.8% (95% CI: 2.4–3.2%) (23,24). This risk is significantly lower than the risk of operating on symptomatic carotid stenosis, for which the average risk of perioperative stroke or death is 5.1% [(95% CI: 4.6–5.6%), odds ratio (OR) 1.62 (95% CI: 1.45–1.81)] (23,25,26).

Based on these data, one in 36 patients undergoing carotid endarterectomy for asymptomatic carotid stenosis experiences a perioperative stroke or dies in the perioperative period. However, this risk cannot be generalized from the literature to one's own institution, surgeons, or patients. A local prospective audit of a large number of patients undergoing carotid endarterectomy is required, and referring doctors (and patients) should have access to the perioperative stroke and death rate of their prospective surgeon(s), derived from such an independent and rigorous audit (24,27). However, interpretation of unusually high or low operative risks must take into account the effects of chance and case-mix (28). Otherwise, over-simplistic interpretation of crude results may lead to unjustified criticism of individual surgeons, and not to improvements in patient care. The decision to operate should be taken after considering all the important prognostic factors for stroke and perioperative stroke and death.

5.2. Prognostic Factors for Perioperative Stroke or Death

There is little reliable data in patients with asymptomatic carotid stenosis, but among patients undergoing carotid endarterectomy for symptomatic carotid stenosis, the risks of perioperative stroke and death are highly dependent on several patient and surgical factors.

5.2.1. Patient Factors

As stated above, the risks of perioperative stroke are greater in patients with symptomatic carotid stenosis than asymptomatic carotid stenosis, but it is not as simple as that. Patients with *symptoms* of ocular ischemia due to carotid stenosis (e.g., amaurosis fugax) have a non-significantly *lower* risk of perioperative stroke or death than patients undergoing carotid endarterectomy for asymptomatic carotid stenosis (23).

Other patient factors which have been associated with an increased risk of perioperative stroke and death in trials of carotid endarterectomy for symptomatic carotid stenosis (and which may be valid for patients undergoing carotid endarterectomy for asymptomatic stenosis) are:

- female gender (perhaps because of smaller carotid arteries; perhaps more difficult to operate on);
- systolic blood pressure >180mmHg (perhaps increased risk of reperfusion injury and cerebral hemorrhage);
- peripheral arterial disease (a marker of atherosclerotic plaque burden);
- occlusion of the contralateral internal carotid artery (indicates poor collateral cerebral circulation);
- stenosis of the ipsilateral external carotid artery (poor collateral circulation) (29); the risk of perioperative stroke or death associated with carotid endarterectomy does not appear to be related to the degree of ipsilateral internal carotid stenosis; and
- poor intracranial collaterals (anterior communicating artery).

5.2.2. Surgical Factors

The surgical factors which may be associated with an increased risk of perioperative stroke or death are inexperience of the surgeon and low hospital case volumes (30), undertaking carotid endarterectomy in the very acute phase of stroke in evolution and crescendo TIAs (23), and during coronary artery surgery for patients with angina whose carotid stenosis was discovered during preparation for coronary artery surgery.

5.3. Prognostic Factors for Perioperative Cranial Nerve Palsy

Patients undergoing carotid endarterectomy for recurrent carotid stenosis have an increased risk of cranial nerve injury and wound hematoma (23).

The risk of functionally disabling bilateral vagal and hypoglossal nerve palsies is increased in patients who have already had an endarterectomy on one side or are undergoing bilateral carotid endarterectomies.

6. BALANCE OF BENEFITS AND RISKS (EFFECTIVENESS) OF CAROTID ENDARTERECTOMY FOR NEUROLOGICALLY ASYMPTOMATIC CAROTID STENOSIS—EVIDENCE FROM UNCONFOUNDED RANDOMIZED CONTROLLED TRIALS

There have been five unconfounded published randomized controlled trials (RCTs) of carotid endarterectomy vs. best medical therapy for patients with neurologically asymptomatic carotid stenosis—the Walter Reed Army Centre Study (WRAMC) (31), the Mayo Asymptomatic Carotid Endarterectomy Study (MACE) (32), the Veterans Affairs Cooperative Study (VA) (33), and the Asymptomatic Carotid Atherosclerosis Study (ACAS) (34). The Carotid Artery Stenosis with Asymptomatic Narrowing: Operation Vs. Aspirin (CASANOVA) study (35) was not included in these analyses because the randomization process was complicated, precluding direct comparison of the results with the other four studies (36,37). The fifth trial, the Asymptomatic Carotid Surgery Trial (ACST), was recently published with interim 5-year results (38).

The ACST trial will be discussed below, but the first four unconfounded randomized trials will be reviewed first. In two trials, all patients received best medical therapy (including aspirin) (33,34), and in two trials aspirin was only given to patients allocated to the medical group (31,32). Three of the trials measured the degree of carotid stenosis by the same method as the NASCET trial (17). The method of angiographic measurement of the degree of carotid stenosis was not defined in the WRAMC trial (31); patients were randomized on the basis of cervical bruits and abnormal oculoplethysmography (OPG), but angiography was then performed in those randomized to carotid endarterectomy.

A total of 2203 patients were randomized (males 1614; females 592). The mean age was about 66 years. The mean duration of follow-up varied from 23.6 to 47.9 months. Overall, there were 6473 person-years of follow-up. There were no patients lost to follow-up in WRAMC or MACE, and only three patients (0.2%) lost to follow-up and excluded from the analysis in ACAS. In the VA trial, however, 35 patients (7.9% overall; 20 patients allocated carotid endarterectomy and 15 medical therapy) withdrew or were lost to follow-up, but substantial follow-up data were available for these patients. Outcomes were assessed by a neurologist, and a blinded review committee adjudicated on outcomes in three of the trials (except WRAMC).

6.1. Risks of Perioperative Stroke or Death

Among patients allocated carotid endarterectomy, the perioperative stroke or death rate was 3.1%, compared with 0.4% among patients allocated best medical therapy alone and followed-up for the same time period (36). This is a relative risk of 6.5 (95% CI: 2.7–16.0, $P < 0.0001$) and an absolute risk excess of 2.7% (Table 1). These data include complications from any angiography performed after, but not before, randomization. Based on these data, one in 37 patients experiences a perioperative stroke or death (36).

6.2. Perioperative Stroke, Death, or Subsequent Ipsilateral Stroke

Among patients allocated carotid endarterectomy, the rate of perioperative stroke or death or subsequent ipsilateral stroke over the 2–4 years of follow-up was 4.9%, compared with 6.8% among patients allocated best medical therapy alone. This is a relative risk of 0.73 (95% CI: 0.52–1.02, $P=0.06$) and an absolute risk reduction of 1.9% over a mean follow-up of almost 3 years. Based on these data, the number of patients with asymptomatic carotid stenosis who need to be treated with carotid endarterectomy to prevent one ipsilateral stroke over the next 3 years is about 53.

6.3. Any Stroke or Perioperative Death

Among patients allocated carotid endarterectomy, the rate of any stroke or perioperative death over the 2–4 years of follow-up was 8.1%, compared with 10.4% among patients allocated best medical therapy alone. This is a relative risk of 0.79 and an absolute risk reduction of 2.3% over a mean follow-up of almost 3 years. Based on these data, the number of patients with asymptomatic carotid stenosis who need to be treated with carotid endarterectomy to prevent one stroke or perioperative death over the next 3 years is about 43.

6.4. Any Stroke or Death

Among patients allocated carotid endarterectomy, the rate of any stroke or death over the 2–4 years of follow-up was 20.2%, compared with 23.2% among patients allocated best medical therapy alone. This is a relative risk of 0.89 (95% CI: 0.76–1.04; $P=0.13$), and an absolute risk reduction of 3.0% over a mean follow-up of almost 3 years. Based on these data, the number of patients with asymptomatic carotid stenosis who need to be treated with carotid endarterectomy to prevent one stroke or death over the next 3 years is about 33. There was a negligible change in the results after omitting the two trials in which aspirin was given only to patients in the medical group.

7. ASYMPTOMATIC CAROTID SURGERY TRIAL

The ACST is the largest and most recently published of the randomized studies pertaining to carotid endarterectomy for asymptomatic stenosis (38). The ACST was a randomized study of immediate carotid endarterectomy vs. indefinite deferral of carotid endarterectomy at 126 centers in 30 countries. Stenosis was measured by carotid ultrasound and expressed as the percentage of diameter reduction. Eligibility included carotid artery diameter reduction of at least 60% on ultrasound and no symptoms within the past 6 months. Enrollment began in 1993 and continued until 2003 and a 10-year follow-up is planned. A total of 3120 patients were randomized, 1560 into each group.

Surgeons were required to provide evidence of an operative risk of 6% or less for their last 50 patients having an endarterctomy for asymptomatic stenosis, but in contrast to ACAS, none were excluded on the basis of their operative risk during the trial. Selection of patients was based on the "uncertainty principle", with very few exclusion criteria and with stenosis assessed by Doppler ultrasonography. There was neither an evaluation of the ultrasonographer's training nor a centralized audit of their performance (38,39). Medical treatment was fairly aggressive in ACST. By 2002–2003, 90% were

Table 1 Summary of the Net Effects of Carotid Endarterectomy for Asymptomatic Carotid Stenosis (36)

Outcome event	Intervention		Relative risk (95% CI)	Absolute risk change (%)	NNT
	Medical (%)	Carotid surgery (%)			
Perioperative stroke or death	0.4	3.1	6.5 (2.7–16.0)	+2.7	37[a]
Perioperative stroke, death, or ipsilateral stroke	6.8	4.9	0.73 (0.52–1.02)	−1.9	53[b]
Any stroke or perioperative death	10.4	8.1	0.79 (0.52–1.02)	−2.3	43[b]
Any stroke or death	23.2	20.2	0.89 (0.76–1.04)	−2.3	33[b]

[a]Indicates that for every 37 patients who underwent carotid endarterectomy for asymptomatic carotid stenosis in these trials, one patient experienced a perioperative stroke or death.
[b]Indicates the number of patients with asymptomatic carotid stenosis who need to be treated with carotid endarterectomy to prevent one outcome event over the next 3 years.

on antiplatelet therapy, 81% on antihypertensives, and 70% on lipid-lowering treatment.

Despite the differences in methods, the results of ACST and ACAS were quite similar. Although the 5-year risk of any stroke or perioperative death in the non-surgical group was lower in ACST (11.8%) than in ACAS (17.5%), the absolute reductions in 5-year risk with surgery were not substantially different (5.4%, 95% CI: 3.0–7.8% vs. 5.1%, 95% CI: 0.9–9.1%, respectively). The main differences between the trials were in the 30-day operative risks of death (0.14%, 95% CI: 0–0.4% in ACAS vs. 1.11%, 95% CI: 0.6–1.8% in ACST; $P=0.02$), and stroke and death combined (1.5%, 95% CI: 0.6–2.4% in ACAS vs. 3.0%, 95% CI: 2.1–4.0% in ACST; $P=0.04$). Combining the perioperative events (stroke and death within 30 days) and the non-perioperative strokes in ACST, the net 5-year risks were 6.4% (immediate carotid endarterectomy) vs. 11.8% (deferred carotid endarterectomy) for all strokes [net gain 5.4% (95% CI, 3.0–7.8) $P<0.0001$].

Apart from replicating the results of ACAS in a more pragmatic setting, what else have the results of ACST added? In ACAS, there was a non-significant ($P=0.26$) 2.7% reduction in the absolute risk of disabling or fatal stroke with surgery. The ACST reported a statistically significant ($P=0.004$) 2.5% (95% CI: 0.8–4.3%) absolute reduction. This observation is important because carotid endarterectomy is a potentially dangerous intervention and having a precise assessment of its benefits in terms of those outcomes that are of most importance to patients is essential before surgery is recommended to otherwise healthy asymptomatic individuals. The ACST has provided this evidence (although the number to treat to prevent one disabling or fatal stroke after 5 years remains about 40).

In contrast to the results of randomized trials of endarterectomy for symptomatic stenosis (40), neither ACST nor ACAS showed an increasing benefit from surgery with an increasing degree of stenosis within the 60–99% range. This counter-intuitive observation was assumed to be due to a lack of statistical power in ACAS, but cannot be dismissed with the additional data provided by ACST. Part of the explanation may be that measurement of the exact degree of stenosis is less accurate with Doppler ultrasound scanning than with catheter angiography. For example, neither ACAS nor ACST identified near-occlusions—situations in which there is very low post-stenotic flow associated with distal narrowing or collapse of the ICA (40,41). This is paradoxically associated with a low risk of stroke on medical treatment in both symptomatic (40,41) and asymptomatic patients (42), and no clear benefit from endarterectomy (at least in symptomatic cases) (40). The prevalence of near-occlusions on angiography increases with the degree of stenosis, and in the pooled analysis of the randomized trials of endarterectomy for symptomatic carotid stenosis, the higher proportion of near-occlusions in the upper deciles of stenoses diluted the benefit of endarterectomy, and a clear increase in benefit with degrees of stenosis between 70 and 99% was only apparent when near-occlusions were analyzed separately (40).

Although some subgroup analyses were reported in ACAS, the trial had insufficient power to reliably analyze subgroup–treatment effect interactions. Because of its larger sample size, ACST had greater power to evaluate subgroups, although no analyses were pre-specified in detail in the trial protocol (39). The ACST did perform some subgroup analyses, but only reported results for the reduction in risk of non-perioperative stroke (i.e., the benefit) and the perioperative risk (i.e., the harm) separately (38). The overall balance of hazard and benefit, which is of most importance to patients and clinicians, was not reported, although the data can be extracted from the web-tables that accompanied the ACST report. Sex-based differences in the overall results of endarterectomy are of particular interest. Due to a higher operative risk in women and a lower risk of stroke without surgery, carotid endarterectomy for *symptomatic* stenosis is less beneficial for 70–99% stenosis in women than in men, and of no benefit in women with 50–69% stenosis (overall interaction: $P=0.003$) (43). The same trend was found in ACAS, with a statistically borderline sex–treatment effect interaction. Figure 1 shows a meta-analysis of the effect of endarterectomy on the 5-year risk of any stroke and perioperative death in ACAS and ACST. Surgical benefit is greater in men than in women (pooled interaction $P=0.01$), and it remains uncertain whether there is any worthwhile benefit at all in women. Subgroup analyses can be unreliable, and the overall benefit from surgery might well accrue in women with longer follow-up, as is planned

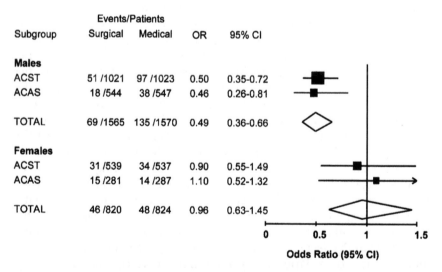

Figure 1 The effect of endarterectomy for asymptomatic carotid stenosis on the risk of any stroke and operative death by sex in the ACST and the ACAS.

for the ACST, but current evidence does not appear to justify the high rates of CEA for asymptomatic stenosis in women in some countries.

8. HOW SHOULD NEUROLOGICALLY ASYMPTOMATIC CAROTID STENOSIS BE MANAGED?

8.1. Screening

Given the low prevalence of severe carotid stenosis in the general population, routine screening (and treatment) of asymptomatic people for carotid stenosis is not recommended because it is likely to be very costly and, more importantly, result in more perioperative strokes than it prevents (44).

8.2. Assessment of the Likely Net Effectiveness of Carotid Endarterectomy for an Individual Patient

The data from randomized controlled trials indicate that for most people with asymptomatic carotid stenosis, the balance of risk and benefit from carotid surgery is quite even overall, and may not favor carotid surgery until several years have passed, and even then the absolute benefit is small.

For an individual patient in whom asymptomatic carotid stenosis has been detected, the net effectiveness of carotid endarterectomy is determined by the following:

- The patient's absolute risk of an ipsilateral carotid-territory ischemic stroke (which can be prevented by carotid endarterectomy): This is generally about 1–2% per year, but may be higher in the presence of irregular plaque surface morphology, impaired collateral flow, and cerebral perfusion reserve.
- The surgical perioperative stroke and death rate: The benefit of carotid endarterectomy for asymptomatic carotid stenosis is also highly dependent on the surgical risk. This is about 3% on average in other centers, and likely to be higher in women, and patients with systolic hypertension, peripheral arterial disease, and occlusion of the contralateral internal carotid artery and ipsilateral external carotid artery. However, the experience of the surgeon and hospital are also crucial factors, and the results of a recent prospective audit of local surgical perioperative stroke and death rates should be widely available.
- The patient's risk of other disabling and fatal events, and life-expectancy.
- The cost of the diagnostic assessment, carotid endarterectomy, and post-operative care (45,46).

- The cost of the adverse outcomes of carotid endarterectomy (perioperative stroke or death, cranial nerve palsy, wound infection, or hematoma).
- The cost of the favorable outcomes of carotid endarterectomy [strokes (non-disabling, disabling, fatal) prevented].
- The generalizability of the results of the trials of carotid endarterectomy to all patients with asymptomatic carotid stenosis and all surgeons performing carotid endarterectomy.
- The effectiveness compared with best medical therapy alone, and compared with best medical therapy combined with other alternative strategies of recanalizing the carotid stenosis, such as carotid angioplasty and stenting.

9. SUMMARY

Carotid endarterectomy is rarely indicated for asymptomatic severe carotid stenosis because of the small absolute benefit. About 40 patients need to undergo the risk, inconvenience, and cost of a carotid endarterectomy in order to prevent one major stroke at 5 years. Although the risk of perioperative stroke or death from carotid endarterectomy for people with asymptomatic carotid stenosis seems to be lower (~3%) than for people with symptomatic carotid stenosis (generally about 6–8%), the risk of stroke or death without carotid surgery in neurologically asymptomatic people is substantially lower. The disease and the operation are both quite benign. Therefore, for most people, the balance of risk and benefit from carotid surgery is quite even overall, and may not favor carotid surgery until several years have passed, and that only in a small minority of patients.

REFERENCES

1. Sandercock PAG, Warlow CP, Jones LN, Starkey I. Pre-disposing factors for cerebral infarction: the Oxfordshire Community Stroke Project. Br Med J 1989; 298:75–80.
2. Norris JW, Rothwell PM. Noninvasive carotid imaging to select patients for endarterectomy. Is it really safer than conventional angiography? Neurology 2001; 56:990–901.
3. Hankey GJ, Warlow CP, Sellar RJ. Cerebral angiographic risk in mild cerebrovascular disease. Stroke 1990; 21:209–222.
4. Rothwell PM, Gibson RJ, Slattery JM, Sellar RJ, Warlow CP. Equivalence of measurements of carotid stenosis: a comparison of three methods of 1001 angiograms. Stroke 1994; 25:2435–2439.
5. Ricci S, Flamini FO, Celani MG, Marini M, Antonini D, Bartolini S, Ballatori E. Prevalence of internal carotid stenosis in subjects older than 49 years: a population study. Cerebrovasc Dis 1991; 1:16–19.

6. Prati P, Vanuzzo D, Casaroli M, Di Chiara A, De Biasi F, Feruglio GA, Touboul PJ. Prevalence and determinants of carotid atherosclerosis in a general population. Stroke 1992; 23:1705–1711.
7. O'Leary DH, Polak JF, Kronmal RA, Kittner SJ, Bond MG, Wolfson SK, Bommer W Jr, Price TR, Gardin JM, Savage PJ. Distribution and correlates of sonographically detected carotid artery disease in the Cardiovascular Health Study: the CHS Collaborative Research Group. Stroke 1992; 23:1752–1760.
8. Fine-Edelstein JS, Wolf PA, O'Leary DH, Poehlman H, Belanger AJ, Kase CS, D'Agostino RB. Precursors of extracranial carotid atherosclerosis in the Framingham Study. Neurology 1994; 44:1046–1050.
9. Norris JW, Zhu CZ, Bornstein NM, Chambers BR. Vascular risks of asymptomatic carotid stenosis. Stroke 1991; 22:1485–1490.
10. Ogren M, Hedblad B, Isacsson S-O, Janzon L, Jungquist G, Lindell S-E. Ten year cerebrovascular morbidity and mortality in 68 year old men with asymptomatic carotid stenosis. Br Med J 1995; 310:1294–1298.
11. Hobson RW, Weiss DG, Fields WS, Goldstone J, Moore WS, Towne JB, Wright CB, and the Veterans Affairs Cooperative Study Group. Efficacy of carotid endarterectomy for asymptomatic carotid stenosis. N Engl J Med 1993; 328:221–227.
12. Executive Committee for the Asymptomatic Carotid Atherosclerosis Study. Endarterectomy for asymptomatic carotid stenosis. JAMA 1995; 273: 1421–1428.
13. Nadareishvili ZG, Rothwell PM, Beletsky V, Pagniello A, Norris JW. Long-term risk of stroke and other vascular events in patients with asymptomatic carotid artery stenosis. Arch Neurol 2002; 59:1162–1166.
14. Barnett HJM, Gunton RW, Eliasziw M, Fleming L, Sharpe B, Gates P, Meldrum H. Causes and severity of ischemic stroke in patients with internal carotid artery stenosis. JAMA 2000; 283:1429–1436.
15. Inzitari D, Eliasziw M, Gates P, Sharpe BL, Chan RKT, Meldrum HE, Barnett HJM (for the North American Symptomatic Carotid Endarterectomy Trial Group). The causes and risk of stroke in patients with asymptomatic internal-carotid-artery stenosis. N Engl J Med 2000; 342:1693–1700.
16. Barnett HJM, Taylor DW, Eliasziw M, Fox AJ, Ferguson GG, Haynes RB, Rankin RN, Clagett GP, Hachinski VC, Sackett DL, Thorpe KE, Meldrum HE (for the North American Symptomatic Carotid Endarterectomy Trial collaborators). Benefit of carotid endarterectomy in patients with symptomatic moderate or severe carotid stenosis. N Engl J Med 1998; 339:1415–1425.
17. European Carotid Surgery Trialists' Collaborative Group. Randomized trial of endarterectomy for recently symptomatic carotid stenosis: final results of the MRC European Carotid Surgery Trial (ECST). Lancet 1998; 351:1379–1387.
18. Rothwell PM, Warlow CP. Prediction of benefit from carotid endarterectomy in individual patients: a risk-modelling study. Lancet 1999; 353:2105–2110.
19. Dippel DWJ, Koudstaal PH, van Urk H, Habbema JDF, van Gijn J, Slattery J, Rothwell PM, Warlow CP, (on behalf of the European Carotid Surgery Trialists' Collaborative Group). After successful endarterectomy for symptomatic carotid stenosis, should any contralateral but asymptomatic carotid stenosis be operated on as well? Cerebrovasc Dis 1997; 7:34–42.

20. Mackey AE, Abrahamowicz M, Langlois Y, Battista R, Simard D, Bourque F, Leclerc J, Cote R and the Asymptomatic Cervical Bruit Study Group. Outcome of asymptomatic patients with carotid disease. Neurology 1997; 48: 896–903.

21. Chimowitz MI, Weiss DG, Cohen SL, Starling MR, Hobson RW, and the Veterans Affairs Cooperative Study 167. Cardiac prognosis of patients with carotid stenosis and no history of coronary artery disease. Stroke 1994; 25:759–765.

22. CAVATAS investigators. Endovascular vs. surgical treatment in patients with carotid artery stenosis in the Carotid and Vertebral Artery Transluminal Angioplasty Study (CAVATAS): a randomised trial. Lancet 2001; 357:1729–1737.

23. Bond R, Rerkasem K, Rothwell PM. Systematic review of the risks of carotid endarterectomy in relation to the clinical indication for and timing of surgery. Stroke 2003; 34:2290–2303.

24. Rothwell PM, Warlow CP. Is self-audit reliable? Lancet 1995; 346:1623.

25. Rothwell PM, Slattery J, Warlow CP. A systematic comparison of the risk of stroke and death due to carotid endarterectomy. Stroke 1996; 27:260–265.

26. Rothwell PM, Slattery J, Warlow CP. A systematic comparison of the risk of stroke and death due to carotid endarterectomy for symptomatic and asymptomatic carotid stenosis. Stroke 1996; 27:266–269.

27. Goldstein LB, Moore WS, Robertson JT, et al. Complication rates for carotid endarterectomy: a call for action. Stroke 1997; 28:889–890.

28. Rothwell PM, Warlow CP (on behalf of the European Carotid Surgery Trialists' Collaborative Group). Interpretation of operative risks of individual surgeons. Lancet 1999; 353:1325.

29. Rothwell P, Slattery J, Warlow C. Clinical and angiographic predictors of stroke and death from carotid endarterectomy: systematic review. Br Med J 1997; 315:1571–1577.

30. Feasby TE, Quan H, Ghali WA. Hospital and surgeon determinants of carotid endarterectomy outcomes. Arch Neurol 2002; 59:1877–1881.

31. Clagett GP, Youkey JR, Brigham RA, Orecchia PM, Salander JM, Collins GJ Jr, Rich NM. Asymptomatic cervical bruit and abnormal ocular pneumoplethysmography: a prospective study comparing two approaches to management. Surgery 1984; 96:823–830.

32. Mayo Asymptomatic Carotid Endarterectomy Study Group. Results of a randomised controlled trial of carotid endarterectomy for asymptomatic carotid stenosis. Mayo Clin Proc 1992; 67:513–518.

33. Hobson RW, Weiss DG, Fields WS, Goldstone J, Moore WS, Towne JB, Wright CB, and the Veterans Affairs Cooperative Study Group. Efficacy of carotid endarterectomy for asymptomatic carotid stenosis. N Engl J Med 1993; 328:221–227.

34. Executive Committee for the Asymptomatic Carotid Atherosclerosis Study. Endarterectomy for asymptomatic carotid stenosis. JAMA 1995; 273: 1421–1428.

35. The CASANOVA Study Group. Carotid surgery versus medical therapy in asymptomatic carotid stenosis. Stroke 1991; 22:1229–1235.

36. Chambers BR, You RX, Donnan GA. Carotid endarterectomy for asymptomatic carotid stenosis (Cochrane Review). In: The Cochrane Library, Issue 3. Oxford: Update Software, 2003.
37. Benavente O, Moher D, Pham B. Carotid endarterectomy for asymptomatic carotid stenosis: a meta-analysis. Br Med J 1998; 317:1477–1480.
38. MRC Asymptomatic Carotid Surgery Trial (ACST) Collaborative Group. Prevention of disabling and fatal strokes by successful carotid endarterectomy in patients without recent neurological symptoms: randomised controlled trial. Lancet 2004; 363:1491–1502.
39. Halliday AW, Thomas D, Mansfield A. The Asymptomatic Carotid Surgery Trial (ACST). Rationale and design. Eur J Vasc Surg 1994; 8:703–710.
40. Rothwell PM, Eliasziw M, Gutnikov SA, Fox AJ, Taylor DW, Mayberg MR, Warlow CP, Barnett HJ. Analysis of pooled data from the randomised controlled trials of endarterectomy for symptomatic carotid stenosis. Lancet 2003; 361:107–116.
41. Rothwell PM, Warlow CP. Low risk of ischaemic stroke in patients with collapse of the internal carotid artery distal to severe carotid stenosis: cerebral protection due to low post-stenotic flow? Stroke 2000; 31:622–630.
42. Norris JW, Zhu CZ. Stroke risk and critical carotid stenosis. J Neurol Neurosurg Psychiatr 1990; 53:235–237.
43. Rothwell PM, Eliasziw M, Gutnikov SA, Warlow CP, Barnett HJM. Effect of endarterectomy for symptomatic carotid stenosis in relation to clinical subgroups and to the timing of surgery. Lancet 2004; 363:915–924.
44. Whitty C, Sudlow C, Warlow C. Investigating individual subjects and screening populations for asymptomatic carotid stenosis can be harmful. J Neurol Neurosurg Psychiatr 1998; 64:619–623.
45. Benade M, Warlow CP. Cost of identifying patients for carotid endarterectomy. Stroke 2002; 33:435–439.
46. Benade M, Warlow CP. Costs and benefits of carotid endarterectomy and associated preoperative arterial imaging. A systematic review of health economic literature. Stroke 2002; 33:629–638.

15

Surgical Controversies

A. Ross Naylor

The Department of Vascular Surgery, Leicester Royal Infirmary, Leicester, U.K.

Carotid endarterectomy (CEA) is one of the few surgical procedures to be subjected to level I scientific scrutiny (1–3). Yet, despite this, there remain a number of controversial issues to be resolved. This chapter reviews the evidence regarding the relationship between volume of surgery and outcome, generalizability of trial data to current clinical practice, choice of anesthesia, shunt and patch usage, technique of endarterectomy, the role of perioperative monitoring, optimal perioperative antiplatelet therapy, and the role of surveillance and intervention for recurrent carotid stenosis.

1. GENERALIZABILITY OF TRIAL RESULTS

1.1. What is the Controversy?

Are the results of large multi-center trials generalizable to routine clinical practice?

1.2. What is the Underlying Debate?

In order to participate in the European Carotid Surgery Trial (ECST), the North American Symptomatic Carotid Endarterectomy Trial (NASCET), and the Asymptomatic Carotid Atherosclerosis Study (ACAS), individual surgeons had to submit a track record of past performance. In the case of NASCET, a minimum of 50 CEAs had to have been performed in the preceding 2 years with a 30-day death/any stroke rate of ≤6%. In the ACAS study, 40% of surgeon applicants for participation were rejected after a review of their track record (4).

Following the publication of the major trials, CEA numbers increased dramatically with seemingly little regard for outcomes in the "real world." What is now often overlooked is the fact that <0.5% of all CEAs performed during 1989 in the United States and Canada were actually randomized into NASCET (5), fuelling suspicions that the final trial results were only generalizable to a highly select group of patients and surgeons. Moreover, with the seemingly indiscriminate implementation of the trial findings (especially in asymptomatic patients following the publication of the ACAS clinical alert), in conjunction with advances in what now constitutes "best medical therapy," an increasing number of neurologists and stroke physicians are beginning to question (again) the overall appropriateness and generalizability of carotid surgery in the third millennium.

1.3. What Randomized Trial Data are Available for Analysis?

The principal operative risks for ECST, NASCET, and ACAS are detailed in Table 1. These have become the "gold-standards" against which individual surgeons, institutions, and national statistics are compared.

1.4. What Non-Randomized Trial Data are Available for Analysis?

There is an increasing body of evidence that national and community-based audits of operative outcome may be inferior to those reported in the general literature. This observation is not unique to carotid endarterectomy. In a recent review of the *published* literature, Anyanwu and Treasure (6) observed that the median operative mortality following coronary artery bypass was 1.5%, increasing to 3.4% for aortic valve replacement, and

Table 1 Summary of 30-Day Risks of Death and/or Stroke in ECST, NASCET, and ACAS

	ECST			NASCET		ACAS
	<30%[a]	30–69%[a]	70–99%[a]	30–69%[a]	70–99%[a]	60–99%[a]
Operative mortality	1.5%	1.1%	0.9%	1.2%	0.6%	0.1%
Death +/− disabling stroke	2.3%	3.8%	3.7%	2.8%	2.1%	1.5%
Death +/− any stroke	4.6%	7.9%	7.5%	6.7%	5.8%	2.3%[b]

[a]Degree of stenosis.
[b]The ACAS trial morbidity of 2.3% included a 1.2% death/stroke rate following angiography

4.7% for mitral valve replacement. These results were lower than the 2.9, 4.0, and 6.0% (respectively) derived from national outcome registries in the United States and 2.6, 4.5, and 6.3% from the National Cardiothoracic Registry in the United Kingdom (6).

Accordingly, one must be cautious about which trials one selects to determine whether results are comparable to international trial outcomes. This was amply demonstrated in a systematic review of published outcomes following 16,046 CEAs in 51 studies (7). What made this study unique was that outcome was stratified according to authorship of the paper. As can be seen in Table 2, the best results were published in papers with a single surgeon authorship. The worst outcomes, though not that different from ECST and NASCET, were observed in studies where a neurologist assessed the patient. To the surgeon's annoyance, this paper has (unintentionally or not) fuelled the neurologists' worst fears that responsibility for auditing CEA outcome should not be left in the hands of the surgeons themselves.

How fair is this opinion? That surgical outcomes vary is nothing new. By definition, 50% of surgeons will, inevitably, perform "below average." The first evidence that the NASCET results may not be generalizable to *routine* practice came as early as 1992 (8). Hsia audited operative mortality following CEA in Medicare beneficiaries between 1985 and 1988 (i.e., while NASCET was actively recruiting). The stroke risk was not reported but the operative mortality rate was 3.0%, i.e., five times higher than that observed in NASCET. When this study was repeated for 1989–1996 (9), the mortality, though reduced to 1.6%, was still twice that reported in NASCET.

Table 2 Systematic Review of Published Operative Risks Following Carotid Endarterectomy Relative to Authorship[a]

Study characteristic	Number of CEAs	Operative mortality (%) (95% CI)	Death and/or any stroke (%) (95% CI)
Prospective	6591	1.9 (1.3–2.6)	5.6 (3.9–7.3)
Retrospective	9455	1.5 (1.2–1.8)	5.1 (4.3–5.8)
Single surgeon author	1849	0.7 (0.4–1.0)	2.3 (1.8–2.7)
Multi-surgeon authors	8375	1.7 (1.4–1.9)	5.5 (4.8–6.1)
Neurologist author included	3217	1.8 (1.2–2.5)	6.4 (4.6–8.1)
Neurologist assessor	2605	1.4 (0.2–2.7)	7.7 (5.0–10.2)

[a]Adapted from Ref. (7)

Few randomized trials involving symptomatic patients have been reported since 1991, with the exception of the Carotid and Vertebral Artery Transluminal Angioplasty Trial (CAVATAS). The CAVATAS trial randomized >500 symptomatic patients to either angioplasty or CEA. Angioplasty was associated with a 30-day death/stroke rate of 10.0%, while the equivalent risk after CEA was 9.9% (10). To put this into context, centers (or surgeons) with a 2% operative risk will prevent 112 ipsilateral strokes per 1000 CEAs. This falls to 72 if the operative risk is 6%. If CAVATAS is indeed a true reflection of current clinical practice, only 32 ipsilateral strokes will be prevented at 3 years for every 1000 CEAs (11).

Evidence that the results in asymptomatic patients may not be as good as reported in ACAS has come from several community-based audits in the United States and Canada. Wong et al. performed a retrospective review of outcomes following CEA in 174 asymptomatic patients undergoing CEA in Edmonton, Canada (12). In this study, the death and/or stroke rate was 5.2%. A similar study was undertaken in Toronto by Kucey et al. (13). Here the death and/or stroke rate was 4.0%. More recently, the SAPPHIRE study randomized patients to CEA or carotid angioplasty (14). Approximately 70% of patients in this study were asymptomatic. In this latter subgroup, the 30-day death/any stroke rate was 6.1% for CEA and 5.8% for angioplasty. These procedural risks exceed the threshold above which CEA or angioplasty confers any long-term benefit at all (15).

1.5. Summary

The international trials have established "gold standards" for assessing the role of CEA in patients with symptomatic and asymptomatic carotid artery disease. Fundamental to the reduction of long-term stroke is the initial operative risk. As the above studies have shown, there are concerns about the generalizability of the trial results to current practice. It is indisputable that many centers are capable of reproducing (or bettering) the operative risks from ECST, NASCET, and ACAS. However, surgeons cannot indiscriminately quote the results from the international trials to justify clinical practice irrespective of their own operative risk. It is therefore essential that each surgeon and institution maintains an accurate audit of outcome. Where the risk exceeds national guidelines (<5% for symptomatic patients and <3% for asymptomatic patients), a careful review must audit each stage in the process from patient selection through performance of the operation.

2. VOLUME OF SURGERY AND OUTCOME

2.1. What is the Controversy?

Does the number of carotid endarterectomies performed by an individual surgeon or institution influence outcome?

2.2. What is the Underlying Debate?

There is an intuitively held belief that surgeons and/or hospitals performing higher annual volumes of CEA achieve better results, regarding operative stroke or death, than surgeons or centers performing fewer procedures. The implication being that in order to achieve the greatest benefit for the patient and community, CEA should be concentrated in centralized or higher volume institutions.

2.3. What Non-Randomized Trial Data are Available for Analysis?

This is one of the most enduring and controversial subjects regarding the performance of carotid surgery. As was noted in the section on generalizability, there is a wide variation in published outcomes following carotid endarterectomy, and inappropriately drawn conclusions could have far-reaching medico-legal implications.

Despite being a relatively simple question (in concept), the relationship between volume and outcome remains a remarkably difficult problem to resolve. A number of studies have addressed this issue, but each has been beset by methodological problems. In a comprehensive review of the available literature, Shackley et al. (16) performed a systematic review of 17 studies that evaluated the relationship between volume and outcome in 290,966 patients undergoing CEA. They observed that meaningful interpretation of the data was confounded by a number of factors including: (i) a failure to correct for case-mix, e.g., symptomatic, asymptomatic, high-risk cases, (ii) varying definitions of what "volume" actually meant, e.g., <3, <5, <10, <25, (iii) the differing methods of reporting outcome, e.g., mortality, stroke, death, and/or stroke, and (iv) the fact that all were retrospective reviews. Other factors include the inevitable tendency for small-volume centers with good results to publish outcomes (poorly performing units seldom do) and a general recognition of the fact that health systems around the world are generally poor at actually recording the data required for such an analysis to be undertaken properly.

In view of these limitations, especially the type of patient undergoing surgery, Shackley et al. attempted to analyze the available data relative to whether some correction was made for case-mix. In their analysis, full adjustment was defined as correcting for "demographic factors, co-morbidity, and severity/stage of the illness." The latter was defined as having differentiated asymptomatic from symptomatic patients. Studies categorized as having made a partial correction adjusted data for demographics and case-mix but not disease severity.

Table 3 presents a simplified overview of their findings. As can be seen, the results are highly conflicting and any surgeon or institution could choose a paper that best suits their particular stance. Notwithstanding this, the

Table 3 Is there a Relationship Between Surgeon or Hospital Volume of CEA and Outcome Relative To Correction for Case-Mix[a]

Level of adjustment for case-mix	Total number of patients in studies	Operative stroke				Operative mortality			
		Physician		Hospital		Physician		Hospital	
		Yes	No	Yes	No	Yes	No	Yes	No
None	10,392	2	1						
Partial	274,635	3	1	1	1	1	2	5	2
Full	5,939	2	2	1	3	2	1	1	2

[a]That is, do surgeons or hospitals doing a low volume of CEAs incur a higher operative risk. Adapted from Shackley et al. (16). Please see text for definition of adjustments for case-mix adopted by Shackley et al.

authors concluded that if one takes all of the available data into considera-tion, "the weight of evidence is supportive of there being a positive volume–outcome relationship for both operative stroke and death at the individual surgeon level." There was less evidence that hospital volume influenced risk. However, if one only included studies making a full correction for case-mix, Shackley concluded that there was *no* evidence to support the hypothesis that low-volume surgeons and institutions were associated with poorer outcomes after CEA (16).

One further study is worthy of mention. Irvine et al. undertook an analysis of how difficult it can be to recognize the surgeon whose perfor-mance is sub-standard relative to the number of CEAs performed each year (17). In order to determine whether a surgeon had a death/stroke rate *twice* the 6% generally accepted for operating upon symptomatic patients, they would need to operate upon at least 130 patients. A similar analysis indi-cated that at least 280 CEAs would have to be performed to determine accurately whether a surgeon's operative risk was twice the 3% recom-mended for asymptomatic patients. Simple maths reveals that for a surgeon performing only 10 CEAs per year, it would take between 13 and 28 years (depending upon case-mix) to determine whether they were performing in a sub-standard manner.

2.4. Summary

Neither the constituent papers nor the systematic review has been able to answer this question. Surely it is time for the recording of accurate and national outcome data to become a priority with governments and health authorities. In this increasing era of increasingly accessible surgeon-specific outcomes (already occurring in cardiothoracic surgery), it is only fair that individual surgeons can rely on information technology to provide accurate and comparable data regarding case-mix. However, it is important to rem-ember what was observed by Irvine et al. regarding the difficulties in deter-mining whether surgeons performing small numbers of CEAs are out with accepted guidelines. This has important implications for clinical governance and fairness to the surgeon and patient. No comparable data are available for the United Kingdom, but in the United States, 60% of *hospitals* perform <17 CEAs per annum on Medicare patients, indicating that the individual surgeons concerned must be doing very small numbers indeed (18).

3. OPTIMAL PERIOPERATIVE ANTIPLATELET THERAPY

3.1. What is the Controversy?

Does the dose of aspirin influence the perioperative risk?

3.2. What is the Underlying Debate?

Although there is a general consensus that antiplatelet therapy should be continued throughout the perioperative period, there has always been controversy about the optimal dose of aspirin. Clearly any risk–benefit analysis must take into account the theoretical benefits of increased antiplatelet activity mediated by high-dose aspirin against the increased risk of side effects. This controversy was highlighted by the findings of a secondary analysis from the NASCET database that suggested that higher-dose aspirin conferred a lower operative risk.

3.3. What Non-Randomized Trial Data are Available for Analysis?

In an unplanned secondary analysis, NASCET observed that patients taking 0–325 mg aspirin daily had a 30-day risk of death/stroke of 6.9% as compared with 1.8% in patients receiving 650–1300 mg aspirin (19). It was hypothesized that the exposed collagen surface following endarterectomy predisposed toward enhanced platelet aggregation and deposition so as to require higher doses of aspirin to counteract it.

3.4. What Randomized Trial Data are Available for Analysis?

As a consequence of this finding, the Aspirin and Carotid Endarterectomy (ACE) trial thereafter randomized 2849 patients undergoing CEA to 81, 325, 650, and 1300 mg of aspirin daily throughout the perioperative and follow-up period (20). Patients receiving 81 or 325 mg aspirin were combined as "low-dose" while those receiving 650 or 1300 mg were classified as "high-dose" in subsequent analyses.

Low-dose aspirin conferred a non-significant reduction in the risk of hemorrhagic stroke. For the purposes of analysis, "stroke, myocardial infarction (MI), and death" were thereafter combined as a single end-point and analyzed at 30 days and 3 months. The risk of stroke, MI, or death at 30 days was lower in patients randomized to low-dose aspirin (5.4% vs. 7.0%, $P = 0.07$) and was 6.2 and 8.4% ($P = 0.03$) at 3 months (low dose vs. high dose respectively). However, the authors noted that some of the results may have been biased by the inclusion of patients who had been receiving >650 mg aspirin daily before randomization or who had been randomized only the day before surgery. In a subsequent efficacy analysis that excluded these patients, the combined morbidity/mortality rates were 3.7% (low dose) and 8.2% (high dose) at 30 days ($P = 0.002$), and 4.2 and 10.0% ($P = 0.0002$) at 3 months (low dose vs. high dose respectively).

3.5. Summary

The available data suggest that the optimal aspirin dose in patients undergoing CEA is <325 mg daily. There is no evidence that aspirin should be stopped before surgery. No trials have evaluated whether alternative antiplatelet therapies confer an advantage over aspirin. There are, however, anecdotal reports that patients on long-term clopidogrel therapy (75 mg daily) may have an increased problem with intra-operative hemostasis. It is worth noting that clopidogrel trebles the bleeding time while a combination of aspirin and full-dose clopidogrel increases the bleeding time by a factor of five as compared with aspirin alone (21). This subject is worthy of scrutiny, as an increasing proportion of cardiovascular patients receive this type of combination antiplatelet therapy.

4. CHOICE OF ANESTHESIA

4.1. What is the Controversy?

Does surgery under locoregional anesthesia (LRA) confer any benefit over general anesthesia (GA)?

4.2. What is the Underlying Rationale for this Debate?

Advocates of GA propose that carotid endarterectomy under GA:

- reduces overall cerebral metabolic requirements;
- provides a motionless environment in which to operate;
- facilitates a less stressful environment for teaching and training surgeons;
- is less likely to be associated with intra-operative hypertension; and
- involves no need for urgent intubation of the restless patient after failure with LRA.

Proponents of LRA propose that carotid endarterectomy under LRA:

- preserves cerebral autoregulation;
- avoids phases of intra-operative hypotension often associated with GA;
- is the gold standard for determining who needs a shunt following carotid clamping;
- is associated with a lower risk of post-operative cardiovascular complications;
- is associated with fewer perioperative strokes;
- facilitates early discharge and optimization of resources;
- is well tolerated by patients.

4.3. What Non-randomized Trial Data are Available for Analysis?

Tangkanakul et al. identified 17 non-randomized studies evaluating CEA under LRA and GA (22). The principal observations (Table 4) were that CEA under LRA conferred significant benefits in terms of a reduced risk of (i) any stroke (0.8 vs. 1.2%), (ii) death/any stroke (2.2 vs. 6.1%), (iii) myocardial infarction (0.6 vs. 1.3%), (iv) pulmonary complications (0.6 vs. 0.9%), and (v) need for shunting (10.8 vs. 44.3%).

One must, however, be cautious about uncritical interpretation of these data. Many of the differences may, simply, be attributable to patient selection in the non-randomized studies. A clue possibly lies in the higher risk of cranial nerve injury following procedures done under GA (3.4% after LRA vs. 5.5% after GA) in this meta-analysis. This could be explained by the fact that patients with suspected distal disease extension were preferentially submitted to CEA under GA.

Several non-randomized trials have indicated that CEA under LRA is well tolerated by patients and the need for conversion to GA is low. Although some centers have reported cost savings and reductions in hospital stay beneficial to LRA (23), these should be interpreted with caution as patient selection, the use of historical controls, and a retrospective review of costs can introduce considerable bias.

Table 4 Systematic Review of Outcomes in Non-randomized Trials of CEA Under General Anesthetic or Locoregional Anesthesia[a]

	LRA	GA	P
Operative death	17/2070 (0.8%)	40/3447 (1.2%)	NS
Any operative stroke	41/2070 (2.0%)	183/3447 (5.3%)	<0.05
Any operative stroke or death	42/1891 (2.2%)	201/3295 (6.1%)	<0.05
Operative myocardial infarction	11/1823 (0.6%)	39/3090 (1.3%)	<0.05
Neck hematoma	18/757 (2.4%)	76/2594 (2.9%)	NS
"Pulmonary" complications	5/696 (0.6%)	23/2451 (0.9%)	<0.05
Cranial nerve injury	20/582 (3.4%)	128/2326 (5.5%)	NS
Requirement for shunting	206/1907 (10.8%)	1407/3178 (44.3%)	<0.05

[a]Adapted from Ref. (22).

4.4. What Randomized Trial Data are Available for Analysis?

Tangkanakul et al. also undertook the only published systematic review on this subject (21), but only three randomized trials were identified for inclusion (24–26). These were all extremely small (total number of patients in the three studies = 143) and all were published prior to 1990.

The systematic review concluded that there were insufficient outcome events in the three randomized trials (even when combined) to determine whether either anesthetic technique conferred any benefit (Table 5).

The randomized trials reported conflicting results regarding perioperative cardiovascular morbidity. Forssell (24) observed that GA patients were more likely to have intra-operative hypotension than LRA patients (25 vs. 7%), while CEA under LRA was associated with a higher risk of catecholamine release and intra-operative hypertension (especially following carotid clamping). These findings were either not corroborated or not evaluated in the remaining studies. However, Pluskwa and Prough reported an increased risk of hypotension in the early post-operative period in patients undergoing CEA with LRA (25,26).

4.5. Summary

There is no doubt that CEA under LRA is the undisputed "gold standard" for determining who requires a shunt following carotid clamping. Locoregional anesthesia will not, however, prevent operative strokes due to thromboembolism. Non-randomized studies suggest a possible benefit for CEA under LRA regarding a reduction in operation-related strokes and overall cardiovascular morbidity. However, this has never been corroborated in

Table 5 Systematic Review of Outcomes in Randomized Trials of CEA Under General Anesthetic or Locoregional Anesthesia[a]

	LRA	GA	P
Operative death	0/79 (0.0%)	1/75 (1.3%)	NS
Any operative stroke	4/79 (5.1%)	3/75 (4.0%)	NS
Any operative death/stroke	4/79 (5.1%)	4/75 (5.3%)	NS
Operative myocardial infarction	2/79 (2.5%)	1/75 (1.3%)	NS
Neck hematoma	1/56 (1.8%)	6/55 (10.9%)	<0.05
Requirement for shunting	5/56 (8.9%)	25/55 (45.5%)	<0.05

Adapted from Ref. (22).

any randomized trial. The GALA (general anesthetic vs. local anesthetic) trial is currently underway in the United Kingdom and will be the largest randomized study of its kind. It will be better placed to evaluate health economics, patient acceptability, and outcomes (stroke, cardiovascular) than any systematic review of non-randomized and usually retrospective trials. Until GALA is published, there is no systematic evidence that anesthetic technique influences outcome. Surgeons and anesthetists can therefore continue to employ whatever anesthetic technique they prefer.

5. SINUS NERVE BLOCKADE

5.1. What is the Controversy?

Does infiltration of the sinus nerve with local anesthetic prevent intra-operative hypotension?

5.2. What is the Underlying Debate?

Baroreceptors are located at the carotid bifurcation and their role is to maintain normotension. Stretch receptors in the carotid sinus send afferent signals via the glossopharyngeal nerve to the vasomotor center in the medulla. The efferent limb comprises a balancing outflow involving the parasympathetic and sympathetic nervous systems. Stimulation of the sympathetic nervous system increases the heart rate and causes peripheral vasoconstriction. Stimulation of the parasympathetic nervous system, via the vagus nerve, reduces heart rate and blood pressure.

   Hypotension is a relatively common problem during carotid dissection, particularly if the procedure is carried out under GA. It has, therefore, been hypothesized that blockade of the sinus nerve with local anesthetic (usually 1% lignocaine or 0.25% bupivacaine) will prevent fluctuations in blood pressure (particularly hypotension). The worry, however, is that there might be rebound hypotension or hypertension in the early post-operative period when the nerve blockade recedes.

5.3. What Randomized Trial Data are Available for Analysis?

Four randomized trials have been performed (27–30). Only one observed that the infiltration of the sinus nerve with LA significantly reduced intra-operative variations in blood pressure (28). Unfortunately, only 40 patients were randomized in this study and no observations were made in the post-operative period. The three remaining studies have reported broadly similar results. None found any evidence that there was any significant reduction in the incidence of intra-operative hypotension requiring treatment. Interestingly, the lowest blood pressures were observed in patients undergoing sinus nerve excision (30). Of most concern was the observation in two studies (235

CEAs) that patients randomized to sinus nerve blockade were more likely to suffer hypertension in the early post-operative period (27,29).

5.4. Summary

There is no systematic evidence that carotid sinus nerve blockade reduces the prevalence of intra-operative hypotension during carotid endarterectomy. There is, however, evidence that such a practice may be associated with an increased risk of post-operative hypertension, presumably due to re-innervation. To date, there is no evidence to support the routine practice of sinus nerve blockade. Sinus nerve excision/division should be avoided wherever possible.

6. SHUNT DEPLOYMENT

6.1. What is the Controversy?

Is there any evidence as to whether shunt policy (routine, selective, never) influences outcome?

6.2. What is the Underlying Debate?

Following carotid clamping, the Circle of Willis may be unable to maintain adequate cerebral perfusion in the hemisphere of the ipsilateral clamped carotid artery. Without a shunt to restore blood flow during the endarterectomy phase, the patient faces an increased risk of suffering a hemodynamic stroke.

Surgeons fall into three camps, usually determined by the policy of their mentor or trainer. "Routine" shunters employ a shunt in every patient on the basis that unless CEA under LRA is employed, there is no infallible method for determining who needs a shunt. The presence of a shunt facilitates an unhurried operation and allows the senior surgeon to supervise trainees more thoroughly. There is anecdotal evidence in the United Kingdom that CEA under LRA tends to be performed by a consultant surgeon to the detriment of any training program. Routine shunters observe that familiarity with a shunt means that it tends to be less in the way in difficult situations; e.g., high carotid dissections, and that the shunt can act as an efficient stent for closure, so minimizing the risk of causing a distal stenosis.

"Selective" shunters believe that shunts are definitely beneficial but that they get in the way and may be potentially dangerous (intimal injury, embolism) and should only be used in patients with inadequate collateralization following clamping. Evidence from the meta-analysis in Table 4 suggests that only about 10% of patients actually need a shunt following carotid clamping. Unfortunately, unless the surgeon chooses to use LRA, there is no infallible monitoring technique (e.g., transcranial

Doppler, EEG, SSEP, transcranial oximetry, stump pressure) for predicting who needs a shunt when the procedure is performed under GA. The question about the potential for shunts to cause intimal injuries and embolization is unresolved. The published incidence varies from 0.002 to 5% (31).

"Never" shunters believe that the operation can be done in such a short period of time and with little risk of suffering a hemodynamic stroke that there is no need to ever employ a shunt at all. As far as the latter surgeons are concerned, shunts compromise the surgeon's ability to ensure a technically excellent result. In short, they are generally of the opinion that shunts probably cause as many strokes as they prevent.

6.3. What Non-Randomized Trial Data are Available for Analysis?

This remains one of the most enduring controversies in carotid surgery. Accordingly, you pay your money and take your choice! Depending upon which stance you wish to adopt, the literature contains supporting and conflicting evidence in a proliferation of uncontrolled and usually retrospective studies. It is inevitable, therefore, that there is no consensus to guide those seeking to modify practice based on evidence.

In a secondary review of surgical outcomes in NASCET, Ferguson et al. observed that shunt policy did not influence the operative risk (32). In a recent debate on this topic, Malone and Ballard reviewed the pooled outcomes from 17 published series comprising 8323 patients undergoing CEA (31). The data indicated no significant difference in outcome relative to shunt policy. Routine shunters incurred a total neurological deficit rate of 2.5% following 3366 procedures as compared with 3.4% after 2131 CEAs treated with a selective shunt policy, and 3.9% in 2826 patients where shunts were never used. As was wryly observed by one of the authors in this debate (who was actively promoting a routine shunting position), much the same data was also interpreted by another colleague who this time used the published data to advocate his position that shunting was never necessary! The one exception for the "never shunt group" is the patient with a severe stenosis and contralateral occlusion who also has a stump pressure < 50 mmHg on carotid clamping (indicative of poor collateralization via the Circle of Willis). Baker's experience (an advocate of never shunting) is that the risk of stroke increases from 0.9 to 11% in these patients (33). Accordingly, most of the "never" shunters would probably recommend shunting patients with contralateral occlusion.

6.4. What Randomized Trial Data are Available for Analysis?

The Cochrane Collaboration has undertaken a systematic review of the literature (34). Two randomized trials (total 590 patients) were identified. In these two trials, routine shunting was compared with no shunting (35,36).

The review observed that although there was a 25% reduction in deaths and strokes within 30 days of surgery (in favor of routine shunting), this did not reach statistical significance.

One must, however, be careful about how one interprets these results. Firstly, relatively small numbers were involved. A definitive trial to address the problem would probably require in excess of 5000 patients. Second, the shunted group in Gumerlock's series had more severe disease in the contralateral carotid artery (35). This could bias any likelihood towards suffering adverse events towards the shunt group. Third, the shunted group in Sandmann's study (36) were more likely to be closed with a patch as opposed to primary closure (57 vs. 39%). As will be seen, this might predispose to more adverse events occurring in the primary closure group. Fourth, there were 10 patients in Sandmann's series who were randomized to no shunting, but who were subsequently shunted because neuromonitoring showed evidence of ipsilateral cerebral ischemia following clamping.

Only one randomized trial has addressed the issue as to whether one type of shunt is preferable to another (37). Wilkinson observed that there were higher flow rates in the larger caliber, tapered Javid shunt compared with the non-tapered, smaller-caliber, balloon-held Pruitt shunts. Javid shunts were associated with a significantly higher number of emboli upon restoration of flow. Neither shunt type, however, influenced the operative stroke risk. In practical terms, the principal limitation of the Javid shunt is the need for proximal and distal external retaining clamps. In the majority of patients this is probably not a problem; however, it assumes greater importance when dissection extends into the upper reaches of the carotid artery and overall access is limited.

6.5. Summary

Shunting is one of the "single-issue" subjects (along with patching and anesthesia) that have dominated discussions about the performance of carotid endarterectomy over the last five decades. No data (randomized or otherwise) has conclusively shown that any one shunt policy is preferable. There is, however, a growing consensus that a policy of "never shunting" anyone is inappropriate. In the absence of level I evidence, advocates of each policy must accept the limitations and benefits of each shunt strategy. It is almost certain that no further large-scale randomized trials will ever again address this issue.

One should, however, remain aware of just what a shunt is meant to do. It will only protect against hemodynamic stroke and, only then, if it is working. Hemodynamic failure accounts for about 20% of all intra-operative strokes (38). The majority of the remaining intra-operative strokes (and most of the post-operative ones) are thromboembolic. Second, about 3% of shunts malfunction (39). This is usually due to undetected impaction of the shunt lumen against the distal carotid wall or a vessel coil. Unless some monitoring modality is available (LRA, TCD), this will go unnoticed and lend further support to the notion that intra-operative strokes still occur despite using a shunt.

The Leicester Vascular Unit advocates a policy of routine shunting. As will be seen later (monitoring and quality control), the rate of intra-operative stroke plummeted once completion angioscopy was introduced which enabled us to remove small portions of luminal thrombus prior to restoration of flow (40). Our experience (in >1200 audited CEAs) has been that shunt-related injuries are extremely rare causes of operation-related stroke.

7. EVERSION OR TRADITIONAL ENDARTERECTOMY?

7.1. What is the Controversy?

Does eversion endarterectomy confer improvements in early and late rates of stroke and restenosis as compared with traditional endarterectomy?

7.2. What is the Underlying Debate?

During traditional endarterectomy, the plaque is removed via a longitudinal arteriotomy. A plane of endarterectomy (somewhere in the media) is developed proximally using a Watson–Cheyne dissector. The intima/media/plaque is then transected and the plaque removed by cephalad extension of the endarterectomy plane until either the lesion feathers off or the intimal step is transected. In the eversion method, the endarterectomy is performed by first transecting the proximal internal carotid artery (ICA) at the bifurcation. A circumferential plane of endarterectomy is then developed in the distal ICA. The adventitia/residual media is everted and the tube of atheroma expelled as the dissection plane continues in a cephalad direction. Distal endarterectomy then continues until the tube of atheroma feathers off. The distal common carotid artery is then endarterectomized in the normal manner. The bulb of the internal carotid artery is then re-anastomosed to the bifurcation, having been shortened as necessary.

Advocates of eversion endarterectomy have cited the following advantages with this technique: (i) the rates of late restenosis are low, (ii) there is no need to patch the artery, (iii) the technique enables shortening of any redundant segment of internal carotid artery to prevent kinking, and (iv) the procedure takes a shorter time to perform. Disadvantages include: (i) the distal intimal step may not be clearly visualized and intimal flaps may be missed, (ii) tacking sutures cannot be readily inserted, (iii) the surgeon cannot insert a shunt until the plaque has been removed, and (iv) if unexpected high mural disease is encountered at operation (e.g., the posterior tongue of the plaque that often extends beyond the main stenosis), distal mobilization and plaque dissection is rendered more difficult (especially as a shunt cannot be placed) and a technically less than satisfactory result may result.

The principal advantages of traditional endarterectomy include: (i) there is more widespread experience with the technique so that trainees can always be supervised in a less stressful, controlled environment, (ii) a shunt can be inserted from the outset, (iii) the distal intimal step is always visualized and tacking sutures can be inserted as required, and (iv) in the event that the surgeon encounters unexpected distal disease, further mobilization can be performed (with a shunt in place) so that (in theory) a more technically perfect outcome can be achieved. Potential disadvantages of traditional endarterectomy include: (i) the procedure takes longer unless the artery is closed primarily; however this increases the risk of late restenosis (see later); (ii) the available evidence suggests that traditional endarterectomy is best completed with patch closure (see later). Patching prolongs the operation; vein patches are prone to a small risk of rupture while prosthetic patches carry a 0.5–1% risk of late infection. Finally, (iii) traditional endarterectomy almost always produces a degree of functional elongation of the endarterectomy zone (especially in patients with large bulky plaques or if the bifurcation is "skeletonized" during the mobilization phase). Functional elongation of the plaque predisposes to rotation of the bifurcation and/or kinking of the distal ICA following restoration of flow and may promote early post-operative thrombosis.

7.3. What Randomized Trial Data are Available for Analysis?

Cao et al. (41) have performed a systematic review of the results of five randomized trials of eversion vs. traditional endarterectomy (42–46) involving 2465 patients and 2590 operated arteries (Table 6).

As with all systematic reviews, the reader must bear in mind the fact that the quality of performing and reporting the component studies varies significantly. For example, some studies randomized arteries rather than patients (i.e., patients undergoing staged bilateral CEA may have been randomized to both treatment arms!), while the "traditional" group contained patients who underwent primary closure or patching. Notwithstanding these limitations, Table 6 summarizes the principal results from this review (40). For the whole study group, there were no statistically significant differences regarding: (i) 30-day risk of stroke/death, (ii) 30-day risk of thrombosis, (iii) perioperative cardiovascular or neck wound complications, and (iv) late stroke. However, patients randomized to eversion endarterectomy had significantly lower rates of late restenosis as compared to those with traditional endarterectomy [OR 0.3 (95% CI: 0.1–0.8)].

The reviewers observed that the latter beneficial effect (relative to eversion endarterectomy) may have been confounded by the inclusion of

Table 6 Systematic Review of the Randomized Trials on Eversion Vs. Traditional Endarterectomy[a]

	Eversion (%)	Traditional (%)	OR (95% CI)
Eversion vs. all traditional			
30 day death/stroke	1.7	2.6	0.44 (0.1–1.8)
30 day occlusion	0.7	1.1	0.70 (0.2–1.6)
Late restenosis >50%	2.5	5.2	0.30 (0.1–0.8)
Late stroke + perioperative death	2.0	2.4	0.75 (0.3–1.9)
Eversion vs. traditional patched[b]			
30 day death/any stroke	1.7	2.4	0.50 (0.1–4.0)
Late stroke + perioperative death	2.0	1.9	0.75 (0.2–2.5)
Late restenosis >50%	2.5	3.9	0.52 (0.2–1.7)

[a]Adapted from Ref. (41).
[b]Only includes patients randomized to traditional endarterectomy who were patched for any analysis to be statistically beneficial in favor of eversion endarterectomy; the OR and the 95% CI must be <1.0.

patched and primarily closed arteries in the traditional endarterectomy group. Accordingly, a second analysis was performed wherein eversion endarterectomy was compared with traditional CEA and *patch* closure. As can be seen in Table 6, the data showed no statistical differences relative to any early or late outcomes.

7.4. Summary

The available data suggest that commendably good outcomes were observed in the randomized trials irrespective of endarterectomy technique. Surgeons can therefore use either method of performing the endarterectomy bearing in mind that equivalent results were only observed in patients undergoing the traditional method provided patch closure had been used.

8. PATCH OR PRIMARY CLOSURE?

8.1. What is the Controversy?

Does a policy of patch closure of the arteriotomy confer any benefit over primary closure?

8.2. What is the Underlying Debate?

Most carotid endarterectomies are performed via a longitudinal arteriotomy (see Sec. 7). There are two methods for closing the arteriotomy: primary closure and patch angioplasty. The principal advantage of primary closure is that it is quicker than patching. The main disadvantage is that it inevitably results in some degree of narrowing of the artery, especially at the most distal aspect of the arteriotomy. This could predispose towards early postoperative thrombosis and late restenosis. The rationale underlying patching is that it widens the bulb, minimizes the risk of distal stenosis formation, and promotes better flow hemodynamics within the endarterectomy zone. Opponents of patching cite the 1% risk of vein patch "blow-out", which usually occurs on the 5–7th post-operative day (47), and the 1% risk of prosthetic patch infection (48).

Accordingly, patching has become another of the "single-issue" subjects in carotid surgery, and surgeons tend to be "routine, selective, or never" patchers. As with shunt deployment, the policy adopted by the surgeon is rarely based on evidence and usually reflects the policy of their trainer.

8.3. What Randomized Trial Data are Available for Analysis?

The Cochrane Collaboration (49) have undertaken a systematic review of six randomized trials (soon to be upgraded). The principal results are summarized in Table 7. Routine primary closure was associated with a 3-fold increase in the 30-day risk of ipsilateral stroke and a 6-fold increase in the risk of early post-operative thrombosis. In terms of late follow-up, primary closure was associated with a 3-fold increase in late stroke and restenosis. No randomized trials have ever evaluated routine vs. selective patching.

Table 7 Systematic Review of Six Randomized Trials Comparing Routine Patch Vs. Primary Closure of the Arteriotomy[a]

	Routine patching (%)	Primary closure (%)[b]	Odds ratio of increased risk with primary closure
30-day outcomes			
Ipsilateral stroke	1.3	3.9	2.9 (95% CI 1.3–6.7)
All strokes	1.6	4.2	2.6 (95% CI 1.1–6.7)
Carotid thrombosis	0.3	3.9	5.9 (95% CI 2.2–17)
Long-term outcomes			
Ipsilateral stroke	1.6	4.4	2.6 (95% CI 1.1–6.3)
All strokes	2.2	5.9	2.6 (95% CI 1.2–5.9)
50–100% restenosis	4.5	13	3.1 (95% CI 1.9–5.3)

[a]Adapted from Ref. 49.
[b]For primary closure to be associated with a significantly worst risk of adverse events compared with primary closure, the OR and both CIs have to be > 1.0.

The Cochrane Collaboration also observed that patch type (vein, prosthetic) did not influence early or late outcome. Despite this, surgeons intuitively believe that prosthetic patches are more thrombogenic than vein patches. In a recent randomized trial of 276 patients, Hayes observed that there was no difference in the magnitude of post-operative embolization (a marker of increased predisposition to thrombosis) between vein and Dacron patched patients (50).

8.4. Summary

The available evidence therefore suggests that a policy of routine patching is preferable to one of routine primary closure, the exception being the patient with a very large-caliber artery. This evolving change in practice is supported by two sequential community-based audits which demonstrated that increasing usage of patch angioplasty was associated with a reduction in the operative risk (51). The choice of patch is at the discretion of the surgeon. Prosthetic patches are not associated with an increased risk of thrombosis and their use preserves the long saphenous vein for future cardiovascular operations. However, for surgeons preferring to use vein, it is important that this is harvested from the groin. Saphenous vein harvested from the ankle has a higher risk of rupture because of its weaker tensile strength (47). There is no randomized trial evidence to guide the surgeon regarding the role of selective patching. As a rule, surgeons adopting a policy of selective patching tend to reserve this for females (narrower caliber ICA), patients whose arteriotomy extends for >2 cm into the ICA, and patients whose ICA diameter is <5 mm.

9. SHOULD HEPARIN BE REVERSED WITH PROTAMINE?

9.1. What is the Controversy?

Prior to carotid clamping, the patient usually receives 3–5000 units of intravenous heparin to minimize the risks of distal thrombus formation. Following the restoration of flow, some surgeons have recommended reversing the effects of heparin so as to minimize the risks of neck hematoma formation in the early post-operative period.

9.2. What is the Underlying Debate?

Neck hematoma formation can predispose towards asphyxiation through compression of the larynx by the adjacent hematoma. Quite apart from the immediate risk to the patient, the presence of a large hematoma also makes re-intubation more difficult. However, many surgeons prefer not to give protamine because of the theoretical benefits conferred by heparin in reducing the risk of early post-operative thrombosis.

9.3. What Non-randomized Trial Data are Available for Analysis?

In 1994, 54% of US surgeons and 26% of European surgeons routinely reversed the effects of heparin with protamine following the restoration of flow (52). There are conflicting results in the literature concerning the effect of protamine and hematoma formation and stroke. Treiman et al. (53) observed an increased incidence of hematoma in non-reversed patients (1.2 vs. 6.2%, $P = 0.0013$) and a similar trend was noted by Levison et al. (54). Mauney et al. (55), however, found no difference in the incidence of hematoma formation requiring re-exploration (1.0 vs. 1.9%). One non-randomized study observed no increase in stroke risk following protamine administration (53), while two noted an increase in stroke risk in protamine-reversed patients (54,55).

Surgeons and anesthetists should also be aware of the principal side-effects associated with protamine administration. In their review of practice in the United States and Europe, Wakefield obtained data on 38,121 patients undergoing a range of vascular procedures. Systemic hypotension was recorded in 1704 patients, pulmonary artery hypotension in 73, anaphylaxis in 62, and death in 9 (52).

9.4. What Randomized Trial Data are Available for Analysis?

Only one randomized trial has been performed and this was abandoned after recruiting only 65 patients (56). In this study, neck drain losses were significantly reduced in reversed patients (35 vs. 69 mL, $P < 0.001$). However, the study was suspended because of three strokes following early post-operative carotid thrombosis in whom no technical error was identified at re-exploration. Although one of these strokes occurred in a non-randomized patient, the authors felt that it was unethical to continue with the study.

9.5. Summary

There is no systematic evidence that a policy of routine protamine reversal of heparin improves outcome after carotid endarterectomy. It may in fact be associated with an increased risk of early thrombotic stroke. Routine protamine reversal cannot, therefore, be recommended on the basis of the available (albeit limited) evidence.

10. IS THERE A ROLE FOR PERIOPERATIVE MONITORING?

10.1. What is the Controversy?

Does a policy of perioperative monitoring and quality control reduce the operative stroke risk?

10.2. What is the Underlying Debate?

Two-thirds of all operative strokes are attributable to some form of inadvertent technical error (57). Yet, despite the fact that most surgeons perform some form of completion assessment after femoro-distal bypass, few surgeons apply the same principles following carotid surgery. Various direct and indirect monitoring methods have been available, some for decades (stump pressure, back flow assessment, awake testing, EEG, SSEP, transcranial Doppler, xenon blood flow measurements, infrared spectroscopy, completion angiography, completion angioscopy, and completion Duplex assessment).

Three principle factors have dogged this important issue (58). First, most of the monitoring techniques have been developed primarily for determining who needs a shunt. This is despite the fact that only 20% of all intraoperative strokes (i.e., apparent upon recovery from anesthesia) are due to hemodynamic failure during carotid clamping (38). Second, there is the flawed assumption that one method alone is infallible and superior to all others. Third, and most important, the simple reason why monitoring and quality control techniques have never reached their maximum potential is a failure to ask the right questions (58).

If you want to know who needs a shunt, perform CEA under locoregional anesthesia. If you want to know who has an unstable plaque with ongoing embolization during carotid dissection, this information can only be provided by transcranial Doppler ultrasound. As was stated earlier, 3% of shunts fail. This can be recognized by a variety of on-line techniques, TCD being the easiest. The EEG and SSEP techniques are useful at informing the surgeon that something has gone wrong, *but not why*. Remember that the EEG and SSEP become isoelectric when cerebral blood flow falls below the threshold for maintaining neuronal electrical activity. The blood flow threshold for neuronal death is much lower. Accordingly, the presence of an isoelectric or abnormal EEG or SSEP recording does *not* mean the patient has suffered a neurological deficit.

There are a number of quality control techniques aimed at identifying technical errors (angiography, Duplex, and angioscopy). Each have their advocates and many surgeons have achieved very good results with each of them. The principal abnormalities to be identified are intimal flaps, but more importantly, retained luminal thrombus despite irrigation with heparinized saline. These thrombi are derived from bleeding from the vasa vasorum onto the endarterectomized surface (40).

Finally, TCD is the only proven method for predicting patients at risk of progressing onto carotid thrombosis. Five centers around the world have now shown that high grade or sustained embolization precedes progression onto thrombosis and stroke (59–65). Recognition of this high-risk subgroup enables therapeutic intervention to be commenced to prevent further thrombus accumulation.

10.3. What Randomized Trial Data are Available for Analysis?

No randomized trials have been performed.

10.4. What Non-randomized Trial Data are Available for Analysis?

The literature abounds with claims and counter-claims regarding the effectiveness of monitoring and quality control assessment. One oft-quoted phrase is that "a stroke occurred despite TCD or EEG and therefore the monitoring technique is useless". It should be clear from the above summary that unless the right questions are asked of each monitoring method, no effective reduction in operative morbidity can be expected.

The Leicester group have undertaken a series of sequential studies to evaluate the role of perioperative monitoring. The rate of intra-operative stroke fell from 4% prior to 1992 to 0.25% after 1200 CEAs following the introduction of TCD monitoring and completion angioscopy. Transcranial Doppler monitoring warns the surgeon of embolization during the dissection phase, and ensures that the shunt is functioning and mean flow velocities remain >15 cm/s throughout; it remains the only method capable of diagnosing the very rare cases of on-table thrombosis (41). This is diagnosed by the presence of increasing embolization following restoration of flow and a decline in middle cerebral artery velocities to that observed during carotid clamping. Completion angioscopy diagnoses intimal flaps >3 mm in about 3–4% of patients. These will not cause intra-operative strokes, but may predispose to thrombus accumulation and secondary embolization post-operatively. The most important role for completion angioscopy, however, is the identification of luminal thrombus *before* flow restoration (41). This can then be carefully aspirated without the need to reopen the anastomosis.

The Leicester group were, however, surprised that the exclusion of technical errors did not prevent early post-operative thrombosis. Subsequent research suggested that this phenomenon is probably patient-mediated. For example, post-operative embolization was unrelated to patch type (66) or aspirin usage (67), and patients undergoing staged, bilateral endarterectomies had similar rates of embolization after each operation (68). However, the main finding was that the platelets of patients with higher rates of embolization were more sensitive to ADP (67). A subsequent randomized trial has shown that embolization can be significantly reduced by the pre-operative administration of one 75 mg tablet of the ADP inhibitor clopidogrel (69). This opens the way for developing novel therapeutic strategies for preventing thrombosis and so obviate the need for post-operative monitoring. Until then, we continued with our protocol of 3 h of TCD monitoring following surgery. Patients with >25 emboli in any 10 minutes period receive a bolus of 20–30 mL of Dextran 40 and then an incremental dose infusion of dextran until the embolization is controlled. In our experience, only 5% of all patients require dextran (41). Since implementing this final protocol change in 1995, >1000 CEAs have been performed and no patient has suffered a stroke due to post-operative carotid thrombosis. Overall, there has been a 60% sustained reduction in the operative risk following implementation of the monitoring program.

10.5. Summary

In the absence of randomized trial data, surgeons must adopt a pragmatic approach to monitoring. Many will feel that their own complication rates are so low that no change in practice is necessary. Others with higher operative risks should first analyze when they occur. If most events occur intra-operatively, then those techniques specifically designed to help (e.g., a combination of TCD and angioscopy) might reduce complications due to technical error. If the principal problem is early post-operative thrombosis, surgeons might wish to consider extending TCD monitoring into the post-operative period so as to recognize and treat those with high-grade embolization before they progress onto thrombosis.

11. SURVEILLANCE AND MANAGEMENT OF RESTENOSIS

11.1. What is the Controversy?

Does serial surveillance and intervention for recurrent stenosis influence the risk of long-term ipsilateral stroke?

11.2. What is the Underlying Debate?

This remains a highly contentious subject. As with most other controversial issues relating to carotid surgery, attitudes usually reflect the prejudices and experience of the trainer. The simple rationale is that recurrent stenosis increases the risk of late ipsilateral stroke. This increased risk can be reduced by serial ultrasound imaging of the operated ICA followed by secondary endarterectomy or angioplasty of any severe stenosis. However, for this strategy to be effective, a number of questions must be answered (70). First, ipsilateral stroke must be an important cause of long-term morbidity and mortality. Second, the incidence of ipsilateral stroke must be high enough to justify a program of surveillance. Third, restenosis must be an important cause of late ipsilateral stroke. Fourth, redo CEA or angioplasty must be a safe and effective mode of treatment.

11.3. What Randomized Trial Data are Available?

No randomized trials have addressed this issue.

11.4. What Non-randomized Trial Data are Available?

Each of the four assumptions in the rationale need to be addressed in turn. It is indisputable that late ipsilateral stroke is an important cause of morbidity and mortality following CEA. However, the overall incidence is relatively low following successful endarterectomy. In the ECST, the 5-year risk of ipsilateral stroke (including operative death and stroke) was 10.5% at 5 years. In NASCET, the 3-year risk of ipsilateral stroke (including the operative risk) was 8.9%. Thus from the outset, the annual risk of ipsilateral stroke following successful surgery is no more than 1% (11).

The third assumption is that restenosis is an important cause of late, ipsilateral stroke. A large number of studies have undertaken serial surveillance of the operated and non-operated contralateral ICA (71,72). Published rates of restenosis >50% and/or occlusion in Duplex screened cohorts range from 2% at 3 years (73) to 36% at 6 years (74). In a recent systematic review, Frericks et al. observed that the risk of recurrent stenosis was about 10% in the first year, 3% in the second, and 2% in the third (72). Thus, the available evidence suggests that restenosis is quite a common phenomenon. However, the key issue in this debate is whether restenosis is associated with an increased risk of ipsilateral stroke long-term. Most early restenoses are due to neo-intimal hyperplasia, which produces a smooth fibrotic narrowing within the endarterectomy zone. The pathology of this lesion is totally different from secondary atherosclerotic disease which tends to occur many years after CEA. Frericks et al. identified 10 published series where stroke risk was correlated with the presence or absence of a recurrent stenosis (72). Overall, the 3-year risk of ipsilateral stroke in patients with a restenosis >50% was about 5.5%. This compares with a stroke risk of 3.1% in patients with no evidence of any restenosis. Accordingly, even if redo CEA or angioplasty could be performed with zero risk (a highly improbable scenario), it is doubtful if any overall clinical benefit could be achieved.

One other cited reason for recommending serial surveillance is disease progression in the non-operated artery. However, the available evidence suggests that the risk of late stroke in the contralateral hemisphere is <2% per annum and that most of the strokes that do occur are not associated with any significant underlying stenosis (75).

11.5. Summary

The role of surveillance and re-intervention for recurrent stenosis is one of the few carotid controversies that varies intensely on a geographical basis. This practice has been widely adopted (and vigorously defended) in the

United States and mainland Europe, but virtually not at all in the United Kingdom and Scandinavia. Although the rationale is attractive in concept, the available data suggest that the risk of late ipsilateral stroke is very low. Patients with restenosis were approximately twice as likely as those with no recurrent disease to suffer a late ipsilateral stroke, but the absolute risk difference at 3 years was very small (about 2–3%). Accordingly, there is relatively little evidence to support the practice of serial surveillance and secondary intervention, particularly as an increasing proportion of arteriotomies are now patched. It would, therefore, seem reasonable to discharge patients early with the strict proviso that they should return immediately if they suffer recurrent symptoms.

12. SUMMARY

As will have been seen, although many of the controversies seem unrelated at first sight, the underlying theme throughout has been the reduction of the initial operative risk and the optimization of long-term stroke prevention. This aim cannot be seen in the context of one parameter only (e.g., patching or choice of anesthesia). The prevention of operative stroke is multi-factorial and the practising surgeon must direct their attention to a number of issues relating to patient selection and performance of the operation.

REFERENCES

1. European Carotid Surgery Trialists' Collaborative Group. Randomized trial of endarterectomy for recently symptomatic carotid stenosis: final results of the MRC European Carotid Surgery Trial (ECST). Lancet 1998; 351:1379–1387.
2. Barnett HJM, Taylor DW, Eliasziw M, Fox AJ, Ferguson GG, Haynes RB, et al. Benefit of carotid endarterectomy in patients with symptomatic moderate or severe stenosis. N Engl J Med 1998; 339:1415–1425.
3. Executive Committee for the Asymptomatic Carotid Atherosclerosis Study. Endarterectomy for asymptomatic carotid artery stenosis. JAMA 1995; 273:1421–1428.
4. Moore WS, Young B, Baker WH, Robertson JT, Toole JF, Vescera CL, Howard VJ. Surgical results: a justification of the surgeon selection process for the ACAS trial. The ACAS investigators. J Vasc Surg 1996; 23:323–328.
5. Barnett HJM, Barnes RW, Clagett GP, Ferguson GG, Robertson JT, Walker PM. Symptomatic carotid artery stenosis: a solvable problem. The NASCET trial. Stroke 1992; 23:1050–1053.
6. Anyanwu AC, Treasure T. Unrealistic expectations arising from mortality data reported in cardiothoracic journals. J Thor Cardiovasc Surg 2002; 123:16–20.
7. Rothwell PM, Slattery J, Warlow CP. A systematic review of the risk of stroke or death due to endarterectomy for symptomatic carotid stenosis. Stroke 1996; 27:260–265.

8. Hsia DC, Krushat WM, Moscoe LM. Epidemiology of carotid endarterectomies among healthcare Medicare beneficiaries. J Vasc Surg 1992; 16:201–208.
9. Hsia DC, Moscoe LM, Krushat WM. Epidemiology of carotid endarterectomy among Medicare beneficiaries: 1985–1996 update. Stroke 1998; 29:346–350.
10. CAVATAS Investigators. Endovascular vs. surgical treatment in patients with carotid stenosis in the Carotid and Vertebral Artery Transluminal Angioplasty Study (CAVATAS): a randomised trial. Lancet 2001; 357:1729–1737.
11. Naylor AR, Rothwell PM, Bell PRF. Overview of the principal results and secondary analyses from the European and the North American randomised trials of carotid endarterectomy. Eur J Vasc Endovasc Surg 2003; 26:115–129.
12. Wong JH, Findlay JM, Suarez-Almazor ME. Regional performance of carotid endarterectomy: appropriateness, outcomes and risk factors for complications. Stroke 1997; 28:891–898.
13. Kucey DS, Bowyer B, Iron K, et al. Determinants of outcome after carotid endarterectomy. J Vasc Surg 1998; 28:1051–1058.
14. Ouriel K, Yadav J, Wholey M, Katzen B, Fayad P. The SAPPHIRE randomised trial of carotid stenting vs. endarterectomy: a subgroup analysis. Proceedings of the Annual Meeting of the Society for Vascular Surgery and the American Association of Vascular Surgeons, Chicago, 8–11 June, 2003.
15. Barnett HJM, Eliasziw M, Meldrum HE, Taylor DW. Do the facts and figures warrant a tenfold increase in the performance of carotid endarterectomy in asymptomatic patients? Neurology 1996; 466:603–608.
16. Shackley P, Slack R, Booth A, Michaels J. Is there a positive volume–outcome relationship in peripheral vascular surgery? Results of a systematic review. Eur J Vasc Endovasc Surg 2000; 20:326–335.
17. Irvine CD, Grayson D, Lusby RJ. Clinical governance and the surgeon. Brit J Surg 2000; 87:766–770.
18. Wennberg DE, Lucas FL, Birkmeyer JD, Bredenberg CE, Fisher ES. Variation in carotid endarterectomy mortality in the Medicare population. JAMA 1998; 279:1278–1281.
19. Barnett HJM, Taylor DW, Eliasziw M, et al. (on behalf of the North American Symptomatic Carotid Endarterectomy Trial Collaborators). Benefit of carotid endarterectomy in patients with symptomatic moderate or severe stenosis. New Engl J Med 1998; 339:1415–1425.
20. Taylor DW, Barnett HJM, Haynes GG, et al. Low dose and high dose salicylic acid for patients undergoing carotid endarterectomy: a randomised trial. Lancet 1999; 353:2179–2184.
21. Payne DA, Hayes PD, Jones CI, Belham P, Naylor AR, Bell PRF, Goodall AH. Combined effects of aspirin and clopidogrel on platelet function in-vivo and in-vitro: implications for use in open vascular surgery. J Vasc Surg 2002; 35:1204–1209.
22. Tangkanakul C, Counsell C, Warlow CP. Local versus general anaesthesia in carotid endarterectomy: a systematic review of the evidence. Eur J Vasc Endovasc Surg 1997; 13:491–499.
23. McCarthy RJ, Walker R, McAteer P, Budd JS, Horrocks M. Patient and hospital benefits of local anaesthesia for carotid endarterectomy. Eur J Vasc Endovasc Surg 2001; 22:13–18.

24. Forssell C, Takolander R, Bergqvist D, Johansson A, Persson NH. Local versus general anaesthesia in carotid surgery: a prospective randomised study. Eur J Vasc Surg 1989; 3:503–509.

25. Pluskwa F, Bonnet F, Abhay K, et al. Blood pressure profiles during carotid endarterectomy: comparing flunitrazepan/fentanyl/nitrous oxide with epidural anaesthesia. Ann Fr Anesth Reanim 1989; 8:26–32.

26. Prough DS, Scuderi PE, McWhorter JM, Balestrieri FJ, Davis CH, Stullken EH. Haemodynamic status following regional and general anaesthesia for carotid endarterectomy. J Neurosurg Anesth 1989; 1:35–40.

27. Elliott BM, Collins GJ, Youkey JR, Donohue HJ, Salander JM, Rich NM. Intra-operative local anaesthetic injection of the carotid sinus nerve: a prospective randomised study. Am J Surg 1986; 152:695–699.

28. Welch M, Tait WF, Durrans D, Carr HM, Jackson PW, Walker MG. Role of topical lignocaine during carotid endarterectomy. Brit J Surg 1992; 79: 1035–1037.

29. Gottlieb A, Satariano-Hayden P, Schoenwald P, Ryckman J, Piedmonte M. The effects of carotid sinus nerve blockade on haemodynamic stability after carotid endarterectomy. J Cardiothorac Vasc Anesth 1997; 11:67–71.

30. Fearn SJ, Mortimer AJ, Faragher EB, McCollum CN. Carotid sinus nerve blockade during carotid surgery: a randomised controlled trial. Eur J Vasc Endovasc Surg 2002; 24:480–484.

31. Malone JM, Ballard JL. Carotid artery shunt: argument for its routine use. In: Moore, WS, eds. Surgery for Cerebrovascular Disease 2nd ed. Philadelphia: WB Saunders, 1996:347–354.

32. Ferguson CG, Eliasziw M, Barr HWK, Clagett GP, Barnes RW, Wallace C, et al. WB Saunders The North American Symptomatic Carotid Endarterectomy Trial: surgical results of 1415 patients. Stroke 1999; 30:1751–1758.

33. Baker WH, Littooy FN, Hayes AC. Carotid endarterectomy without a shunt: the control series. J Vasc Surg 1984; 1:50.

34. Counsell C, Salinas R, Warlow CP, Naylor AR. The role of carotid artery shunting during carotid endarterectomy: a systematic review of the randomised trials of routine and selective shunting and the different methods of intra-operative monitoring. In: Warlow CP, van Gijn J, Sandercock P, eds. Stroke Module of the Cochrane Database of Systematic Reviews, Issue 2. London: BMJ Publishing Group, 1996.

35. Gumerlock MK, Neuwelt EA. Carotid endarterectomy: to shunt or not to shunt. Stroke 1988; 19:1485–1490.

36. Sandmann WF, et al. In: Veith FJ, ed. Current Critical Problems in Vascular Surgery, Vol. 5. St. Louis, Missouri: Quality Medical Publishing Inc., 1993:434–440.

37. Wilkinson JM, Rochester JR, Sivaguru A, Cameron IC, Fisher R, Beard JD. Middle cerebral artery blood velocity, embolisation and neurological outcome during carotid endarterectomy: a prospective comparison of the Javid and Pruitt-Inahara Shunts. Eur J Vasc Endovasc Surg 1997; 14:399–402.

38. Krul JM, van Gijn J, Ackerstaff RG, Eikelboom BC, Theodorides T, Vermeulen FE. Site and pathogenesis of infarcts associated with carotid endarterectomy. Stroke 1989; 20:324–328.

39. Ghali R, Palazzo EG, Rodriguez DI, Zammit M, Loudenback DL, DeMuth RP, Spencer MP, Sauvage LR. Transcranial Doppler intra-operative monitoring during carotid endarterectomy: experience with regional or general anaesthesia, with and without shunting. Ann Vasc Surg 1997; 11:9–13.

40. Naylor AR, Hayes PD, Allroggen H, Lennard N, Gaunt ME, Thompson MM, London NJM, Bell PRF. Reducing the risk of carotid surgery: a seven year audit of the role of monitoring and quality control assessment. J Vasc Surg 2000; 32:750–759.

41. Cao P, De Rango P, Zannetti S. Eversion versus conventional carotid endarterectomy: a systematic review. Eur J Vasc Endovasc Surg 2002; 23:195–201.

42. Balzer K, Guds I, Heger J, Jahnel B. Conventional thrombo-endarterectomy with carotid patch plasty versus eversion endarterectomy: technique, indications and results. Zentralb Chir 2000; 125:228–238.

43. Vanmaele RG, van Schil PE, Demaeseneer MG, et al. Division endarterectomy anastomosis of the internal carotid artery: a prospective randomised comparative study. Cardiovasc Surg 1994; 2:573–578.

44. Ballotta E, Da Giau G, Saladini M, et al. Carotid endarterectomy with patch closure versus carotid eversion endarterectomy and reimplantation: a prospective randomised study. Surgery 1999; 125:271–279.

45. Ballotta E, Renon L, Da Giau G, et al. A prospective randomised study on bilateral carotid endarterectomy: patching versus eversion. Ann Surg 2000; 232:119–125.

46. Cao P, Giordano G, De Rango P, et al. (on behalf of the collaborators of the EVEREST study group). A randomised study on eversion versus standard endarterectomy. Study design and preliminary results: the Everest Study. J Vasc Surg 1998; 27:595–605.

47. Archie JP, Green JJ. Saphenous vein rupture pressure, rupture stress and carotid endarterectomy vein patch reconstruction. Surgery 1990; 107:389–396.

48. Naylor AR, Payne D, Thompson MM, London NJM, Sayers RD, Dennis MS, Bell PRF. Prosthetic patch infection after carotid endarterectomy. Eur J Vasc Endovasc Surg 2002; 23:11–16.

49. Counsell CE, Salinas R, Naylor R, Warlow CP. A systematic review of the randomised trials of carotid patch angioplasty in carotid endarterectomy. Eur J Endovasc Surg 1997; 13:345–354.

50. Hayes PD, Allroggen H, Steel S, Thompson MM, London NJM, Bell PRF, Naylor AR. A randomised trial of vein versus dacron patching during carotid endarterectomy: influence of patch type on post-operative embolisation. J Vasc Surg 2001; 33:994–1000.

51. Kresowik TF, Bratzler DW, Kresowik RA, Hendel ME, Grund SL, Brown KR, et al. Multi-state improvement in process and outcomes of carotid endarterectomy. J Vasc Surg 2004; 39:372–380.

52. Wakefield TW, Lindblad B, Stanlet TJ, et al. Heparin and protamine use in peripheral vascular surgery: a comparison between surgeons of the Society for Vascular Surgery and the European Society for Vascular Surgery. Eur J Vasc Surg 1994; 8:193–198.

53. Treiman RL, Cossman DV, Foran RF, Levin PM, Cohen JL, Wagner WH. The influence of neutralizing heparin after carotid endarterectomy on post-operative stroke and wound haematoma. J Vasc Surg 1990; 12:445–446.

54. Levison JA, Faust GR, Halpern VJ, et al. Relationship of protamine dosing with post-operative complications of carotid endarterectomy. Ann Vasc Surg 1999; 13:67–72.

55. Mauney MC, Buchanan SA, Lawrence WA, et al. Stroke rate is markedly reduced after carotid endarterectomy by avoidance of protamine. J Vasc Surg 1995; 22:264–270.

56. Fearn SJ, Parry AD, Picton AJ, Mortimer AJ, McCollum CN. Should heparin be reversed after carotid endarterectomy: a randomised prospective trial. Eur J Vasc Endovasc Surg 1997; 13:394–397.

57. Riles TS, Imparato AM, Jacobowitz GR, Lamparello PJ, Giangola G, Adelman MA, Landis R. The cause of perioperative stroke after carotid endarterectomy. J Vasc Surg 1994; 19:206–214.

58. Naylor AR. Prevention of operation related stroke: are we asking the right questions? Cardiovasc Surg 1999; 7:155–157

59. Gaunt ME, Smith J, Martin PJ, Ratliff DA, Bell PRF, Naylor AR. On-table diagnosis of incipient carotid artery thrombosis during carotid endarterectomy using transcranial Doppler sonography. J Vasc Surg 1994; 20:104–107.

60. Gaunt ME, Smith JL, Martin PJ, Ratliff DA, Bell PRF, Naylor AR. A comparison of quality control methods applied to carotid endarterectomy. Eur J Vasc Endovasc Surg 1996; 11:4–11.

61. Spencer MP. Transcranial Doppler monitoring and causes of stroke from carotid endarterectomy. Stroke 1997; 28:685–691.

62. Levi CR, O'Malley HM, Fell G, Roberts AK, Hoare MC, Royle JP, et al. Transcranial Doppler detected cerebral embolism following carotid endarterectomy: high microembolic signal loads predict post-operative cerebral ischaemia. Brain 1997; 120:621–629.

63. Spencer MP. Transcranial Doppler monitoring and causes of stroke from carotid endarterectomy. Stroke 1997; 28:685–691.

64. Cantelmo NL, Babikian VL, Samaraweera RN, Gordon JK, Pochay VE, Winter MR. Cerebral microembolism and ischaemia changes associated with carotid endarterectomy. J Vasc Surg 1998; 27:1024–1030.

65. Laman DM, Wieneke GH, van Duijn H, van Huffelen AC. High embolic rate after carotid endarterectomy is associated with early cerebrovascular complications. J Vasc Surg 2002; 36:278–284.

66. Hayes PD, Allroggen H, Steel S, Thompson MM, London NJM, Bell PRF, Naylor AR. A randomised trial of vein versus dacron patching during carotid endarterectomy: influence of patch type on post-operative embolisation. J Vasc Surg 2001; 33:994–1000.

67. Hayes PD, Box H, Tull S, Gaunt ME, Bell PRF, Goodall AH, Naylor AR. The patient's thrombo-embolic response following carotid endarterectomy is related to enhanced platelet sensitivity to ADP. J Vasc Surg 2003; 38:1226–1231.

68. Hayes PD, Patel F, Bell PRF, Naylor AR. Patients' thrombo-embolic potential between bilateral carotid endarterectomies remains stable over time. Eur J Vasc Endovasc Surg 2001; 22:496–498.

69. Payne DA, Jones CI, Hayes PD, Thompson MM, London NJM, Bell PRF, Goodall AH, Naylor AR. Beneficial effects of clopidogrel combined with

aspirin in reducing cerebral emboli in patients undergoing carotid endarterectomy. Circulation 2004; 109:1476–1481.

70. Beard JD. Does serial clinical or Duplex surveillance reduce the long-term risk of stroke? In: Naylor AR, Mackey WC, eds. Carotid Artery Surgery: A Problem Based Approach. London: WB Saunders, 2000.

71. Lattimer CR, Burnand KG. Recurrent stenosis after carotid endarterectomy. Brit J Surg 1997; 84:1206–1219.

72. Frericks H, Kievit J, van Baalen JM, van Bockel JH. Carotid recurrent stenosis and risk of ipsilateral stroke: a systematic review of the literature. Stroke 1998; 29:244–250.

73. Katz D, Snyder SO, Gandhi RH, et al. Long term follow-up for recurrent stenosis: a prospective randomised study of expanded PTFE patch angioplasty versus primary closure after carotid endarterectomy. J Vasc Surg 1994; 198–203.

74. Norrving B, Nilsson B, Olsson JE. Progression of carotid disease after endarterectomy: a Doppler ultrasound study. Ann Neurol 1982; 12:548–552.

75. Naylor AR, John T, Howlett J, Gillespie I, Allan P, Ruckley CV. Fate of the non-operated carotid artery after contralateral endarterectomy. Br J Surg 1995; 82:44–48.

16

Symptomatic Carotid Artery Occlusion: Extracranial Intracranial Bypass and Other Treatment Options

Catharina J. M. Klijn and L. Jaap Kappelle
University Department of Neurology, University Medical Center Utrecht and Rudolf Magnus Institute of Neuroscience, Utrecht, The Netherlands

Patients with transient or moderately disabling symptoms of ischemia of the brain or eye who are found to have an ipsilateral occlusion of the internal carotid artery (ICA) are at risk of further stroke and other vascular events. A meta-analysis showed that the risk of recurrent stroke in these patients is about 5–6% per year (1), about half to two-thirds of which occur in the hemisphere ipsilateral to the ICA occlusion. The etiology of stroke in patients with ICA occlusion is still a matter of debate. Thromboembolism is a potential cause, with emboli either from the distal or proximal ICA stump or from atherosclerotic plaques in the common carotid artery or external carotid artery (ECA), which find their way to the ipsilateral hemisphere or retina via collateral pathways involving the ECA (2–4). Even transhemispheric passage of micro-emboli via the anterior communicating artery has been suggested to cause ischemic events ipsilateral to the ICA occlusion (5). In addition to thromboembolism, a compromised cerebral blood flow has been suggested to play an important role in causing transient ischemic attacks (TIAs) and stroke in patients with ICA occlusion (6). Prevention of recurrent ischemic stroke by extracranial to intracranial (EC/IC) bypass surgery in patients with symptomatic ICA occlusion is based on the notion that in some patients, ischemic stroke is caused by a failure of blood flow towards the brain rather than by embolism. In patients with occlusion of the ICA, other treatment options such as carotid endarterectomy or angioplasty are not feasible.

The efficacy of EC/IC bypass surgery for the prevention of recurrent ischemic stroke was evaluated in the International EC/IC Bypass Study. In this international randomized trial, patients with symptomatic ICA occlusion or intracranial ICA stenosis, or MCA stenosis or occlusion were treated either with an anastomosis between the superficial temporal artery (STA) and a cortical branch of the middle cerebral artery (MCA) in addition to best medical therapy or with best medical treatment alone (7). In 1985, after randomization of 1377 patients (960 patients with a symptomatic ICA occlusion and 417 with an intracranial ICA stenosis or MCA stenosis or occlusion) over a period of 8 years, the study showed that the operation was not effective, despite good operative results (8). Moreover, subgroup analysis failed to show any trends toward a benefit of the operation in any of the pre-specified subgroups, such as patients with ongoing symptoms after demonstration of the occlusion of the ICA, or patients with frequent transient ischemic attacks (≥ 6) and poor collateral blood supply (8,9). As a result, the operation has been largely abandoned throughout the world (10). Proponents of the hemodynamic theory, however, commented that the EC/IC Bypass Study did not restrict the inclusion of patients to those who were at high risk of recurrent stroke, i.e., in whom a compromised blood flow to the hemisphere ipsilateral to the occluded carotid artery had been demonstrated (11–15). If such patients at high risk can indeed be identified, the role of the EC/IC bypass operation needs reappraisal.

1. HOW TO IDENTIFY PATIENTS AT HIGH RISK OF RECURRENT ISCHEMIC STROKE?

In patients with an occlusion of the carotid artery who had never had any symptoms at all, the risk of recurrent ischemic stroke is low ($\sim$1–2% per year) (16,17). In these patients, collateral pathways probably are sufficient. The same applies to patients who had had symptoms only before the occlusion of the carotid artery was found, but never thereafter (15,18). One might speculate that in these patients, symptoms arose as a result of thromboembolism before the carotid artery became occluded and that collateral pathways could adequately sustain blood flow to the brain once the occlusion had occurred. Also patients who have only retinal symptoms and never symptoms of cerebral ischemia are at a relatively low risk of stroke; none of 16 such patients in one study (19) and none of 24 in another (15) had an ischemic stroke during follow-up of more than 2 years.

It is unlikely that in any of these patient groups, the potential benefit of any type of surgical intervention would be larger than the risk of the procedure.

In contrast, several studies have demonstrated that patients with recurrent symptoms associated with an ICA occlusion in whom a compromised cerebral blood flow has been demonstrated have a risk of recurrent ischemic stroke of approximately 9–18% per year (18–25). It should be noted, however, that several other studies, using similar techniques, could not confirm the association between a decreased hemodynamic reserve and recurrent ischemic stroke (15,26–28). Some of these studies can be criticized because the study population was not homogenous in that asymptomatic patients were also included (20–22,26,27), or patients with intracranial carotid artery or middle cerebral artery lesions or extracranial carotid artery stenosis were included (18,23–28), or because some patients were censored (15,26) or excluded (25) owing to surgical intervention. At this moment it remains unclear whether the different techniques identify the same patients to be at a high risk of recurrent ischemic stroke and which technique can most accurately predict the occurrence of a future stroke. Correlations between different hemodynamic measures such as the oxygen extraction fraction by PET and transcranial Doppler ultrasonography (TCD) CO_2-reactivity (29) or changes in regional blood flow velocity and volumetric flow after acetazolamide (30) have been disappointingly low. Studies comparing the predictive value of the measurement of oxygen extraction fraction and cerebral blood volume by PET, TCD, stable xenon or (133) xenon-inhalation techniques, or (123) I-labeled IMP single photon emission computed tomography before and after vasodilatory stimuli (by means of breath-holding, carbogen inhalation, or acetazolamide) in the same patients have not been performed. Magnetic resonance (MR) techniques such as MR perfusion, diffusion, and spectroscopy may provide new prognostic indicators in the near future (31). The mean transit time measured with perfusion-weighted MR imaging was recently shown to correlate well with the mean transit time, cerebral blood flow, vascular reactivity, and the oxygen extraction fraction measured with PET (32).

Typical features from the literature that have classically been associated with hemodynamic compromise, such as limb-shaking or precipitation of symptoms by rising or exercise, were found to be associated with a relatively high risk of recurrent cerebral ischemic events (HR 5.0; 95% CI: 1.4–17.2; P=0.01) (15). However, such symptoms occur in only a minority of patients (~14–20%) (15,33). The presence of leptomeningeal pathways on angiography was associated with a worse outcome in one study (15) but not in another (19). The number of collateral pathways was inversely related to the risk of ischemic stroke in a single study (20).

Accumulating evidence leads to the tentative conclusion that patients with symptomatic ICA occlusion who are at a high risk of recurrent ischemic stroke can be distinguished from those at a relatively low risk by means of a number of methods that give information on the hemodynamic status of the hemisphere at risk.

2. TREATMENT OPTIONS

2.1. Extracranial Intracranial Bypass

The current evidence shows that STA–MCA bypass does not prevent recurrent stroke better than medical treatment alone in patients with symptomatic carotid artery occlusion in general (8). Whether or not the EC/IC bypass confers benefit in a subgroup of patients with clinical or technical evidence for a hemodynamically compromised hemisphere on the side of the carotid artery occlusion remains as yet unknown. Many studies have reported the improvement of cerebral hemodynamic measurements after STA–MCA bypass operation (34–37) but comparisons with similar patients who were not operated on are not available. Others found that improvement of hemodynamic measures did not occur after operation (38) or was not consistent (39,40). Improvement of hemodynamic measures has been shown especially in patients in whom such measures were most disturbed before operation (41–43). A caveat is that improvement of cerebral blood flow shortly after STA–MCA bypass surgery may not last over time (42,44) and that cerebral hemodynamic measures may improve spontaneously (22,26,45).

If STA–MCA bypass surgery is considered in the subgroup of patients with carotid artery occlusion who are at a high risk of recurrent ischemic stroke, it should be kept in mind that the number of complications of surgery in this subgroup may be higher than that reported in the EC/IC Bypass Study. One study reported a complication rate of STA–MCA bypass surgery close to 12% in patients who were considered neurologically unstable (46). Patients who on theoretical grounds have the most to gain by EC/IC bypass surgery may also carry the highest perioperative risk.

Recently the Carotid Occlusion Surgery Study (COSS) was started in the United States (14). Patients with ICA occlusion will be eligible for inclusion in this prospective multicenter randomized trial if they have suffered a cerebral TIA or ischemic stroke in the previous 4 months and have an increased PET oxygen extraction fraction in the hemisphere ipsilateral to the ICA occlusion. Patients are randomized to either STA–MCA bypass surgery in addition to best medical therapy or to best medical therapy alone. The COSS is powered to detect a reduction in the risk of recurrent ipsilateral ischemic stroke after 2 years from 40 to 24% (absolute risk reduction of 16%), including a surgical morbidity and mortality rate of 12% (COSS, manual of operations; courtesy of H. P. Adams, Jr.). Screening of 930 patients by PET should identify 372 patients with increased oxygen extraction fraction between 2002 and 2007. Hopefully this tremendous effort will result in an answer to the clinically important question of the potential benefit of STA–MCA bypass surgery for patients with symptomatic ICA occlusion at a high risk of recurrent ischemic stroke.

Over the last few years, a new technique of the EC/IC bypass operation has been developed, the so-called high flow EC/IC bypass, or Excimer laser-assisted non-occlusive anastomosis (ELANA) (47,48). Instead of connecting the STA to a small artery at the brain convexity, in this procedure the STA (or the ECA) is connected to the intracranial, distal part of the ICA or the proximal part of the MCA by means of a venous (or arterial) transplant. The intracranial anastomosis is made with the Excimer laser, which obliterates the need to temporarily clamp the recipient artery. This allows the construction of an anastomosis with one of the large arteries proximal to the vascular tree (49). The amount of flow that can be obtained through this bypass is higher than that reported for the conventional STA–MCA bypass (50). The increase in blood flow towards the hemisphere at risk that can be obtained with a high flow EC/IC bypass may therefore be larger than can be accomplished by means of the STA–MCA bypass. However, direct comparisons of such measures in patients with symptomatic carotid artery occlusion are not yet available. Preliminary results have shown that the Excimer laser-assisted EC/IC bypass operation is a potentially promising procedure for revascularization of the brain in patients with symptomatic carotid artery occlusion at a high risk of recurrent stroke, but carries a substantial risk in these patients (51).

2.2. Other Treatment Options

2.2.1. Medical Treatment

All patients with symptomatic ICA occlusion should be treated with an antiplatelet agent, aspirin in most patients, with rigorous control of vascular risk factors such as hyperlipidemia, diabetes mellitus, smoking, and obesity. It should be noted that this recommendation is based on extrapolation of the results of studies on secondary prevention of stroke in general. If patients have ongoing transient ischemic attacks despite aspirin, oral anticoagulation may be prescribed instead (1) but again evidence from randomized controlled trials is not available. Furthermore, in our experience, the change from aspirin to oral anticoagulants rarely results in cessation of symptoms, especially in patients with clinical features suggesting a hemodynamic cause. The treatment of hypertension should be performed prudently because aggressive treatment may actually induce cerebral ischemic symptoms in patients with symptomatic carotid artery occlusion (52).

2.2.2. Tapering of Antihypertensive Treatment and Bed-Rest

In patients with ICA occlusion in whom a hemodynamic cause seems likely either because of specific clinical features, such as limb-shaking or precipitation of symptoms by rising, or because of investigations that show that the cerebral blood flow in the hemisphere at risk is compromised, temporary tapering of antihypertensive drugs and bed-rest may be considered. It seems pathophysiologically plausible that the induction of a relatively high blood flow and avoidance of orthostatic drops in blood pressure could be beneficial in patients with an ICA occlusion and a compromised cerebral blood flow. In our experience and in that of others (53), these interventions have resulted in cessation of symptoms in some patients, but we would like to stress again that there is no evidence from randomized trials on the efficacy of these interventions.

2.2.3. Endarterectomy or Endovascular Treatment of Severely Stenosed Cerebropetal Collateral Pathways

Patients with symptomatic ICA occlusion who also have a severe (70–99%) stenosis of the contralateral ICA that is asymptomatic, may be advised to undergo endarterectomy (or endovascular treatment) of this stenosis if there is evidence for collateral blood supply via the anterior communicating artery. Similarly, treatment of severely stenosed other collateral pathways such as the ipsilateral ECA or the vertebral arteries may be considered. In our experience an important stenosis in a collateral cerebropetal vessel other than the contralateral ICA is a rare finding.

Again, we acknowledge that for these treatment options, there is no evidence from controlled studies, and the considerations are based on pathophysiological plausibility—admittedly a shaky basis.

3. CONCLUDING REMARKS

Patients with symptomatic carotid artery occlusion who are at a high risk of recurrent ischemic stroke may benefit from treatment with an EC/IC bypass, but presently there is insufficient evidence to support this.

Patients with ICA occlusion who have never been symptomatic and patients who have only had symptoms of the eye, but never of the brain, appear to have a good prognosis and in them the risk of EC/IC bypass is unlikely to be outweighed by their potential benefit from the procedure. This probably also holds for patients who never had symptoms after the occlusion of the ICA has been documented. Identification of patients at a high risk of ischemic stroke can be obtained by several methods that assess the hemodynamic status of the hemisphere at risk.

At present it is unclear whether an EC/IC bypass results in significantly more improvement of the hemodynamic state of the hemisphere at risk than is observed over time without surgical intervention. In addition no information is available on the comparison of the STA–MCA bypass and the Excimer laser-assisted high flow EC/IC bypass with respect to the potential improvement of the cerebral blood flow to the hemisphere at risk, the risk of the procedure, or their potential benefit in the prevention of recurrent stroke in patients with ICA occlusion who are at high risk of recurrent ischemic stroke.

Recently a randomized controlled trial has been commenced, testing whether STA–MCA bypass surgery in addition to optimal medical treatment can reduce the risk of recurrent ischemic stroke in patients with recently symptomatic ICA occlusion and a high oxygen extraction measured by PET. Results are expected at the end of 2007.

ACKNOWLEDGMENTS

CJM Klijn is supported by grants from the Niels Stensen Foundation and the Dr. Jan Meerwaldt Foundation.

REFERENCES

1. Klijn CJM, Kappelle LJ, Algra A, van Gijn J. Outcome in patients with symptomatic occlusion of the internal carotid artery or intracranial arterial lesions: a meta-analysis of the role of baseline characteristics and type of antithrombotic treatment. Cerebrovasc Dis 2001; 12:228–234.
2. Barnett HJM. Delayed cerebral ischemic episodes distal to occlusion of major cerebral arteries. Neurology 1978; 28:769–774.
3. Barnett HJM, Peerless SJ, Kaufmann JCE. "Stump" of internal carotid artery—a source for further cerebral embolic ischemia.
4. Finklestein S, Kleinman GM, Cuneo R, Baringer JR. Delayed stroke following carotid occlusion. Neurology 1980; 30:84–88.
5. Georgiadis D, Grosset DG, Lees KR. Transhemispheric passage of microemboli in patients with unilateral internal carotid artery occlusion. Stroke 1993; 24:1664–1666.
6. Klijn CJM, Kappelle LJ, Tulleken CAF, van Gijn J. Symptomatic carotid artery occlusion. A reappraisal of hemodynamic factors. Stroke 1997; 28:2084–2093.
7. The EC/IC bypass study group. The international cooperative study of extracranial/intracranial arterial anastomosis (EC/IC bypass study): methodology and entry characteristics. Stroke 1985; 16:397–406.
8. The EC/IC bypass study group. Failure of extracranial–intracranial arterial bypass to reduce the risk of ischemic stroke. Results of an international randomized trial. N Engl J Med 1985; 313:1191–1200.
9. Barnett HJM, Sackett D, Haynes B, Peerless SJ, Meissner I, Hachinski V, Fox A. Are the result extracranial–intracranial bypass trial generalizable? N Engl J Med 1987; 316:820–824.
10. Caplan LR, Piepgras DG, Quest DO, Toole JF, Samson D, Futrell N, Millikan C, Flamm ES, Heros RC, Yonekawa Y, Eguchi T, Yonas H, Rothbart D, Spetzler RF. EC-IC bypass 10 years later: is it valuable? Surg Neurol 1996; 46:416–423.
11. Ausman JI, Diaz FG. Critique of the extracranial–intracranial bypass study. Surg Neurol 1986; 26:218–221.
12. Day AL, Rhoton AL, Little JR. The extracranial–intracranial bypass study. Surg Neurol 1986; 26:222–226.
13. Sundt TM Jr. Was the international randomized trial of extracranial–intracranial arterial bypass representative of the population at risk? N Engl J Med 1987; 316:814–816.

14. Adams HP Jr, Powers WJ, Grubb RL Jr, Clarke WR, Woolson RF. Preview of a new trial of extracranial-to-intracranial anastomosis. The carotid occlusion surgery study. Neurosurg Clin N Am 2001; 36:613–624.
15. Klijn CJM, Kappelle LJ, van Huffelen AC, Visser GH, Algra A, Tulleken CAF, van Gijn J. Recurrent ischemia in symptomatic carotid occlusion: prognostic value of hemodynamic factors. Neurology 2000; 56:1806–1812.
16. Powers WJ, Derdeyn CP, Fritsch SM, Carpenter DA, Yundt KD, Videen TO, Grubb RL Jr. Benign prognosis of never-symptomatic carotid occlusion. Neurology 2000; 54:878–882.
17. Vernieri F, Pasqualetti P, Passarelli F, Rossini PM, Silvestrini M. Outcome of carotid artery occlusion is predicted by cerebrovascular reactivity. Stroke 1999; 30:593–598.
18. Yamauchi H, Fukuyama H, Nagahama Y, Nabatame H, Ueno M, Nishizawa S, Konishi J, Shio H. Significance of increased oxygen extraction fraction in five-year prognosis of major cerebral arterial occlusive diseases. J Nucl Med 1999; 40:1992–1998.
19. Grubb RL Jr, Derdeyn CP, Fritsch SM, Carpenter DA, Yundt KD, Videen TO, Spitznagel EL, Powers WJ. Importance of hemodynamic factors in the prognosis of symptomatic carotid occlusion. JAMA 1998; 280:1055–1060.
20. Vernieri F, Pasqualetti P, Matteis M, Passarelli F, Troisi E, Rossini PM, Caltagirone C, Silvestrini M. Effect of collateral blood flow and cerebral vasomotor reactivity on the outcome of carotid artery occlusion. Stroke 2001; 32:1552–1558.
21. Kleiser B, Widder B. Course of carotid artery occlusions with impaired cerebrovascular reactivity. Stroke 1992; 23:171–174.
22. Widder B, Kleiser B, Krapf H. Course of cerebrovascular reactivity in patients with carotid artery occlusions. Stroke 1994; 25:1963–1967.
23. Webster MW, Makaroun MS, Steed DL, Smith HA, Johnson DW, Yonas H. Compromised cerebral blood flow reactivity is a predictor of stroke in patients with symptomatic carotid artery occlusive disease. J Vasc Surg 1995; 21: 338–345.
24. Ogasawara K, Gawa A, Yoshimoto T. Cerebrovascular reactivity to acetazolamide and outcome in patients with symptomatic internal carotid or middle cerebral artery occlusion: a xenon-133 single-photon computed tomography study. Stroke 2002; 33:1857–1862.
25. Kuroda S, Houkin K, Kamiyama H, Mitsumori K, Iwasaki Y, Abe H. Long-term prognosis of medically treated patients with internal carotid or middle cerebral artery occlusion. Can acetazolamide test predict it? Stroke 2001; 32: 2110–2116.
26. Yokota C, Hasegawa Y, Minematsu K, Yamaguchi T. Effect of acetazolamide reactivity and long-term outcome in patients with major cerebral artery occlusive diseases. Stroke 1998; 29:640–644.
27. Hasegawa Y, Yamaguchi T, Tsuchiya T, Minematsu K, Nishimura T. Sequential change of hemodynamic reserve in patients with major cerebral artery occlusion or severe stenosis. Neuroradiology 1992; 34:15–21.

28. Powers WJ, Tempel LW, Grubb RL Jr. Influence of cerebral hemodynamics on stroke risk: one-year follow-up of 30 medically treated patients. Ann Neurol 1989; 25:325–330.
29. Sugimori H, Ibayashi S, Fujii K, Sadoshima S, Kuwabara Y, Fujishima M. Can transcranial Doppler really detect reduced cerebral perfusion states? Stroke 1995; 26:2053–2060.
30. Demolis P, Tran Dinh YR, Giudicelli J-F. Relationships between cerebral regional blood flow velocities and volumetric blood flows and their respective reactivities to acetazolamide. Stroke 1999; 27:1835–1839.
31. Klijn CJM, Kappelle LJ, van der Grond J, Algra A, Tulleken CAF, van Gijn J. Magnetic resonance techniques for the identification of patients with symptomatic carotid artery occlusion at high risk of cerebral ischemic events. Stroke 2000; 31:3001–3007.
32. Mihara F, Kuwubara Y, Tanaka A, Yoshira T, Sasaki M, Yoshida T, Masuda K, Matsushima T. Reliability of mean transit time obtained with perfusion-weighted MR imaging; comparison with positron emission tomography. Magn Reson Imaging 2003; 21:33–39.
33. Klijn CJM, van Buren PA, Kappelle LJ, Tulleken CAF, Eikelboom BC, Algra A, van Gijn J. Outcome in patients with symptomatic occlusion of the internal carotid artery. Eur J Vasc Endovasc Surg 2000; 19:579–586.
34. Iwama T, Hashimoto N, Hayashida K. Cerebral hemodynamic parameters for patients with neurological improvements after extracranial-intracranial arterial bypass surgery: evaluation using positron emission tomography. Neurosurgery 2001; 48:504–512.
35. Takagi Y, Hashimoto N, Iwama T, Hayashida K. Improvement of oxygen metabolic reserve after extracranial-intracranial bypass surgery in patients with severe haemodynamic insufficiency. Acta Neurochir (Wien) 1997; 139:52–56.
36. Karnik R, Valentin A, Ammerer H, Donath P, Slany J. Evaluation of vasomotor reactivity by transcranial Doppler and acetazolamide test before and after extracranial-intracranial bypass in patients with internal carotid artery occlusion. Stroke 1992; 23:812–817.
37. Yamashita T, Kashiwagi S, Nakano S, Takasago T, Abiko S, Shiroyama Y, Hayashi M, Ito H. The effect of EC–IC bypass surgery on resting cerebral blood flow and cerebrovascular reserve capacity studies with stable Xe-CT and acetazolamide test. Neuroradiology 1991; 33:217–222.
38. De Weerd AW, Veering MM, Mosmans PCM, van Huffelen AC, Tulleken CAF, Jonkman EJ. Effect of the extra-intracranial (STA–MCA) arterial anastomosis on EEG and cerebral blood flow. A controlled study on patients with unilateral cerebral ischemia. Stroke 1982; 13:674–679.
39. Vorstrup S, Lassen NA, Henriksen L, Haase J, Lindewald H, Boysen G, Paulson OB. CBF before and after extra-intracranial bypass surgery in patients with ischemic cerebrovascular disease studied with (133)Xe inhalation tomography. Stroke 1985; 16:616–626.
40. Ishikawa T, Yasui N, Suzuki A, Hadeishi H, Shishido F, Uemura K. STA–MCA bypass surgery for internal carotid artery occlusion. Comparative follow-up study. Neurol Med Chir (Tokyo) 1992; 32:5–9.

41. Laurent JP, Lawner PM, O'Connor M. Reversal of intracerebral steal by STA–MCA anastomosis. J Neurosurg 1982; 57:629–632.
42. Yonekura M, Austin G, Hayward W. Long-term evaluation of cerebral blood flow, transient ischemic attacks, and stroke after STA–MCA anastomosis. Surg Neurol 1982; 18:123–130.
43. Powers WJ, Martin WRW, Herscovitch P, Raichle ME, Grubb RL Jr. Extra-cranial–intracranial bypass surgery: hemodynamic and metabolic effects. Neurology 1984; 34:1168–1174.
44. Tanahashi N, Stirling Meyer J, Rogers RL, Kitagawa Y, Mortel KF, Kandula P, Levinthal R, Rose J. Long term assessment of cerebral perfusion following STA–MCA by-pass in patients. Stroke 1985; 16:85–91.
45. Derdeyn CP, Videen TO, Fritsch SM, Carpenter DA, Grubb RL Jr, Powers WJ. Compensatory mechanisms for chronic cerebral hypoperfusion in patients with carotid occlusion. Stroke 1999; 30:1019–1024.
46. Sundt TM Jr, Whisnant JP, Fode NC, Piepgras DG, Houser OW. Results, com-plications, and follow-up of 415 bypass operations for occlusive disease of the carotid system. Mayo Clin Proc 1985; 60:230–240.
47. Tulleken CAF, Verdaasdonk RM, Mansvelt Beck RJ, Mali WPThM. The mod-ified Excimer laser-assisted high-flow bypass operation. Surg Neurol 1996; 46:424–429.
48. Tulleken CAF, van der Zwan A, Verdaasdonk RM, Mansvelt Beck RJ, Moreira Pereira Ramos L, Kappelle LJ. High-flow Excimer laser-assisted extra-intracranial and intra-intracranial bypass. Oper Tech Neurosurg 1999; 2:142–148.
49. Streefkerk HJ, van der Zwan A, Verdaasdonk RM, Beck GJ, Tulleken CAF. Cerebral revascularization. Adv Tech Stand Neurosurg 2003; 28:145–225.
50. van der Zwan A, Tulleken CAF, Hillen B. Flow quantification of the non-occlusive Excimer laser-assisted EC–IC bypass. Acta Neurochir (Wien) 2001; 143:647–654.
51. Klijn CJM, Kappelle LJ, van der Zwan A, van Gijn J, Tulleken CAF. Excimer laser-assisted high-flow EC/IC bypass in patients with symptomatic carotid artery occlusion at high risk of recurrent cerebral ischemia: safety and long-term outcome. Stroke 2002; 33:695–701.
52. Hankey GJ, Gubbay SS. Focal cerebral ischaemia and infarction due to antihy-pertensive therapy. Med J Aust 1987; 146:412–414.
53. Leira EC, Ajax T, Adams HP. Limb-shaking carotid transient ischemic attacks successfully treated with modification of the antihypertensive regimen. Arch Neurol 1997; 7:904–905.

17

Stenting for Symptomatic Stenosis

Lucy Coward and Martin M. Brown

Institute of Neurology, University College London, London, U.K.

1. INTRODUCTION

Most strokes are caused by cerebral infarction in the territory of the carotid arteries, and significant ipsilateral carotid stenosis is found in 20–30% of these cases (1). This observation has led to a search for the most effective form of secondary prevention of stroke in these patients. Large randomized trials have shown that carotid endarterectomy significantly reduces the risk of stroke from severe, recently symptomatic stenosis but this benefit is dependent on a low perioperative complication rate. In recent years, endovascular techniques have been routinely used to treat coronary and peripheral arterial disease. The low complication and high success rates of angioplasty and stenting at these sites mean that they have become the treatment of choice in many patients. There has been some resistance to treating carotid artery disease in the same way because of concern over distal embolization at the time of the procedure. Endovascular equipment and techniques have been developed to combat this problem and are being used increasingly.

In line with the data from surgical trials which show differential efficacy and complication rates for carotid endarterectomy in symptomatic and asymptomatic patients, we review the data on stenting for symptomatic carotid artery disease.

2. RISKS ASSOCIATED WITH CAROTID ENDARTERECTOMY

Results from two large randomized trials have shown that carotid endarterectomy combined with best medical treatment significantly reduces the risk of recurrent stroke in recently symptomatic patients (2,3). In the European Carotid Surgery Trial (ECST), 30-day outcomes following surgery were associated with a death or major stroke rate of 7.5%. The corresponding rate in the North American Symptomatic Carotid Endarterectomy Trial (NASCET) was 6.5%. These complications rates, whilst acceptable, leave room for improvement. The NASCET study also reported an 8.9% risk of wound complication, 7.5% risk of cranial nerve injury, and 0.9% risk of myocardial infarction. It is difficult to generalize the results from large multicenter trials to everyday clinical practice in individual centers where there may be much less experience with the technique of carotid endarterectomy (4). This is particularly important as the benefit of carotid surgery relies on the balance between stroke prophylaxis and the risk of stroke or death at the time of the procedure.

3. THE BENEFITS OF ENDOVASCULAR TREATMENT

Endovascular intervention has the advantage of being performed under local anesthesia, avoiding the effects of anesthetic drugs and intubation. The risk of potentially fatal complications such as myocardial infarction and pulmonary embolism are also reduced. The use of local anesthesia also means a faster recovery for patients treated endovascularly, reducing the length of hospital stay and potentially reducing costs.

Another advantage of endovascular treatment is the avoidance of an incision in the neck. Carotid endarterectomy incisions may be complicated by infection or hematoma which may occasionally lead to life-threatening airway obstruction. In addition, cutaneous and cranial nerves may be damaged by a surgical incision in the neck. Although nerve injury is usually temporary, in some patients, serious cranial nerve injury or uncomfortable neck and facial numbness may be more debilitating than stroke. Complications at the site of endovascular access in the groin are rare and not usually a cause for concern.

4. PROBLEMS WITH ENDOVASCULAR TREATMENT

Difficulty arises in comparing the well-established technique of carotid endarterectomy with the newer endovascular techniques. There are very few interventionists with extensive experience of angioplasty and stenting in the carotid artery in contrast to the large number of vascular surgeons and neurosurgeons who regularly perform carotid endarterectomy. In centers where endovascular treatment of carotid artery stenosis takes place, there has been a move away from simple balloon angioplasty of the artery towards stenting with or without prior angioplasty. One reason for this is that stents are thought to limit the consequences of carotid dissection and improve the anatomic result compared to balloon angioplasty alone, reducing the subsequent thromboembolic risk at the time of the procedure (5). However, embolization will still occur during the passage of the device across the stenosis prior to deployment, and from dislodgement of plaque debris or thrombosis through the struts of the stent. Transcranial Doppler studies have confirmed that embolization frequently occurs during deployment of the stent and post-stent balloon dilatation (6). A variety of devices have therefore been developed to provide cerebral protection against embolization during endovascular treatment. These include filters and occlusive balloons which are deployed via the endovascular route distal to the stenosis prior to stent deployment. A recent review of the literature suggests that these devices significantly reduce the 30-day risk of stroke or death when compared with procedures carried out without cerebral protection (7).

Following simple balloon angioplasty, there is a significant incidence of restenosis of the treated artery, although it remains uncertain how often this leads to recurrent symptoms. Stents are possibly associated with less restenosis after treatment.

The standard endovascular technique used now involves the use of a stent, often with a cerebral protection device. These devices are expensive and therefore the overall cost of endovascular treatment may now be greater than surgery, despite the likelihood of a reduced length of stay in hospital after stenting.

5. CASE SERIES

Early reports of endovascular treatment for carotid artery stenosis were derived from small case series using simple balloon angioplasty (8,9). Later, stents became available and there are now at least 30 series reporting experience of at least 10 carotid stenting procedures (Table 1) (10–39). Analysis of these data is limited by the fact that most series were small and were studied retrospectively. There are also considerable differences between studies in the technique employed, in particular whether or not a cerebral protection device was used. There is a lack of long-term follow-up data with most series only reporting the 30-day outcomes. Perhaps most importantly, although it is well established that outcome following carotid endarterectomy depends on whether the patient is symptomatic or not, most of these series did not present separate early complication rates for symptomatic and asymptomatic patients. Analysis of the data where this information is available shows a combined stroke and death rate within 30 days of stenting that is significantly higher in symptomatic compared with asymptomatic patients (6.4 vs.

Table 1 Case-Series of Carotid Stenting Procedures

Author	Year published	Reference	Number of treated arteries	Percentage of patients who were symptomatic
AbuRahma	2001	10	25	72
Adami	2002	11	30	50
Al-Mubarak	2002	12	164	47
Bonaldi	2002	13	71	100
Cremonesi	2000	14	119	24
Criado	2002	15	135	40
Diethrich	1996	16	129	35
Dietz	2001	17	43	100
Guimaraens	2002	18	194	89
Gupta	2000	19	100	85
Henry	1999	20	184	44
Hobson	2002	21	54	35
Jaeger	2001	22	20	65
Jordan	1998	23	312	27
Kastrup	2003	24	100	63
Kaul	2000	25	15	100
Kirsch	2001	26	57	68
Lanzino	1999	27	18	50
Malek	2000	28	18	100
Mericle	1999	29	21	57
Paniagua	2001	30	69	84
Pappada	2001	31	27	93
Parodi	2000	32	46	39
Qureshi	2002	33	73	38
Reimers	2001	34	88	36
Roubin	2001	35	604	46
Shawl	2000	36	192	61
Vozzi	1997	37	19	55
Waigand	1998	38	53	26
Whitlow	2002	39	75	100
			Total 3055	Mean 61%

1%; $P < 0.01$) (7). Higher complication rates of carotid endarterectomy in symptomatic patients have also been reported (40). The stroke and death rate in symptomatic patients is comparable to the reported complication rates of endarterectomy in NASCET and ECST, and justifies the evaluation of stenting for carotid artery disease within the context of large multicenter randomized trials.

6. RANDOMIZED TRIALS

To date, four randomized trials of endovascular treatment compared with carotid endarterectomy for carotid artery stenosis have been reported. The first trial of carotid stenting was a single center study based in Leicester, England (41). All patients were symptomatic and had severe (70–99%) stenosis. The trial was stopped after 23 patients had been randomized to treatment (although only 17 patients had received their allocated treatment). Ten carotid endarterectomies proceeded without complication, but five of the seven patients who underwent stenting had a stroke at the time of the procedure.

    The Wallstent study was a multicenter randomized trial based in the United States. All patients had >60% carotid artery stenosis with ipsilateral symptoms of cerebral ischemia in the preceding 120 days. The study was also stopped prematurely after enrolling 219 patients when the 30-day rate of any stroke or death was noted to be 12.1% in the stented group compared with 4.5% in the surgical group ($P = 0.049$) (42).

    In contrast to these studies, another single center study based in Kentucky, USA, randomized 104 patients with symptomatic carotid stenosis of >70% to stenting or surgery and reported very low complication rates in both groups (43). No patient in either group had a stroke following the procedure although one individual died from an immediate post-operative myocardial infarction following carotid endarterectomy. Whilst these results sound reassuring, they cannot be compared to the 30-day complication rates from the Leicester and Wallstent studies as they are immediate post-procedure results only.

    The largest trial to be reported is the Carotid and Vertebral Artery Transluminal Angioplasty Study (CAVATAS) (44). This study was an international multicenter randomized trial involving 560 patients from 24 centers. Of these, 504 patients with carotid stenosis suitable for surgery were randomized to receive endovascular treatment (251 patients) or surgery (253 patients). The remaining 56 patients had carotid artery stenosis unsuitable for surgery or vertebral artery stenosis and were not included in the main published analysis. Within CAVATAS, investigators used their own protocol to establish the presence of clinically relevant carotid stenosis before treatment. About 88% of patients in the endovascular group and 91% in the surgical group had been symptomatic within 6 months prior to randomization. In total, only 4% of the endovascular group and 3% of the surgical group had no relevant symptoms (Table 2). The common carotid method was used to measure vessel stenosis. Mean stenosis was 86% in the endovascular group and 85% in the group treated with carotid endarterectomy (equivalent to 75% using the NASCET method). The CAVATAS trial began recruiting patients in 1992 before arterial stents were in use and therefore the majority of patients randomized to endovascular treatment received

Table 2 Baseline Characteristics of CAVATAS Patients[a]

	Endovascular treatment ($n = 251$) (%)	Surgical treatment ($n = 253$) (%)
Demography		
Female	30	30
Mean age (years)	67	67
Symptoms leading to randomization		
Amaurosis fugax	24	25
Transient ischemic attack	37	39
Retinal infarct	2	1
Hemisphere stroke	25	26
Symptoms more than 6 months prior to randomization	8	6
Never symptomatic	4	3
Vascular risk factors at randomization		
Hypertension	53	58
Mean SBP (mmHg)	152	152
Mean DBP (mmHg)	84	84
Ischemic heart disease	39	37
Previous history of myocardial infarction	19	17
Peripheral vascular disease	24	20
Diabetes	14	13
Current cigarette smoking	28	27
Ex-smoker	50	50
Cholesterol >6.5 mmol/L	34	32
Atrial fibrillation	5	5
Other cardiac embolic source	1	2
Angiographic characteristics		
Mean percentage ipsilateral carotid stenosis (CC method)	87	86
Contralateral carotid artery occlusion	10	8

[a]Numbers are percentage of patients. Mean SBP = mean systolic blood pressure, mean DBP = mean diastolic blood pressure; mmHg = millimeters of mercury. CC method = common carotid method.

percutaneous transluminal angioplasty with balloon catheters. In the endovascular arm, 55 (22%) patients were treated by stenting.

The analysis of results was by intention to treat. The rate of any stroke lasting for more than 7 days or death from any cause occurring within 30 days of treatment was virtually identical in both groups (9.9% surgical group vs. 10.0% endovascular group; $P = $ NS) (Table 3). Analyses of other complications confirmed that endovascular treatment caused less minor morbidity than surgery. Cranial or peripheral neuropathy was reported

Table 3 Thirty-Day Outcome Events in CAVATAS[a]

	Endovascular arm ($n = 251$) (%)	Surgery arm ($n = 253$) (%)	P
Major outcome events			
Death	2.8	1.6	NS
Disabling stroke	3.6	4.3	NS
Non-disabling stroke	3.6	4.0	NS
Death or disabling stroke	6.4	5.9	NS
Death or any stroke	10.0	9.9	NS
Other outcome events			
Cranial nerve palsy	0	8.7	< 0.0001
Hematoma (requiring surgery or prolonging hospital stay)	1.2	6.7	< 0.0015
Myocardial infarction (non-fatal)	0	1.2	NS
Pulmonary embolus	0	0.8[b]	NS

[a]Only strokes lasting more than 7 days in any territory were included. Numbers are percentage of patients. NS = non-significant.
[b]One fatal, included above.

in 9% of surgical patients but not at all following endovascular treatment ($P < 0.0001$). In addition only 1% of patients treated endovascularly suffered major wound hematoma, prolonging hospital stay or requiring blood transfusion, compared with 7% of surgical patients ($P < 0.00015$). There was also a difference between the groups favoring endovascular treatment in the number of patients who sustained a myocardial infarction (three surgical patients and no endovascular patients) or pulmonary embolism (two surgical patients and no endovascular patients). Around a third of all strokes that occurred in the 30 days following treatment were delayed for up to 3 weeks. This finding emphasizes the importance of interpreting with caution studies reporting only in-hospital morbidity.

There is little doubt that stenting produces superior anatomical results compared with simple balloon angioplasty. This might be expected to be associated with improved safety of endovascular treatment but there is little evidence to support this. Within CAVATAS, post-hoc subgroup analysis was done to examine the rate of stroke associated with stenting. One (2%) of 55 stented patients had a stroke at the time of stent deployment. Within 30 days of treatment, two ischemic and two hemorrhagic strokes occurred (between 2 and 11 days) in this group. There were no further strokes in the stented patients for the duration of follow-up. Hence stenting seemed safer at the time of the procedure but was associated with a similar number of delayed strokes compared to the patients treated with balloon

angioplasty. The CAVATAS trial also found that when results were analyzed by individual center experience, the average rate of stroke in the first
30 patients treated in any center was 11% but fell to 4% once an individual
center had treated more than 50 patients. This is likely to reflect the learning
curve with increasing experience but may be partly due to the increasing use
of stents as the trial progressed.

CAVATAS is the only randomized study to have reported any long-
term results. Patients were followed up for a mean duration of 2 years.
Results from the 3-year survival analyses showed that both surgery and
endovascular treatment were equally effective at preventing stroke (Fig. 1).
The rates of death or disabling stoke in any arterial territory including
treatment-related events was 14.3% in the endovascular group, and 14.2%
in the patients who underwent carotid endarterectomy. Survival analysis
with adjustment for age, sex, and trial center showed no difference between
the two groups with a hazard ratio for any disabling stroke or death
(endovascular/surgery) of 1.03 (95% CI: 0.64–1.64; $P = $ NS).

It is possible to conclude from CAVATAS that endovascular treatment and carotid endarterectomy appear to have similar major risks and
benefits. The 10% 30 day rate of stroke or death in both treatment groups,
whilst relatively high, is not significantly different from the corresponding
reported rate from ECST of 7.5%. This result may have occurred purely

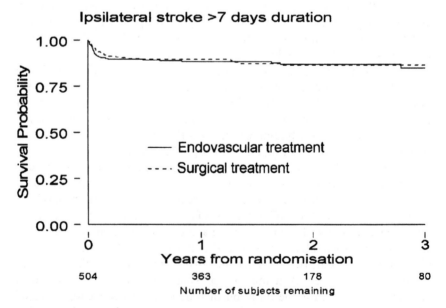

Figure 1 Survival analysis showing number of patients in CAVATAS free of ipsilateral stroke lasting more than 7 days.

due to chance given the wide confidence intervals. However, an analysis of the baseline characteristics of patients included in CAVATAS showed that there were substantially more patients with vascular risk factors assigned to surgery than in ECST and NASCET. This may have been partly because enthusiasm to operate on patients with carotid artery stenosis increased following ECST and NASCET. Also the availability of endovascular techniques may have led to the inclusion in this trial of patients who were less fit for surgery.

The wide confidence intervals surrounding the hazard ratio for any disabling stroke or death imply that a significant difference between endovascular intervention and surgery has not been excluded by CAVATAS. What is clear, however, is that the rate of minor morbidity, for example, from nerve injury and wound hematoma is significantly reduced by endovascular treatment. This may indicate an important advantage over surgery if indeed the major risks and benefits are similar.

Recently, a fifth trial, the Stenting and Angioplasty with Protection in Patients at High Risk for Endarterectomy study (SAPPHIRE), published one year results (45). This trial is a multicenter study based in the United States comparing the safety and efficacy of carotid artery stenting with embolic protection to carotid endarterectomy in high surgical risk patients. All patients had > 50% symptomatic stenosis or > 80% asymptomatic stenosis plus one or more co-morbidity conditions such as congestive heart failure, left ventricular dysfunction, or severe pulmonary disease. There were 334 patients; they were randomized to stenting (167 patients) or surgery (159 patients). Only 30% of patients in the stent group and 28% in the surgery group were symptomatic from their carotid stenosis. The primary endpoint of the study was the cumulative incidence of a major cardiovascular events at one year – a composite of death, stroke or myocardial infection within 30 days after the intervention or death or ipsilateral stroke between 31 days and 1 one year. The primary endpoint occurred in 12.2% of patients randomized to stenting and 20.1% of those randomized to surgery (P = 0.004 for non-inferiority and P = 0.053 for superiority). In the analysis of patients with symptomatic stenosis, the cumulative incidence of the primary end point at one year was 16.8% in the stent group compared with 16.5% in the surgery group (P = 0.95)

7. META-ANALYSIS OF THE RANDOMIZED TRIALS

A meta-analysis of results from these five randomized trials has been performed in a recent systematic review of percutaneous transluminal angioplasty and stenting for carotid artery stenosis (46). The following results are all taken from the 30 day follow-up data for the combined meta-analysis of a total of 1157 patients randomized in the five trials. There was no significant difference in the rate of death or any stroke between the two treatments; 8.6% of all patients allocated endovascular treatment died or had a stroke compared to 7.1% of patients allocated surgery [odds ratio (OR) 1.26, 95% CI: 0.82–1.94; $P = $ NS]. In addition, data from the three trials that provided information on the type of stroke sustained showed that 6.0% of patients treated endovascularly died or had a disabling stroke compared with 5.0% of patients treated surgically [OR 1.22, 95% CI: 0.61–2.41; $P = $ NS]. When the data regarding myocardial infarction (MI) was included in the meta-analysis, there was no significant difference in the rate of death, stroke, or MI, which was virtually identical after either treatment (endovascular group 9.0%; surgical group 9.2%; OR 0.99, 95% CI: 0.66–1.48; $P = $ NS) (Fig. 2). No endovascular patient sustained cranial neuropathy compared with 7.2% of surgical patients [OR 0.12, 95% CI: 0.06–0.25; $P < 0.00001$].

One year follow-up data was only available from CAVATAS and the Wallstent study. There was no significant difference in the rate of death or stroke during follow-up in the meta-analysis from these two trials between the patients treated endovascularly and those who had surgery (13.7 vs. 10.4%, $P = $ NS).

Data on the degree of residual stenosis or restenosis at 1 year following treatment was only available from CAVATAS. Ipsilateral carotid artery stenosis of > 70% was more common after endovascular treatment than carotid endarterectomy (14% compared with 4%, $P < 0.001$) but as mentioned earlier, there was no difference in the rate of ipsilateral stroke in the 3 year survival analysis between the groups. Importantly, the rate of restenosis to > 50% after stenting was only slightly less than after balloon angioplasty alone (42 vs. 52%) although ipsilateral carotid occlusion at 1 year was less common (2% after stenting vs. 5% after balloon angioplasty).

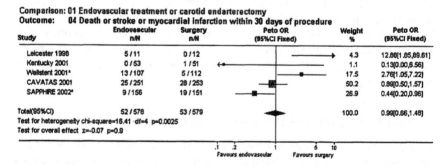

Figure 2 Meta-anaylsis of trials comparing endovascular treatment with surgery for carotid artery stenosis. Outcome is based on death or stroke or myocardial infarction within 30 days of procedure. There is significant heterogeneity between the trials ($P = 0.0025$).

The meta-analysis highlighted significant heterogeneity between the results of the randomized studies. This difference is likely to be the result of the endovascular technique used (stenting vs. balloon angioplasty, and use of cerebral protection or not), patient characteristics (symptomatic vs. asymptomatic, and normal vs. high surgical risk), and status of trial (completed vs. stopped prematurely). The reviewers concluded that carotid angioplasty and stenting had similar major risks and benefits compared with surgery and avoid minor morbidity. This conclusion should be interpreted with caution as two trials were stopped because of concerns over stenting. Furthermore, there remains uncertainty about the potential for restenosis following endovascular treatment to cause recurrent stroke. Moreover, despite analyzing data from over 1100 patients in the meta-analysis, the confidence intervals surrounding the odds ratios for the comparison between events after endovascular treatment and surgery remain wide. Hence, it remains possible that one treatment may be substantially more hazardous or less effective than the other. This meta-analysis will be regularly updated to take into account new data (46).

8. THE ROLE OF CEREBRAL PROTECTION DEVICES

The introduction of cerebral protection devices for use during carotid stenting is a major recent advance, which is expected to improve the safety of stenting. The concept was first described in a series published in 1990 (47). There are now several case series in the literature reporting experience of endovascular treatment with temporary cerebral protection but they have not yet been adequately evaluated within randomized trials. Several devices are available, including filters and occlusion balloons on guidewires, which can be placed distal to the carotid stenosis prior to stent insertion. Initial case series experience confirms that these devices catch embolic debris and suggests that the risk of immediate complications from stenting is reduced (34,48). A recent systematic review of the literature found that in over 3400 reports of carotid stenting, the combined stroke or death rate within 30 days in both symptomatic and asymptomatic patients was 1.8% in patients treated with cerebral protection devices compared with 5.5% in patients treated without cerebral protection ($P < 0.001$) (7). The use of distal protection devices will not prevent stroke while crossing the stenosis to deploy the filter or occlusion balloon. A system developed by Parodi involves inserting an anti-embolism system proximal to the stenosis, which includes two balloons (11,32). These are deployed to occlude the common carotid and external carotid arteries at the same time. The guiding catheter is then externally connected to the contralateral femoral vein with an interposed blood filter. This results in reversal of the direction of flow in the internal carotid artery (ICA), which allows angioplasty and stent insertion to be performed safely so that any debris is washed away from the brain. Despite these advances, it is possible that the use of a protection device will increase hazards in some patients, for example, if the device leads to a significant reduction in cerebral blood flow, or if there is difficulty removing the device. Initial experience suggests that these are rare complications.

9. THE FUTURE OF CAROTID STENTING

The relative high rate of procedural stroke in the surgical and endovascular groups in CAVATAS and the concern over stenting in the Leicester and Wallstent studies argues strongly against the general introduction of stenting as an alternative to surgery. Despite the encouraging findings of the meta-analysis, there remains uncertainty about the relative risks and benefits of endovascular treatment compared to surgery in patients suitable for either procedure. It seems reasonable that there should be a move away from simple balloon angioplasty towards stenting with cerebral protection. However, this endovascular technique requires further evaluation. The ongoing randomized trials of carotid stenting are justified on the basis that there is a definite reduction in minor morbidity in patients who undergo stenting compared to those who have surgery. Future trials need to provide more convincing data regarding the immediate major risks and the long-term benefits of stenting as well as the overall costs of the procedure compared to carotid endarterectomy.

10. ONGOING TRIALS

There are four randomized trials of carotid stenting vs. endarterectomy in progress. The Endarterectomy Vs. Angioplasty in patients with Severe Symptomatic carotid Stenosis (EVA-3S) study is based in France (49). The Carotid Revascularization Endarterectomy vs. Stenting Trial (CREST) is based in the United States (50). The Stent-protected Percutaneous Angioplasty of the Carotid vs. Endarterectomy (SPACE) study is based in Germany (51). The International Carotid Stenting Study (ICSS) is recruiting patients worldwide with the central office based in London, England (52).

11. ENSURING SAFETY—THE INTERNATIONAL CAROTID STENTING STUDY PROTOCOL

The ICSS is the follow-on study to CAVATAS. The protocol has stringent requirements for center enrolment and safety is the major consideration. Centers must have a neurologist or physician with an interest in cerebrovascular disease, a vascular surgeon or neurosurgeon who has performed at least 50 carotid endarterectomies, and a radiologist with training in carotid angiography who has performed at least 50 stenting procedures, 10 of which must have been in the carotid artery. All investigators submit an audit of their recent results, which are assessed by a credentialing committee. Radiologists are required to attend approved courses on carotid stenting and must have their technique approved by an experienced carotid stenting expert.

The ICSS has developed the concept of probationary centers which may join the study if they fulfill all entry criteria but do not have audited data on 10 recent carotid stenting procedures. If patients in these centers are randomized to receive carotid stenting, then this must be performed under the supervision of an experienced carotid stenting expert. When this expert is satisfied that the supervised interventionist has adequate skill and the center results are satisfactory, the probationary center may be fully enrolled. This has the advantage of producing randomized data about the learning curve in carotid stenting, while promoting safety by supervision of the procedure.

Patients in ICSS must have recently symptomatic extracranial, internal, or bifurcation carotid artery stenosis. They must be suitable for both surgery and stenting and give informed consent. Patients who have sustained a major stroke with no useful recovery of function, with stenosis unsuitable for stenting, e.g., because of tortuous anatomy or visible thrombus and those with a life expectancy of < 2 years are excluded from the study.

Randomization is stratified within each center and deploys a computerized program to balance the main risk factors between the arms of the trial. Randomization is also stratified over time to balance for any improvements or change in technology over the course of the trial.

The trial requires stenting or surgery to be performed as soon as possible after randomization. All patients will receive best medical care as deemed appropriate by the randomizing physician. Protection devices and stents used in the trial are required to be CE marked and approved by the steering committee, but otherwise radiologists are not restricted to the use of any one device. Local and general anesthesia may be used for patients randomized to carotid endarterectomy. The outcome measures include the rates of stroke, myocardial infarction, cranial nerve palsy, and hematoma within 30 days of treatment, long-term survival free of stroke, quality of life and economics measures, and restenosis to $>70\%$ on ultrasound at follow-up.

The ICSS plans a sample size of 1500 patients. This has been calculated on the basis of equivalence between the two procedures. Sample size calculations under these circumstances are difficult because one has to estimate what difference between two procedures in risk or benefits would influence clinicians in choosing between the two treatments. The sample size of 1500 will give 95% confidence intervals of ± 3 percentage points for disabling stroke and death within 30 days of treatment, for disabling stroke during follow-up.

Over 40 centers throughout the world including Europe, Australia, and North America have expressed a firm interest in joining ICSS and to date, there are 30 centers enrolled. The trial has set up a web page where further information about progress can be obtained. The current address is www.cavatas.com.

12. CONCLUSION

Stenting for symptomatic carotid artery stenosis is a potential alternative to carotid endarterectomy. Evidence from several case series has shown that it is feasible to perform carotid artery stenting in symptomatic patients but that the complication rate is higher than occurs in asymptomatic patients. Carotid endarterectomy is also known to have similar differential complication rates between symptomatic and asymptomatic patients. Stenting has been reported to be safer than simple balloon angioplasty and indeed evidence from randomized trials support this in terms of a reduced rate of procedural complications. However, data from CAVATAS suggest that the rate of delayed stroke following stenting may be similar to that which occurs following angioplasty.

A meta-analysis of results from five randomized trials of endovascular treatment vs. carotid endarterectomy involving over 1100 patients has shown that endovascular treatment has similar major risks and benefits as surgery whilst avoiding more minor morbidity. Current evidence does not support a widespread change in clinical practice away from recommending carotid endarterectomy as the treatment of choice for symptomatic carotid artery stenosis.

A recent systematic review of case series of stenting with and without cerebral protection has shown that the safety of stenting is improved by the use of cerebral protection devices. In combination with evidence from previous randomized trials, this is a basis on which to design future trials of carotid stenting which should concentrate on producing good data regarding the safety and efficacy of the procedure.

REFERENCES

1. Ricci S, Flamini FO, Celani MG. Prevalence of internal carotid artery stenosis in subjects older than 49 years: a population study. Cerebrovasc Dis 1991; 1: 6–19.
2. European Carotid Surgery Trialists' Collaborative Group. Randomised trial of endarterectomy for recently symptomatic carotid stenosis: final results of the MRC European Carotid Surgery Trial (ECST). Lancet 1998; 351:1379–1387.
3. North American Symptomatic Carotid Endarterectomy Trial Collaborators. Beneficial effect of carotid endarterectomy in symptomatic patients with high-grade carotid stenosis. N Engl J Med 1991; 325:445–453.

4. Chaturvedi S, Aggarwal R, Murugappan A. Results of carotid endarterectomy with prospective neurologist follow-up. Neurology 2000; 55:769–772.

5. Roubin GS, New G, Iyer SS, Vitek JJ, Al-Mubarak N, Liu MW, Yadav J, Gomez C, Kuntz RE. Immediate and late clinical outcomes of carotid artery stenting in patients with symptomatic and asymptomatic carotid artery stenosis: a 5-year prospective analysis. Circulation 2001; 103:532–537.

6. Gaines PA. Carotid angioplasty and stenting. Br Med Bull 2000; 56(2):549–556.

7. Kastrup A, Groschel K, Krapf H, Brehm BR, Dichgans J, Schulz JB. Early outcome of carotid angioplasty and stenting with or without cerebral protection devices. A systematic review of the literature. Stroke 2003; 34(3):813–819.

8. Brockenheimer S, Mathias K. Percutaneous transluminal angioplasty in atherosclerotic internal carotid artery stenosis. Am J Neuroradiol 1983; 4:791–792.

9. Brown MM. Balloon angioplasty. Neurol Res 1992; 14(supp):159–173.

10. Aburahma AF, Bates MC, Stone PA, Wulu JT. Comparative study of operative treatment and percutaneous transluminal angioplasty/stenting for recurrent carotid disease. J Vasc Surg 2001; 34:831–838.

11. Adami CA, Scuro A, Spinamano L, Galvagni E, Antoniucci D, Farello GA, Maglione F, Manfrini S, Mangialardi N, Mansueto GC, Mascoli F, Nardelli E, Tealdi D. Use of the Parodi anti-embolism system in carotid stenting: Italian trial results. J Endovasc Ther 2002; 9:147–154.

12. Al-Mubarak N, Colombo A, Gaines PA, Iyer SS, Corvaja N, Cleveland TJ, Macdonald S, Brennan C, Vitek JJ. Multicenter evaluation of carotid artery stenting with a filter protection system. J Am Coll Cardiol 2002; 39:841–846.

13. Bonaldi G. Angioplasty and stenting of the cervical carotid bifurcation: report of a 4-year series. Neuroradiology 2002; 44:164–174.

14. Cremonesi A, Castriota F, Manetti R, Balestra G, Liso A. Endovascular treatment of carotid atherosclerotic disease: early and late outcome in a non-selected population. Ital Heart J 2000; 1:801–809.

15. Criado FJ, Lingelbach JM, Ledesma DF, Lucas PR. Carotid artery stenting in a vascular surgery practice. J Vasc Surg 2001; 33:1001–1007.

16. Diethrich EB, Ndiaye M, Reid DB. Stenting in the carotid artery: initial experience in 110 patients. J Endovasc Surg 1996; 3:42–62.

17. Dietz A, Berkefeld J, Theron JG, Schmitz-Rixen T, Zanella FE, Turowski B, Steinmetz H, Sitzer M. Endovascular treatment of symptomatic carotid stenosis using stent placement: long-term follow-up of patients with a balanced surgical risk/benefit ratio. Stroke 2001; 32:1855–1859.

18. Guimaraens L, Sola MT, Matali A, Arbelaez A, Delgado M, Soler L, Balaguer E, Castellanos C, Ibanez J, Miquel L, Theron J. Carotid angioplasty with cerebral protection and stenting: report of 164 patients (194 carotid percutaneous transluminal angioplasties). Cerebrovasc Dis 2002; 13:114–119.

19. Gupta A, Bhatia A, Ahuja A, Shalev Y, Bajwa T. Carotid stenting in patients older than 65 years with inoperable carotid artery disease: a single-centre experience. Cath Cardiovasc Interv 2000; 50:1–8.

20. Henry M, Amor M, Henry I, Klonaris C, Chati Z, Masson I, Kownator S, Luizy F, Hugel M. Carotid stenting with cerebral protection: first clinical experience using the PercuSurge GuarWire system. J Endovasc Surg 1999; 6:321–331.

21. Hobson RW, Lal BK, Chakhtoura EY, Goldstein J, Kubicka R, Haser PB, Padberg FTJ, Pappas PJ, Jamil Z. Carotid artery closure for endarterectomy does not influence results of angioplasty-stenting for restenosis. J Vasc Surg 2002; 23:200–207.

22. Jaeger H, Mathias K, Drescher R, Hauth E, Bockisch G, Demirel E, Gissler HM. Clinical results of cerebral protection with a filter device during stent implantation of the carotid artery. Cardiovasc Intervent Radiol 2001; 24: 249–256.

23. Jordan WD, Voellinger DC, Fisher WS, Redden D, McDowell HA. A comparison of carotid angioplasty with stenting versus endarterectomy with regional anesthesia. J Vasc Surg 1998; 28:397–402.

24. Kastrup A, Skalej M, Krapf H, Nägele T, Dichgans J, Schulz JB. Early outcome of carotid angioplasty and stenting versus carotid endarterectomy in a single academic center. Cerebrovasc Dis 2003; 15:84–89.

25. Kaul U, Singh B, Bajaj R, Sapra R, Sudan D, Yadav RD, Garg R, Dixit NS. Elective stenting of extracranial carotid arteries. J Assoc Physicians India 2000; 48:196–200.

26. Kirsch EC, Khangure MS, van Schie GP, Lawrence-Brown MM, Stewart-Wynne EG, McAuliffe W. Carotid arterial stent placement: results and follow-up in 53 patients. Radiology 2001; 220:737–744.

27. Lanzino G, Mericle RA, Lopes DK, Wakhloo AK, Guterman LR, Hopkins LN. Percutaneous transluminal angioplasty and stent placement for recurrent carotid artery stenosis. J Neurosurg 1999; 90:668–694.

28. Malek AM, Higashida RT, Phatouros CC, Lempert TE, Meyers PM, Smith WS, Dowd CF, Halbach VV. Stent angioplasty for cervical carotid artery stenosis in high-risk symptomatic NASCET-ineligible patients. Stroke 2000; 31:3029–3033.

29. Mericle RA, Kim SH, Lanzino G, Lopes DK, Wakhloo AK, Guterman LR, Hopkins LN. Carotid artery angioplasty and use of stents in high-risk patients with contralateral occlusions. J Neurosurg 1999; 90:1031–1036.

30. Paniagua D, Howell M, Strickman N, Velasco J, Dougherty K, Skolkin M, Toombs B, Krajcer Z. Outcomes following extracranial carotid artery stenting in high-risk patients. J Invasive Cardiol 2001; 13:375–381.

31. Pappada G, Marina R, Fiori L, Agostini E, Lanterna A, Cardia A, Ferrarese C, Beghi E, Gaini SM. Stenting of atherosclerotic stenoses of the extracranial carotid artery. Acta Neurochir (Wien) 2001; 143:1005–1011.

32. Parodi JC, La Mura R, Ferreira LM, Mendez MV, Cersosimo H, Schonholz C, Garelli G. Initial evaluation of carotid angioplasty and stenting with three different cerebral protection devices. J Vasc Surg 2000; 32:1127–1136.

33. Qureshi AI, Suri MF, New G, Wadsworth DCJ, Dulin J, Hopkins LN. Multicenter study of the feasibility and safety of using the Memotherm carotid arterial stent for extracranial carotid artery stenosis. J Neurosurg 2002; 96:830–836.

34. Reimers B, Corvaja N, Moshiri S, Sacca S, Albiero R, Di Mario C, Pascotto P, Colombo A. Cerebral protection with filter devices during carotid artery stenting. Circulation 2001; 104:12–15.

35. Roubin GS, New G, Iyer SS, Vitek JJ, Al-Mubarak N, Liu MW, Yadav J, Gomez C, Kuntz RE. Immediate and late clinical outcomes of carotid artery

stenting in patients with symptomatic and asymptomatic carotid artery stenosis: a 5-year prospective analysis. Circulation 2001; 103:532–537.

36. Shawl F, Kadro W, Domanski MJ, Lapetina FL, Iqbal AA, Dougherty KG, Weisher DD, Marquez JF, Shahab ST. Safety and efficacy of elective carotid artery stenting in high-risk patients. J Am Coll Cardiol 2000; 35:1721–1728.

37. Vozzi CR, Rodriguez AO, Paolantonio D, Smith JA, Wholey MH. Extracranial carotid angioplasty and stenting: initial results and short-term follow-up. Tex Heart Inst J 1997; 24:167–172.

38. Waigand J, Gross CM, Uhlich F, Kramer J, Tamaschke C, Vogel P, Luft FC, Dietz R. Elective stenting of carotid artery stenosis in patients with severe coronary artery disease. Eur Heart J 1998; 19:1365–1370.

39. Whitlow PL, Lylyk P, Londero H, Mendiz OA, Mathias K, Jaeger H, Parodi J, Schonholz C, Milei J. Carotid artery stenting protected with an emboli containment system. Stroke 2002; 33:1308–1314.

40. Rothwell PM, Slattery J, Warlow C. A systematic comparison of the risks of stroke and death due to endarterectomy for symptomatic and asymptomatic carotid stenosis. Stroke 1996; 27(2):266–269.

41. Naylor AR, Bolia A, Abbott RJ, Pye IF, Smith J, Lennard N, Lloyd AJ, London NJM, Bell PRF. Randomised study of carotid angioplasty and stenting versus carotid endarterectomy: a stopped trial. J Vasc Surg 1998; 28:326–334.

42. Alberts MJ. Results of a multicentre prospective randomised trial of carotid artery stenting vs. carotid endarterectomy. Stroke 2001; 32:325 (abstract).

43. Brooks WH, McClure RR, Jones MR, Cloeman TC, Breathitt L. Carotid angioplasty and stenting versus carotid endarterectomy: randomised trial in a community hospital. J Am Coll Cardiol 2001; 38:1589–1595.

44. CAVATAS Investigators. Endovascular versus surgical treatment in patients with carotid stenosis in the Carotid and Vertebral Artery Transluminal Angioplasty Study (CAVATAS): a randomised trial. Lancet 2001; 357:1729–1737.

45. Yadav JS, Wholey MH, Kuntz RE, Fayad P, Katzen BT, Mishkel GJ, Bajwa TK, Whitlow P, Strickman NE, Jaff MR, Popma JJ, Snead DB, Cutlip DE, Firth BG, Ouriel K for the stenting and Angioplasty with Protection in Patients at High Risk for Endarterectomy Investigators. Protected Carotid-artery stenting versus endarterectomy in high-risk patients. N Engl J Med 2004; 351(15):1493–1501.

46. Coward LJ, Featherstone RL, Brown MM. Percutaneous transluminal angioplasty and stenting for carotid artery stenosis. The Cochrane Database of Systematic Reviews 2004, Issue 1. Art. No.: CD000515. DOI: 10.1002/14651858.CD000515.pub2.

47. Theron J, Courtheoux P, Alackar F, Bouvard G, Maiza D. New triple coaxial catheter system for carotid angioplasty with cerebral protection. Am J Neuroradiol 1990; 11:869–874.

48. Wholey M. Carotid angioplasty. J Am Coll Cardiol 2002; 39(supp A):66A.

49. www.eva3s.hegp.bhdc.jussieu.fr.

50. Hobson RW. CREST (Carotid Revascularisation Endarterectomy versus Stent Trial): background, design and current status. Semin Vasc Surg 2000; 14:139–143.

51. Ringleb PA, Kunze A, Allenberg JR, Hennerici MG, Jansen O, Maurer PC, Zeumer H, Hacke W, Steering Committee of the SPACE Study. The Stent-Supported Percutaneous Angioplasty of the Carotid Artery vs. Endarterectomy Trial. Cerebrovasc Diseases 2004; 18(1):66–68.
52. Featherstone RL, Brown MM, Coward LJ, ICSS Investigators. International carotid stenting study: protocol for a randomised clinical trial comparing carotid stenting with endarterectomy in symptomatic carotid artery stenosis. Cerebrovasc Diseases. 2004; 18(1):69–74.

18

Stenting for Asymptomatic Stenosis

Mark K. Borsody

Stroke Program and Department of Neurology, Wayne State University, Detroit, Michigan, U.S.A.

Seemant Chaturvedi

Department of Neurology, Detroit Medical Center, Wayne State University, Detroit, Michigan, U.S.A.

1. INTRODUCTION

The use of stents placed by an endovascular approach is a relatively new treatment for carotid artery stenosis. However, the use of carotid artery stenting is growing in popularity as more clinical trials begin to demonstrate its efficacy as an alternative to surgical endarterectomy. Herein we review the evidence behind the use of endovascular stenting in the treatment of asymptomatic carotid stenosis. Other chapters in this volume have discussed stenting for symptomatic carotid stenosis and endarterectomy for asymptomatic stenosis.

2. HISTORICAL BACKGROUND

The application of endovascular procedures to carotid artery atherosclerotic disease was initially limited to patients who were not candidates for surgical endarterectomy. The exclusion criteria for surgical endarterectomy are ideally those laid out in the major clinical trials that originally demonstrated the efficacy of this procedure. Exclusion from the trials or surgical endarterectomy that involved asymptomatic patients was based on such broad criteria as "high surgical risk due to associated medical illness" (1), the "expectation of poor surgical risk . . . or any major life threatening condition" (2), or the presence of "a disorder that could seriously complicate surgery . . . or a condition that could prevent continuing participation or was likely to produce disability or death" (3). Ultimately, because of the breadth of these criteria, only 4 and 22% of screened patients were found eligible for the Asymptomatic Carotid Atherosclerosis Study (ACAS) (3) and Veterans' Affairs trials (1), respectively. Because patients were so carefully chosen for endarterectomy in those trials, the periprocedural (i.e., occurring within 30 days of the procedure) morbidity and mortality in patients with asymptomatic carotid stenosis was found to be 1.9–2.8% [in comparison with the 5.8% measured in patients with symptomatic stenosis (4)], but that figure would likely be much greater in patients who were excluded from the study (5).

Limiting the use of endovascular stenting to patients at high risk for surgical endarterectomy, then, very likely biased early non-concurrent comparisons of the two treatments in favor of surgical endarterectomy since most of the exclusion criteria for the large endarterectomy trials certainly would also increase the risk associated with an endovascular procedure. Despite this handicap, some case series found periprocedural complication rates for carotid stenting that were comparable to the historical rates of endarterectomy, for example, a 2.9% incidence of any stroke or death in the series of Shawl et al. (6), which included 104 symptomatic and 66 asymptomatic patients with an average stenosis of 78%. These patients were followed for 2 years, and exhibited an 11.8% incidence of stroke, myocardial infarction (MI), or death. Similarly, subgroup analysis of the 5261 asymptomatic patients in the ongoing Global Carotid Artery Stent Registry has found only a 3.0% periprocedural rate of stroke or death after stent placement (7). Such results would suggest that endovascular stenting would be competitive against endarterectomy at least in terms of the procedural risk, which is a necessary first step before the two treatments can be directly compared in clinical trials.

Some studies also began to evaluate the use of endovascular stenting in patients who were otherwise candidates for surgical endarterectomy. The Louisianna State University series of 108 patients with >70% stenosis exhibited a periprocedural stroke and death rate of 4.5% after treatment with angioplasty and stent placement (8). Only one-fifth of these patients would have been suitable candidates for surgical endarterectomy and 44% were asymptomatic. All of the periprocedural complications encountered in that patient series occurred in patients with symptomatic carotid stenosis, and more specifically in symptomatic patients with "an atherosclerotic, tortuous aortic arch". Qureshi et al. (9) demonstrated a 2.7% periprocedural stroke rate in 73 patients, 46 of whom were asymptomatic with stenoses of at least 70%. Similarly, Gray et al. (10) found only a 0.7% stroke rate in a group of NASCET- or ACAS-eligible patients with >60% stenosis, of whom about two-thirds were asymptomatic. The 1 year rate of non-procedure-related death was 7.7% and the specific rate of stroke was only 0.8% in that study, but since symptomatic and asymptomatic patients were combined for analysis, it is unclear what this figure should be compared against.

Much of the stroke morbidity encountered in clinical trials of endovascular stenting of the asymptomatic carotid artery involved distal embolization during or shortly after the procedure. A significant degree of embolization seems to be caused directly by the process of guidewire placement and angioplasty (11). As demonstrated by Jordan et al. (12), the number of emboli detected by carotid ultrasonography was about 10 times greater during angioplasty than it was during endarterectomy, which likely accounted for the greater periprocedural stroke rate in patients treated with angioplasty in that study (10 vs. 1.5%). Subgroup analysis showed that the greater incidence of embolic ultrasound signals during angioplasty occurred in both symptomatic and asymptomatic patients, although the former had a greater overall incidence than the latter. Accordingly, the advent of self-expanding stents may reduce the use of angioplasty on the stenosed artery. Madyoon et al. (13) demonstrated that self-expanding stents have a similar periprocedural stroke rate in a group of 49 carotid stenosis patients (35 were asymptomatic) when compared against a historical control group of endarterectomy patients. However, in this case series, patients thought to be at high risk for neurological complications were referred for surgical endarterectomy and not treated with endovascular stenting. The Carotid Artery Stent Trial (CAST) similarly evaluated patients with carotid stenosis >70% who appear to have been good candidates for surgical endarterectomy (14). In that group of 99 patients (57 of whom were asymptomatic), only 2% developed a stroke or died within 30 days of the procedure. This low periprocedural complication rate may, in part, relate to the use of a cervical approach in the majority of these procedures, which avoids passing a catheter through an atherosclerotic aorta that is thought to be a source for many cerebral emboli. More impressive was the 2 year follow-up data from the CAST patients, which identified only one vascular death and that being caused by myocardial infarction.

Uncontrolled case series have suggested that the incidence of stroke from distal embolization may be reduced by the use of modified endovascular catheters that involve downstream devices that can block embolizations [i.e., filter devices (8,15) or distal balloon occlusion followed by aspiration of the stagnant material (Medtronic, Inc., press release, 9/2004)]. Filter devices are most commonly used, and while they likely reduce the frequency of tissue infarction associated with angioplasty (16–19), they are far from perfect in terms of catching all embolic particles (20). In an evaluation of distal embolization protection devices, the Global Carotid Artery Stent Registry reported that the use of distal embolization protection devices is associated with a periprocedural stroke or death rate following stenting of 2.2%, in comparison with 5.3% when they are not used (7). Of the more than 11,000 patients identified by this registry, about a half had asymptomatic carotid stenosis, and the use of distal embolization protection devices in the asymptomatic subgroup also reduced the periprocedural stroke and death rate from 4.0 to 1.8%. A recent review of several smaller case series (21) similarly found that the use of distal embolization protection devices was associated with a periprocedural stroke rate of 1.8% in comparison with a rate of 5.5% in patients treated without protection devices; again, no distinction could be made by the reviewers between the use of these devices in symptomatic and asymptomatic carotid stenosis patients with the available literature.

Furthermore, comparison of patients enrolled in the first two phases of the Acculink for Revascularization of Carotids in High Risk patients (ARCHeR) registries does not show a definite favorable effect of distal embolization protection devices (Society of Interventional Radiology press release, 5/2004). These two non-concurrent groups were composed of approximately 75% asymptomatic patients. The use of any kind of protection device was associated with a rate of periprocedural death or stroke >7 days duration of 3.8%, in comparison to a rate of 2.5% when they were not used. The benefit of distal embolization protection devices is also not clear when using expanded definitions of morbidity: periprocedural rate of any adverse event including myocardial infarction increased from 7.6 to 8.6% with the use of a distal embolization protection device. This difference was not statistically significant and, in fact, a study with adequate power to evaluate the complication rate in patients treated with and without distal protection would require several thousand patients. A significant rate of periprocedural myocardial infarction has also been observed in other case series using self-expanding stents and distal embolization protection devices [accounting for one-third of the 3.9% periprocedural morbidity in the case series of Powell et al. (22), for example]. The value of such devices should be carefully evaluated in future trials of stenting therapy.

3. COMPARATIVE CLINICAL TRIALS

The CAVATAS trial (23) has been discussed in the chapter on symptomatic stenosis. Of the patients enrolled, only 3% were asymptomatic and therefore, it does not have great relevance to the subject of asymptomatic stenosis.

Small studies of stenting after angioplasty without using distal embolization protection devices have provided mixed results about the treatment of asymptomatic carotid stenosis. In a randomized trial involving only 85 asymptomatic patients with >80% stenosis, Brooks et al. (24) found no periprocedural stroke or deaths using angioplasty and stenting; the patients treated with surgical endarterectomy in that study also had no periprocedural stroke or deaths. No long-term follow-up from this trial has yet been made available. Similarly encouraging measures of periprocedural morbidity and mortality were observed in a non-randomized Japanese trial

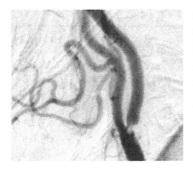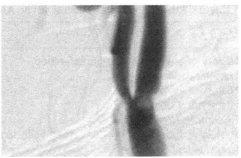

Figure 1 Angiogram showing severe internal carotid artery stenosis and the post-stenting reconstructed vessel.

comparing endarterectomy against endovascular stenting in 565 patients (2.5 vs. 3.4% respectively), in which almost all cases involved a distal embolization protection device (25). An example of angiographic images in an asymptomatic patient who had successful carotid stenting is provided in Figure 1.

All of the aforementioned studies had unregulated use of distal embolization protection devices. The recent Stenting and Angioplasty with Protection in Patients at High Risk for Endarterectomy (SAPPHIRE) trial required the use of a specific protection device—called the Angioguard™ in a randomized comparison of endovascular stenting and surgical endarterectomy (26). Approximately four-fifths of the 334 enrolled patients in that study were considered to have asymptomatic stenoses, and the degree of stenosis in such patients was required to be at least 80% as determined by carotid ultrasonography. In the asymptomatic stenosis subgroup, death or ipsilateral stroke occurring between 30 days and 1 year after the procedure, was reduced by 54% in patients treated with endovascular stenting (9.9% absolute risk vs. 21.5% after surgical endarterectomy). Periprocedural mortality and morbidity including myocardial infarction was 5.4% in patients treated with endovascular stenting in comparison to 10.2% in patients treated with surgical endarterectomy.

The previously mentioned ARCHeR study evaluated a predominantly asymptomatic group of carotid stenosis patients in a series of three separate trials. There was no group randomly assigned to endarterectomy and instead a weighted historical control calculation was derived for an estimated rate of complications for a comparable endarterectomy population. Overall, it was estimated that the combined rate of stroke, death, or myocardial infarction in a comparable cohort undergoing endarterectomy would be 14.5%.

In the three single-arm studies, a total of 581 patients were recruited. Phases II and III of the protocol used the Accunet distal protection device. Patients were enrolled with either >50% symptomatic or >80% asympto-

Table 1 Select Features of Patients in the ARCHeR Trials ($n = 581$)

Mean Age	70.3 years
History of angina/myocardial infarction	66.4%
Diabetes mellitus	37.9%
History of stroke	28.6%
History of TIA	26.2%
Ejection fraction <30%	33.6%
Restenosis following previous carotid endarterectomy	35.1%
Contralateral occlusion	16.5%
Need for open heart surgery within 30 days	15.7%

matic stenosis. Patients could qualify as "high risk" for having either medical comorbidities or unfavorable anatomy for surgical treatment. Examples of high-risk qualifying conditions included ejection fraction <30%, restenosis following a previous carotid endarterectomy, recent myocardial infarction or unstable angina.

Among the patients enrolled, select features are provided in Table 1. Overall, the 30 day rates of stroke, myocardial infarction or death in the three phases of the study were 7.6, 8.6, and 8.3%. For stroke and death alone, they were 6.3, 6.8, and 7.6%. Among patients classified as having a "minor stroke" at day 30, all the patients had a NIH stroke scale score of 0 or 1 at 12 months, suggesting that these did have persisting functional consequences. Between days 31 and 365, only 1.1% of patients in ARCHeR 1 and ARCHeR 2 had an ipsilateral stroke. Fewer than 3% of the patients underwent a repeat revascularization procedure in the first year for the treated vessel.

Overall, based on the fact that the combined rate of stroke, death, and myocardial infarction was lower in ARCHeR compared to the weighted historical control, the Food and Drug Administration approved the ACCU-LINK/ACCUNET device for high-risk patients in the summer of 2004. A post-approval registry has started to assess the results in a broader group of practitioners and patients. This is the Carotid Acculink/Accunet Post-approval Trial to uncover Unanticipated and Rare Events (CAPTURE) study.

Some physicians have criticized the SAPPHIRE and ARCHeR designs for not having a contemporaneous group of patients who were treated with best medical therapy. In both studies, the 30 day rate of stroke and death exceeded 3%. Previous studies such as ACAS have shown that the annual rate of stroke with medical therapy is approximately 2%. Therefore, a future trial comparing stenting versus intensive medical therapy for high-risk carotid stenosis patients would be of interest.

The non-randomized Phase I portion of the Carotid Revascularization Using Endarterectomy or Stenting Systems (CARESS) trial has also been reported (27). The results from 397 patients with carotid stenosis (68%

asymptomatic, with a stenosis of at least 75%) demonstrated equivalent peri-procedural stroke and death rates in patients treated with endarterectomy (2.4%) vs. patients treated with stenting and distal embolization protection (2.1%, using the GuardWire Plus® device). Subgroup analysis from future CARESS trials will hopefully provide a better understanding of the long-term outcome of endovascular stenting in the context of asymptomatic stenosis.

4. TECHNICAL AND ECONOMIC CONSIDERATIONS

The ability to deploy catheters in convoluted carotid arteries or along complex stenoses has been a source of concern in early studies of endovascular therapies such as the CAVATAS trial (23), which had a success rate of only 89% using the relatively simple technique of angioplasty. Procedural failure has not proven to be problematic in recent studies, however. Of the patients treated in the Global Carotid Artery Stent Registry, 99% were considered procedural successes (7) as were 98% of the patients in a prospective case series of 528 patients from three major endovascular centers (28). Similar rates are reported in case series of patients considered to be at high risk for endarterectomy (6), which one would expect to be the most difficult to treat. Additionally, few patients referred for endovascular stenting are actually excluded from it based on readily available pre-procedure information about the stenosed carotid. This was demonstrated in the SAPPHIRE trial (26), where the randomization of a patient first required both the vascular surgeon and the interventionist to agree that the patient was a suitable candidate for either endovascular stenting or endarterectomy. Of the 413 patients who were thought to be unsuitable for one of the procedures, 406 were excluded from endarterectomy whereas only 7 were excluded from endovascular stent placement. Clearly, in this study, there was a greater willingness by the interventionists to consider treatment for a patient with carotid stenosis.

Restenosis of a treated carotid artery can occur after endovascular stenting or surgical endarterectomy. Much of the concern about restenosis following endovascular stenting is extrapolated from studies of simple angioplasty in which restenosis was common [e.g., >70% restenosis occurring within 1 year in 25% of patients in the CAVATAS trial (23)]. Comparison of endovascular stenting against historical controls also initially suggested that restenosis to a degree suitable for a second intervention appears to occur at slightly faster rates after stenting [about 5% over a 1 year period (7,10,29) vs. 2% per year after endarterectomy (3)]. Any difference in these restenosis rates was unlikely to be due to the degree of residual stenosis immediately post-procedure since both stenting and endarterectomy typically reduce the stenosis to <10% of the lumen diameter. However, recent comparative trials have not supported the notion that restenosis occurs at a faster rate after an endovascular procedure. In the SAPPHIRE trial, restenosis to >70% after endovascular stenting occurred at 0.8% per year, in comparison with 4.2% after surgical endarterectomy. Thus, the concern that stenting allows for rapid restenosis of the carotid artery may prove unjustified but it remains to be further substantiated in future trials.

Considering its minimally invasive nature, endovascular stenting would be expected to consume fewer hospital resources and to require shorter postprocedural hospitalizations. Gray et al. (10) report lower costs and shorter hospitalizations (by 1.5 days) in patients treated with endovascular stenting. In the SAPPHIRE trial, patients subjected to endovascular treatments were discharged about 1 day earlier than patients treated with endarterectomy (26). It is unclear how much these differences were due to medical necessity or simply the treating physician's preferences, since in no comparative study of the two treatments were the physicians responsible for the patients' postprocedure management blinded to the patient treatment. Other trials, in fact, show no difference in the length of hospitalization in patients treated with endarterectomy or with endovascular stenting (24,27).

5. FUTURE EXPECTATIONS

Failure to distinguish between symptomatic and asymptomatic carotid stenoses greatly impairs the interpretation of much of the available literature on the use of endovascular therapy. It should, then, be obvious that a clear distinction should be made between patients with symptomatic and asymptomatic carotid stenosis when evaluating the effectiveness of stenting or other endovascular therapies. Symptomatic and asymptomatic carotid stenoses differ in terms of histology (30), natural history [1.9% yearly stroke risk for asymptomatic stenosis >70% (31) vs. 13% for symptomatic stenosis >70% (4)], and responsiveness to medical management [e.g., the lack of efficacy of aspirin in the treatment of asymptomatic carotid stenosis (32) unlike in symptomatic carotid stenosis (33)]. All of these differences likely factor into how the two types of carotid stenoses respond to surgical endarterectomy, and could also affect their responsiveness to endovascular treatments.

Future trials comparing endovascular stenting and surgical endarterectomy may do well to reconsider patients who are at "high risk" for procedural complications as either their primary concern or else as a specific subgroup analysis. High-risk patients are those who would be excluded by the stringent criteria of the large endarterectomy trials. High-risk patients may prove to benefit from an endovascular procedure such as stenting with distal embolization protection particularly if the periprocedural complication rate can be minimized. Conversely, the ongoing efforts to replace cerebral angiography with carotid ultrasonography as the means of defining the degree of carotid stenosis might make endarterectomy more competitive in future trials of high-risk patients (34,35).

Endovascular stenting should also be evaluated in specific subgroups of patients with complex patterns of atherosclerotic disease who are thought to be at increased risk for surgical endarterectomy. An example of such a subgroup would be patients with an asymptomatic carotid stenosis and a contralateral carotid occlusion. In a post-hoc analysis of the patients enrolled in the ACAS trial, Baker et al. (36) found that the presence of a contralateral carotid occlusion eliminated the benefit of the endarterectomy procedure independent of any effect on periprocedural complications. Another condition of potential interest is combined carotid stenosis and coronary artery disease that has considerable mortality when treated simultaneously in a procedure that involves endarterectomy (37). Restenosis of a carotid artery after an initial treatment may also be one of these special situations that deserve specific attention in future trials. When restenosis does occur after endarterectomy, it has generally been considered an indication for treatment with endovascular procedures. As with patients who would be considered ineligible for endarterectomy according to the exclusion criteria of the major endarterectomy trials, the use of stenting in patients with post-endarterectomy restenosis is in reality only the default option given the poor outcome that has been documented with redo endarterectomy (38).

Endovascular stenting and surgical endarterectomy should also be specifically compared in women with asymptomatic carotid stenosis. In the ACAS trial (3), asymptomatic women had more than twice the periprocedural rate of stroke or death after endarterectomy in comparison with men (3.6 vs. 1.7%). In contrast, large case series of endovascular stenting in symptomatic and asymptomatic women show they had less—not more—periprocedural complications in comparison with men [5.9 vs. 8.0% (28)]. If such a distinction proves substantial, perhaps it would provide the basis for a sex-specific treatment paradigm for asymptomatic carotid stenosis.

It would also seem that the risk of stroke associated with various features of an asymptomatic carotid stenosis could be better defined in future trials. Stroke risk with carotid stenosis is apparently increased by plaque ulcerations (39), ultrasonographic detection of embolism signals (40), or by having neuroimaging evidence of infarction in the brain region fed by the affected carotid artery (41). Additionally, poor reactivity of cerebral arteries downstream from an asymptomatic carotid stenosis may increase the patient's risk of stroke and transient ischemic attack (42). Since some of this loss of reactivity may be due to the abnormal function of vasoregulatory nerve fibers that course along the surface of the large arteries (43,44), it could be hypothesized that further damage to such nerve fibers after surgical endarterectomy could be avoided by an endovascular approach. Such patients might then benefit more from endovascular treatment.

Finally, current studies will provide important insights into the role of stenting for asymptomatic stenosis. As an example, the multi-center Carotid

Revascularization Endarterectomy vs. Stent Trial (CREST) recently amended the protocol to include asymptomatic patients with at least 70% stenosis. Since this study is enrolling low-to-medium risk patients, it will provide valuable information regarding whether the role of stenting should be expanded for asymptomatic patients in the future.

REFERENCES

1. Hobson RW 2nd, Weiss DG, Fields WS, Goldstone J, Moore WS, Towne JB, Wright CB. Efficacy of carotid endarterectomy for asymptomatic carotid stenosis. The Veterans Affairs Cooperative Study Group. N Engl J Med 1993; 328:221–227.
2. Halliday A, Mansfield A, Marro J, Peto C, Peto R, Potter J, Thomas D. Prevention of disabling and fatal strokes by successful carotid endarterectomy in patients without recent neurological symptoms: randomised controlled trial. Lancet 2004; 363:1491–1502.
3. Endarterectomy for asymptomatic carotid artery stenosis. Executive Committee for the Asymptomatic Carotid Atherosclerosis Study [see comments]. JAMA 1995; 273:1421–1428.
4. Beneficial effect of carotid endarterectomy in symptomatic patients with high-grade carotid stenosis. North American Symptomatic Carotid Endarterectomy Trial Collaborators [see comments]. N Engl J Med 1991; 325:445–453.
5. Marcinczyk MJ, Nicholas GG, Reed JF 3rd, Nastasee SA. Asymptomatic carotid endarterectomy. Patient and surgeon selection. Stroke 1997; 28:291–296.
6. Shawl F, Kadro W, Domanski MJ, Lapetina FL, Iqbal AA, Dougherty KG, Weisher DD, Marquez JF, Shahab ST. Safety and efficacy of elective carotid artery stenting in high-risk patients. J Am Coll Cardiol 2000; 35:1721–1728.
7. Wholey MH, Al-Mubarek N. Updated review of the global carotid artery stent registry. Catheter Cardiovasc Interv 2003; 60:259–266.
8. Wholey MH, Jarmolowski CR, Eles G, Levy D, Buecthel J. Endovascular stents for carotid artery occlusive disease. J Endovasc Surg 1997; 4:326–338.
9. Qureshi AI, Suri MF, New G, Wadsworth DC Jr, Dulin J, Hopkins LN. Multi-center study of the feasibility and safety of using the memotherm carotid arterial stent for extracranial carotid artery stenosis. J Neurosurg 2002; 96:830–836.
10. Gray WA, White HJ Jr, Barrett DM, Chandran G, Turner R, Reisman M. Carotid stenting and endarterectomy: a clinical and cost comparison of revascularization strategies. Stroke 2002; 33:1063–1070.
11. McCleary AJ, Nelson M, Dearden NM, Calvey TA, Gough MJ. Cerebral haemodynamics and embolization during carotid angioplasty in high-risk patients. Br J Surg 1998; 85:771–774.
12. Jordan WD Jr, Voellinger DC, Doblar DD, Plyushcheva NP, Fisher WS, McDowell HA. Microemboli detected by transcranial Doppler monitoring in patients during carotid angioplasty versus carotid endarterectomy. Cardiovasc Surg 1999; 7:33–38.
13. Madyoon H, Braunstein E, Callcott F, Oshtory M, Gurnsey L, Croushore L, Macbeth A. Unprotected carotid artery stenting compared to carotid endarterectomy in a community setting. J Endovasc Ther 2002; 9:803–809.

14. Bergeron P, Becquemin JP, Jausseran JM, Biasi G, Cardon JM, Castellani L, Martinez R, Fiorani P, Kniemeyer P. Percutaneous stenting of the internal carotid artery: the European CAST I Study. Carotid Artery Stent Trial. J Endovasc Surg 1999; 6:155–159.
15. Macdonald S, Venables GS, Cleveland TJ, Gaines PA. Protected carotid stenting: safety and efficacy of the MedNova NeuroShield filter. J Vasc Surg 2002; 35:966–972.
16. Schluter M, Tubler T, Steffens JC, Mathey DG, Schofer J. Focal ischemia of the brain after neuroprotected carotid artery stenting. J Am Coll Cardiol 2003; 42:1007–1013.
17. Jager HJ, Mathias KD, Drescher R, et al. Cerebral protection with balloon occlusion during carotid artery stent implantation—first experiences. Rofo 2001; 173:139–146.
18. van Heesewijk HP, Vos JA, Louwerse ES, Van Den Berg JC, Overtoom TT, Ernst SM, Mauser HW, Moll FL, Ackerstaff RG. New brain lesions at MR imaging after carotid angioplasty and stent placement. Radiology 2002; 224:361–365.
19. Jaeger HJ, Mathias KD, Hauth E, Drescher R, Gissler HM, Hennigs S, Christmann A. Cerebral ischemia detected with diffusion-weighted MR imaging after stent implantation in the carotid artery. AJNR Am J Neuroradiol 2002; 23:200–207.
20. Order BM, Glass C, Liess C, Heller M, Muller-Hulsbeck S. Comparison of 4 cerebral protection filters for carotid angioplasty: an in vitro experiment focusing on carotid anatomy. J Endovasc Ther 2004; 11:211–218.
21. Kastrup A, Groschel K, Krapf H, Brehm BR, Dichgans J, Schulz JB. Early outcome of carotid angioplasty and stenting with and without cerebral protection devices: a systematic review of the literature. Stroke 2003; 34:813–819.
22. Powell RJ, Schermerhorn M, Nolan B, Lenz J, Rzuidlo E, Fillinger M, Walsh D, Wyers M, Zwolak R, Cronenwett JL. Early results of carotid stent placement for treatment of extracranial carotid bifurcation occlusive disease. J Vasc Surg 2004; 39:1193–1199.
23. Group CaVATAS. Endovascular versus surgical treatment in patients with carotid stenosis in the Carotid and Vertebral Artery Transluminal Angioplasty Study (CAVATAS): a randomised trial. Lancet 2001; 357:1729–1737.
24. Brooks WH, McClure RR, Jones MR, Coleman TL, Breathitt L. Carotid angioplasty and stenting versus carotid endarterectomy for treatment of asymptomatic carotid stenosis: a randomized trial in a community hospital. Neurosurgery 2004; 54:318–324; discussion 324–325.
25. Endo S, Kuwayama N, Hirashima Y. Japan Carotid Atherosclerosis Study: JCAS. Neurol Med Chir (Tokyo) 2004; 44:215–217.
26. Yadav JS, Wholey MH, Kuntz RE, Fayad P, Katzen BT, Mishkel GJ, Bajwa TK, Whitlow P, Strickman NE, Jaff MR, Popma JJ, Snead DB, Cutlip DE, Firth BG, Ouriel K. Protected carotid-artery stenting versus endarterectomy in high-risk patients. N Engl J Med 2004; 351:1493–1501.
27. Carotid revascularization using endarterectomy or stenting systems (CARESS): phase I clinical trial. J Endovasc Ther 2003; 10:1021–1030.
28. Roubin GS, New G, Iyer SS, Vitek JJ, Al-Mubarak N, Liu MW, Yadav J, Gomez C, Kuntz RE. Immediate and late clinical outcomes of carotid artery

stenting in patients with symptomatic and asymptomatic carotid artery stenosis: a 5-year prospective analysis. Circulation 2001; 103:532–537.

29. Moore WS, Kempczinski RF, Nelson JJ, Toole JF. Recurrent carotid stenosis: results of the asymptomatic carotid atherosclerosis study. Stroke 1998; 29: 2018–2025.

30. Spagnoli LG, Mauriello A, Sangiorgi G, Fratoni S, Bonanno E, Schwartz RS, Piepgras DG, Pistolese R, Ippoliti A, Holmes DR, Jr. Extracranial thrombotically active carotid plaque as a risk factor for ischemic stroke. JAMA 2004; 292:1845–1852.

31. Risk of stroke in the distribution of an asymptomatic carotid artery. The European Carotid Surgery Trialists Collaborative Group [see comments]. Lancet 1995; 345:209–212.

32. Cote R, Battista RN, Abrahamowicz M, Langlois Y, Bourque F, Mackey A. Lack of effect of aspirin in asymptomatic patients with carotid bruits and substantial carotid narrowing. The Asymptomatic Cervical Bruit Study Group. Ann Intern Med 1995; 123:649–655.

33. Fields WS, Lemak NA, Frankowski RF, Hardy RJ. Controlled trial of aspirin in cerebral ischemia. Stroke 1977; 8:301–314.

34. Chervu A, Moore WS. Carotid endarterectomy without arteriography. Ann Vasc Surg 1994; 8:296–302.

35. Horn M, Michelini M, Greisler HP, Littooy FN, Baker WH. Carotid endarterectomy without arteriography: the preeminent role of the vascular laboratory. Ann Vasc Surg 1994; 8:221–224.

36. Baker WH, Howard VJ, Howard G, Toole JF. Effect of contralateral occlusion on long-term efficacy of endarterectomy in the asymptomatic carotid atherosclerosis study (ACAS). ACAS Investigators. Stroke 2000; 31:2330–2334.

37. Brown KR, Kresowik TF, Chin MH, Kresowik RA, Grund SL, Hendel ME. Multistate population-based outcomes of combined carotid endarterectomy and coronary artery bypass. J Vasc Surg 2003; 37:32–39.

38. Bartlett FF, Rapp JH, Goldstone J, Ehrenfeld WK, Stoney RJ. Recurrent carotid stenosis: operative strategy and late results. J Vasc Surg 1987; 5:452–456.

39. Troyer A, Saloner D, Pan XM, Velez P, Rapp JH. Major carotid plaque surface irregularities correlate with neurologic symptoms. J Vasc Surg 2002; 35: 741–747.

40. Molloy J, Markus HS. Asymptomatic embolization predicts stroke and TIA risk in patients with carotid artery stenosis. Stroke 1999; 30:1440–1443.

41. el-Barghouty N, Nicolaides A, Bahal V, Geroulakos G, Androulakis A. The identification of the high risk carotid plaque. Eur J Vasc Endovasc Surg 1996; 11:470–478.

42. Silvestrini M, Vernieri F, Pasqualetti P, Matteis M, Passarelli F, Troisi E, Caltagirone C. Impaired cerebral vasoreactivity and risk of stroke in patients with asymptomatic carotid artery stenosis. JAMA 2000; 283:2122–2127.

43. Faraci FM, Heistad DD. Regulation of large cerebral arteries and cerebral microvascular pressure. Circ Res 1990; 66:8–17.

44. Akiguchi I, Fukuyama H, Kameyama M, Koyama T, Kimura H, Maeda T. Sympathetic nerve terminals in the tunica media of human superficial temporal and middle cerebral arteries: wet histofluorescence. Stroke 1983; 14:62–66.

19

Angioplasty and Stenting for Non-atherosclerotic Diseases of the Carotid Artery

Kumar Rajamani

Department of Neurology, Wayne State University, Detroit, Michigan, U.S.A.

Seemant Chaturvedi

Department of Neurology, Detroit Medical Center, Wayne State University, Detroit, Michigan, U.S.A.

1. INTRODUCTION

Other chapters in this book have discussed the role of carotid endarterectomy and stenting for patients with moderate-to-severe internal carotid artery stenosis due to atherosclerosis. Due to the frequency of carotid stenosis, large clinical trials have been performed to evaluate this condition, such as the North American Symptomatic Carotid Endarterectomy Trial (NASCET), European Carotid Surgery Trial (ECST), and the Asymptomatic Carotid Atherosclerosis Study (ACAS).

In addition to carotid atherosclerosis, neurologists, surgeons, and stroke specialists are likely to encounter non-atherosclerotic vasculopathies affecting the internal carotid artery (ICA). These include fibromuscular dysplasia (FMD), post-radiation carotid stenosis, and carotid dissection with or without pseudoaneurysm formation. These conditions were excluded from the multicenter carotid endarterectomy trials and, therefore, there are limited data available regarding the comparative efficacy of various therapeutic options.

Some of these conditions such as radiation-induced carotid stenosis present a formidable challenge for the surgeon in terms of surgical anatomy and consequent complications. Therefore, angioplasty and stenting is a potentially attractive treatment option for some non-atherosclerotic conditions. Since the non-atherosclerotic causes of carotid disease are relatively uncommon, the literature consists of essentially small case series. We shall review the experience to date on the use of angioplasty and stenting for some of these conditions.

2. ANGIOPLASTY AND STENTING FOR CAROTID ARTERY DISSECTION

Carotid artery dissections account for only 2% of all ischemic strokes, but account for 10–25% of ischemic strokes in younger people (1). They often occur spontaneously in apparently healthy vessels often as a result of trauma, which may be trivial. The natural history is quite variable and strokes occur in about 50–95% of individuals with carotid dissection. It is likely that with increasing awareness, more asymptomatic cases and those presenting with non-stroke complaints are increasingly being recognized. In about a third of the cases, pseudoaneurysm formation can occur. Based on the view that the mechanism of strokes is primarily embolic, treatment is often antithrombotic therapy, though controlled studies are lacking. More recently, endovascular procedures have been performed as a therapy for carotid dissection. In addition to stenting of an area of stenosis, some procedures have included coil placement for patients with pseudoaneurysms (2).

Many patients with cervicocephalic arterial dissections will have an improvement in the luminal diameter over a period of weeks to months (3). However, for patients with continued symptoms or patients who develop progressive pseudoaneurysms, stenting can be employed. In one series of seven patients with dissections in which stenting was undertaken, it was found that all patients were free of ischemic symptoms for a mean period of 3.5 years (4). Reopening of a complete internal carotid occlusion due to dissection with subsequent stent placement has also been reported (5).

Binaghi et al. (6) and Albuquerque et al. (7) have reported small series of patients with carotid dissection on whom they have performed angioplasty and stenting successfully. These authors report the excellent safety of the procedure, as well as success in eliminating the pseudoaneurysm, though the anatomy may be sufficiently distorted in some cases precluding the deployment of the microwire over which the stent is threaded.

In an interesting long-term outcome study, Kremer et al. (8) have studied 161 consecutive patients with carotid artery dissections and have shown a relatively low stroke risk of up to 0.7% at the end of the first year; they have questioned the routine use of surgical or endovascular treatments for carotid dissection. Cohen et al. (9) have addressed this issue by advocating carotid angioplasty and stenting only in patients who do not respond to antithrombotic treatment, and have persistent cerebral ischemia based on diffusion–perfusion MRI mismatch. This may help in an appropriate and rational choice of patients who are most likely to benefit based upon radiological demonstration of salvageable brain in the ischemic penumbra, and excluding those with complete and irreversible ischemia.

3. ANGIOPLASTY FOR RADIATION-INDUCED CAROTID STENOSIS

Carotid artery disease is a well-known complication of external beam radiation such as is administered for head and neck cancers. In a long-term follow-up study of 6 years, Cheng et al. (10) estimated a risk of significant carotid artery stenosis in 11.7% patients after external beam radiation to the head and neck area. Another review of 415 patients who received external beam radiation as treatment for Hodgkin's lymphoma reported a 7.4% development of carotid and/or subclavian disease at a mean of 17 years following treatment (11). Radiation induced carotid disease has been classified into three subtypes: (i) acute carotid artery rupture, (ii) early carotid artery occlusion, occurring within months, probably the result of direct arterial wall injury, and (iii) chronic late development of occlusion akin to atherosclerosis (12). Rarely, pseudoaneurysm formation has also been described (13). Although the term "accelerated atherosclerosis" is often used, there are some key differences based on the fact that the lesion often affects the common carotid artery, and that long segments of the artery are commonly involved.

These lesions are challenging to the surgeon as conventional tissue planes are lost due to fibrosis. The site of the lesions in the lower part of the neck and their relatively long length make them less amenable to surgical repairs. In addition, healing is poor in these tissues. Houdart et al. (14) report seven patients with radiation-induced carotid artery stenosis of the common and internal carotid arteries treated with angioplasty and stenting. They had no complications and, after 8 months follow-up, had excellent results with no patient showing restenosis. Ting et al. (15) report on a patient who had successful angioplasty for recurrent carotid stenosis which occurred after a previous CEA for radiation-induced carotid stenosis.

Decidedly, little data exist to guide the clinician who is faced with a patient with radiation-induced carotid stenosis. The natural history of these lesions, and the risk of ischemic events with and without medical treatment alone, is not known. Decisions often need to be individualized based on the availability of local expertise in surgical and endovascular techniques.

4. ANGIOPLASTY FOR FIBROMUSCULAR DYSPLASIA OF THE CAROTID ARTERY

Fibromuscular dysplasia (FMD) is a rare condition of unknown etiology, characterized by a segmental, non-atheromatous, non-inflammatory angiopathy predominantly affecting young white women. It can involve the cervicocephalic arteries, typically the carotid arteries in the neck, but uncommonly can involve the intracranial portions such as the carotid siphon region. The renal arteries and iliac arteries may be more commonly involved, but when the cervicocephalic arteries are affected, patients can present with neck pain, carotid bruit, headaches, transient ischemic attacks, ischemic strokes, and subarachnoid hemorrhage. In some patients, the disease may be bilateral. The affected cervical carotid artery may be more prone to arterial dissection, thrombosis, and occlusion. Diagnosis is made by angiography, with characteristic intimal irregularity giving the artery a "string of beads" appearance.

Whereas the treatment options available are antithrombotic drugs, endarterectomy, or angioplasty, the optimal treatment of cervicocephalic FMD remains controversial. Vascular involvement in FMD tends to be higher in the neck or may involve longer or multifocal segments, compared to atherosclerotic disease. Transluminal dilatation of the carotid artery for FMD has hence been increasingly performed over the last two decades (16). Previously, it was performed by gradual dilatation of the artery using metal dilators, but over the years, the techniques have become more sophisticated with the use of transluminal balloon angioplasty, with stent placement. Manninen et al. (17) describe a patient with both the internal carotid arteries and both the vertebral arteries affected by FMD who was successfully treated by balloon angioplasty and stenting, and, in addition, had detachable coils placed in the pseudoaneurysms with excellent results at 1 year after the procedure. Finsterer et al. (18) describe their experience with a patient with FMD that had affected bilateral internal carotid arteries who remained symptomatic in spite of antithrombotic treatment. The patient received stenting procedures bilaterally, and in spite of a mild transient hemiparesis after the procedure, was asymptomatic after 9 months.

The treatment of a given patient should be individualized based on the presence or absence of symptoms, and the nature of symptoms. In the vast majority of patients with cervicocephalic FMD, the prognosis is probably benign, and antithrombotic treatment may suffice for ischemic symptoms. Failure of medical treatment and presence of pseudoaneurysms, with or without subarachnoid hemorrhage, may necessitate angioplasty with stenting. Coiling to obliterate the aneurysm may be appropriate. Local availability of technical expertise will obviously be important in such decision-making.

5. TAKAYASU'S DISEASE

Takayasu's disease is a chronic inflammatory arteriopathy and typically involves the aorta and its branches (19). The cause is unknown though an autoimmune disorder is suspected. Although more common in Japan and parts of Asia, it is seen in North America among young women of Asian, Mexican, and native Indian ancestry. Clinical presentation can vary depending upon the location and severity of the branches involved, with involvement of brachiocephalic arteries resulting in stroke or transient ischemic attacks and exercise intolerance in the hands. Diagnosis requires a high index of suspicion, and angiography may reveal stenosis or occlusion of parts of the aorta or its major branches.

Several authors have reported encouraging results after treatment with balloon angioplasty with stenting in this progressive condition. Sharma et al. (20) report their experience with carotid angioplasty and stenting in six patients. In one patient the guidewire could not be negotiated through the block. One patient was reported to develop a transient ischemic attack during the procedure. All patients were said to experience "good relief of symptoms" immediately after the procedure. However, two patients developed restenosis and became symptomatic again after 5 months. Maskovic et al. (21) report successful angioplasty in a young woman with stroke, who had good lasting benefit even after 6 months. Takahashi et al. (22) from Japan report a young woman with Takayasu's disease who underwent a two-step procedure for angioplasty and stent placement in both common carotid arteries. Follow-up angiography 2 years later did not reveal any restenosis. In spite of these encouraging results, the general impression is that the rate of restenosis after angioplasty is much higher among patients with Takayasu's disease compared to those with atherosclerosis (23,24). Although further long-term data are needed, angioplasty and stenting may be an attractive option for patients who remain symptomatic.

6. INTRACRANIAL VASCULITIS

We have been able to identify only one report describing the use of angioplasty for intracranial vasculitis. In this article, five patients are described who underwent angioplasty for lesions involving locations such as the distal ICA and middle cerebral artery (25). In one patient, the vasculitis was said to be due to herpes encephalitis but etiologies for the other cases are not described. In this single-center paper, transient angiographic improvement was reported in all patients but the vessels went to occlusion subsequently. The authors felt that angioplasty during the acute phase of vasculitis may be contraindicated due to the risk of iatrogenic dissection or acute vessel closure.

7. CONCLUSIONS

In the scenarios discussed in this chapter, angioplasty with or without stenting has been attempted with mixed results. The clinician should keep in mind that some of the conditions discussed in this chapter are usually benign (FMD) and that for others, such as arterial dissection, the majority of patients can be managed without surgical or endovascular intervention.

Nevertheless, in patients who remain symptomatic despite maximal medical therapy, angioplasty can be considered for certain non-atherosclerotic conditions. The success rate will likely be lower for inflammatory vascular disorders. Conversely, the success rate is likely to be higher in experienced centers and, therefore, referral of patients to tertiary centers for angioplasty of vasculopathies is recommended.

REFERENCES

1. Schievink WI. Spontaneous dissection of the carotid and vertebral arteries. NEJM 2001; 344:898–906.
2. Schievink WI. The treatment of spontaneous carotid and vertebral artery dissections. Curr Opin Cardiol 2000; 15:316–321.
3. Kasner SE, Hankins LL, Bratina P, Morgenstern LB. Magnetic resonance angiography demonstrates vascular healing of carotid and vertebral artery dissections. Stroke 1997; 28:1993–1997.
4. Liu AY, Paulsen RD, Marcellus ML, Steinberg GK, Marks MP. Long-term outcomes after carotid stent placement for treatment of carotid artery dissection. Neurosurgery 1999; 45:1368–1374.
5. DeOcampo J, Brillman J, Levy DI. Stenting: a new approach to carotid dissection. J Neuroimag 1997; 7:187–190.
6. Binaghi S, Chapot R, Rogopoulos A, Houdart E. Carotid stenting of chronic cervical dissecting aneurysm: a report of two cases. Neurology 2002; 59: 935–937.
7. Albuquerque FC, Han PP, Spetzler RF, Zabramski JM, Mcdougall CG. Carotid dissection: technical factors affecting endovascular therapy. Can J Neurol Sci 2002; 29:54–60.
8. Kremer C, Mosso M, Georgiadis D, Stockli E, Benninger D, Arnold M, Baumgartner RW. Carotid dissection with permanent and transient occlusion or severe stenosis, long term outcome. Neurology 2003; 60:271–275.
9. Cohen JE, Leker RR, Gotkine M, Gomori M, Ben-Hur T. Emergent stenting to treat patients with carotid artery dissection, clinically and radiologically directed therapeutic decision making. Stroke 2003; 34: e254–e257.
10. Cheng SW, Wu LL, Ting AC, Lau H, Lam LK, Wei WI. Irradiation induced extracranial carotid stenosis in patients with head and neck malignancies. Am J Surg 1999; 178:323–328.
11. Hull MC, Morris CG, Pepine CJ, Mendendall NP. Valvular dysfunction and carotid, subclavian, and coronary artery disease in survivors of Hodgkin lymphoma treated with radiation therapy. JAMA 2003; 290:2831–2837.
12. Loftus CM, Biller J, Hart MN, Cornell SH, Hiratzka LF. Management of radiation induced accelerated carotid atherosclerosis. Arch Neurol 1987; 44:711–714.
13. Koenigsberg RA, Grandinetti LM, Freeman LP, McCormick D, Tsai F. Endovascular repair of radiation-induced bilateral common carotid artery stenosis and pseudoaneurysms-a case report. Surg Neurol 2001; 55:347–352.
14. Houdart E, Mounayer C, Chapot R, Saint-Maurice JP, Merland JJ. Carotid stenting for radiation induced stenosis. Stroke 2001; 32:118–121.

15. Ting AC, Cheng SW, Cheng PW. Carotid stenting for irradiation associated carotid stenosis 3 years after previous carotid endarterectomy. Hong Kong Med J 2003; 9:51–53.
16. Garrido E, Montoya J. Transluminal dilation of internal carotid artery in fibromuscular dysplasia: a preliminary report. Surg Neurol 1981; 16:469–471.
17. Manninen HI, Koivisto T, Saari T, Matsi PJ, Vanninen RL, Luukonen M, Hernesniemi J. Dissecting aneurysms of all the four craniocervical arteries in fibromuscular dysplasia: treatment with self expanding endovascular stents, coil embolization and surgical ligation. Am J Neuroradiol 1997; 18:1216–1220.
18. Finsterer J, Strassegger J, Haymerle A, Hagmuller G. Bilateral stenting of symptomatic and asymptomatic internal carotid artery stenosis due to fibromuscular dysplasia. J Neurol Neurosurg Psychiatr 2000; 69:683–686.
19. Creager M. Takayasu's disease. Rev Cardiovasc Med 2001; 2:211–214.
20. Sharma BK, Jain S, Bali HK, Jain A, Kumari S. A follow-up study of balloon angioplasty and de novo stenting in Takayasu arteritis. Int J Cardio 2000; 75(suppl) S147–S152.
21. Maskovic J, Jankovic S, Lusic I, Cambj-Sapunar L, Mimica Z, Bacic A. Subclavian artery stenosis caused by non-specific arteritis (Takayasu disease): treatment with Palmaz stent. Eur J Radiol 1997; 31:193–196.
22. Takahashi JC, Sakai N, Manaka H, Iihara K, Sakai H, Sakaida H, Higashi T, Ishibashi T, Nagata I. Multiple supra-aortic stenting for Takayasu arteritis: extensive revascularization and two year follow-up. Am J Neuroradiol 2002; 23:790–793.
23. Joseph S, Mandalam KR, Rao VR, Gupta AK, Unni NM, Rao AS, Neelakandhan KS, Unnikrishnan M, Sandhyamani S. Percutaneous transluminal angioplasty of the subclavian artery in non-specific aortoarteritis: results of long term follow up. J Vasc Interv Radiol 1994; 5:573–580.
24. Tyagi S, Verma PK, Gambhir DS, Kaul UA, Saha R, Arora R. Early and long term results of subclavian angioplasty in aotoarteritis (Takayasu disease). Cardiovasc Interv Radiol 1998; 21:219–224.
25. Mckenzie JD, Wallace RC, Dean BL, Flom RA, Khayata MH. Preliminary results of intracranial angioplasty for vascular stenosis caused by atherosclerosis and vasculitis. Am J Neuroradiol 1996; 17:263–268.

20

Controversies in Endovascular Therapy for Carotid Artery Stenosis

Andrew R. Xavier, Catalina C. Ionita, Jawad F. Kirmani, and Adnan I. Qureshi

Cerebrovascular Program, Department of Neurology and Neurosciences, University of Medicine and Dentistry of New Jersey, Newark, New Jersey, U.S.A.

1. INTRODUCTION

Carotid angioplasty and stenting (CAS) is rapidly evolving as an alternative to carotid endarterectomy (CEA) in the primary and secondary prevention of stroke from carotid atherovascular disease (1–6). Although endovascular treatment of carotid stenosis was first reported 20 years back (7–10), and has undergone rapid development in the last few years (11–16), there are still plenty of controversies surrounding this procedure. There are controversies regarding who should undergo CAS vs. CEA, whether embolic protection devices need to be used every time CAS is performed, what type of antithrombotic agent should be used before, during, and after the procedure, and other procedural details. In this chapter, we address some of these controversies using currently published literature.

2. WHICH ARE THE PATIENTS THAT SHOULD UNDERGO CAROTID ANGIOPLASTY AND STENTING?

Which among the patients with carotid disease should be selected to undergo CAS remains a controversial issue. This issue has been addressed in depth in the previous chapters, but just to summarize, there is now sufficient data to consider CAS instead of CEA in patients with severe coronary artery disease (CAD), radiation-induced carotid stenosis, high carotid bifurcation, tandem lesions, post-CEA restenosis, and severe medical illnesses like chronic obstructive pulmonary disease and congestive heart failure (17).

2.1. Severe Coronary Artery Disease and Congestive Heart Failure

The management of carotid stenosis identified in patients who require coronary artery bypass grafting (CABG) for CAD remains controversial (18,19). Surgical options are rather limited in this situation as published reports on combined CEA and CABG suggest a perioperative risk of stroke or death ranging from 7.4 to 9.4%, which is 1.5–2.0 times the perioperative risk with each operation when performed alone (20). A multi-center review (21) found an unacceptably high rate of stroke or death (18.7%) in patients who had CEA performed in conjunction with CABG. The CEA guidelines published by the American Heart Association report that the incidence of stroke, myocardial infarction (MI), and death is 16.4% for combined CEA and CABG, 26.2% for CEA followed by CABG, and 16.4% for CABG followed by CEA (22). Patients with congestive heart failure (CHF) also have a higher rate of postoperative stroke or death with CEA (21,23)— 8.6% in patients with CHF as opposed to a rate of 2.3% in patients without CHF. In this high-risk subgroup, avoiding a major operation or general anesthesia by performing CAS may be preferred (24,25).

In a recent report on CAS (24) performed on 49 patients prior to undergoing CABG, the 30-day mortality rate for the combined procedure was 8% and the stroke rate for the same period was only 2%. The complication rates appear to be substantially lower compared with combined CABG and CEA. The preliminary results of the SAPPHIRE trial (17) also support the use of CAS as an alternative to CEA in patients with severe CAD and CHF.

2.2. Restenosis After Carotid Endarterectomy

Post-endarterectomy recurrent carotid artery stenosis is becoming an increasingly common long-term complication after CEA (26,27). Repeat surgical revascularization in this group of patients has nearly five times the risk of morbidity and mortality as primary CEA (27,28). Multiple case-series (29,30) have reported much lower peri-procedural complications for CAS performed in individuals with post-CEA recurrent stenosis.

2.3. Contralateral Carotid Occlusion

Patients with recent symptoms referable to severe carotid artery stenosis and coexistent contralateral carotid artery occlusion have a high rate of ipsilateral ischemic stroke (31). In the North American Symptomatic Carotid Endarterectomy Trial (NASCET) (32), CEA was found to significantly reduce the stroke risk in this group of patients; however, the perioperative risk of stroke or death was very high (14.3%). Prior reports (33) have described the performance of CAS with much lower perioperative complications (3.8%) in this group of high-risk individuals.

2.4. Presence of Tandem Lesions and Other Anatomical Factors

Anatomical variations like a high bifurcation, especially in a patient with a short neck, or a long carotid artery stenosis that extends to the skull base can be difficult to manage surgically. The presence of tandem lesions, where the distal lesion is more severe than the proximal lesion, was an exclusion criterion for the NASCET (32). A multi-center review of 1160 CEA procedures (23) found that symptomatic patients with ipsilateral carotid siphon stenosis have a postoperative stroke or death risk of 13.9%, compared with a rate of 7.9% in patients without distal stenosis.

Kim et al. (34) have reported their experience in performing angioplasty with and without stenting in 11 patients with tandem lesions. No perioperative stroke, cardiac event or deaths occurred in their series. Hence, angioplasty with or without stenting could be considered as a viable alternative to CEA in patients with surgically inaccessible tandem carotid artery lesions.

2.5. Radiation-Induced Carotid Stenosis

Patients who develop radiation-induced accelerated carotid stenosis represent a similar high-risk group primarily resulting from difficulties with the surgical approach. The presence of long lesion length, lack of well-defined dissection planes, and scarring around the vessels make the surgery more difficult (35,36), exposing the patients to a higher risk of wound infections and cranial nerve palsies. The CAS technique can provide a more effective method for treatment of carotid stenosis associated with radiation (37).

3. WHAT TYPE OF ANTITHROMBOTIC THERAPY SHOULD BE USED DURING CAROTID ANGIOPLASTY AND STENTING?

Thromboembolic phenomena could potentially complicate the performance of CAS, and it remains controversial how best to prevent these complications. The best pharmacological agent and the duration of therapy are still empirically selected with current evidence coming mostly from the coronary literature.

A morphologically intact arterial endothelium forms a natural protective barrier between blood elements and highly thrombogenic elements of the vessel wall such as collagen, von Willebrand factor, and tissue thromboplastin (coagulation Factor III) (38). Damage to the vessel wall during the performance of CAS exposes these subendothelial elements triggering platelet adhesion (39); the morphological change of platelets with the activation of GPIIb/IIIa receptors mediate platelet aggregation (40); and activated platelets get bound together by fibrinogen. Activated platelets also release adenosine diphosphate (ADP), serotonin, and thromboxane A2, resulting in further recruitment and activation of surrounding platelets (41). Concomitant with platelet activation and aggregation, the plasma coagulation cascade and fibrinolysis get activated (42). Tissue thromboplastin, exposed through vascular injury, forms a complex with Factor VIIa, which activates Factors IX and X. Activated Factor X converts prothrombin to thrombin. Thrombin hydrolyzes fibrinogen into fibrin monomers, which undergo spontaneous polymerization resulting in fibrin clot formation. Endothelial cells synthesize and secrete plasminogen activators and plasminogen-activator inhibitors (43). The plasma fibrinolytic system contains plasminogen, an inactive precursor of the active protease plasmin, which degrades fibrin to soluble degradation products (44). In plasma, the balance between activation and inhibition of fibrinolysis is regulated by plasminogen activator inhibitors and [alpha]2-antiplasmin, which inhibits the active plasmin (45).

The increased prothrombotic state induced by arterial wall injury is markedly reduced 24 h after the injury. However, prolonged expression of tissue thromboplastin accompanied by persistent activation and high levels of thrombin can be detected for up to 72 h (46). Re-endothelization of injured blood vessels starts from areas of intact endothelium and is almost complete 2 weeks after the injury (47). However, the functional capacity of endothelial cells could be impaired up to 4 weeks after injury. Covering areas of extensive denudation or foreign surfaces such as metallic stents might prolong this process from 4 to 6 weeks (48,49).

3.1. Pharmacological Agents Available for Prophylaxis

Pharmacological treatment is aimed at the inhibition of platelet adhesion and aggregation, and tissue thromboplastin-induced activation of thrombin and fibrinogen. The platelet inhibitory effect is based primarily on thromboxane A2 inhibition, ADP release, or GPIIb/IIIa receptors inhibition.

3.2. Anti-platelet Therapy

Aspirin is the most popular antiplatelet agent for coronary artery or cerebrovascular disease; its antiplatelet effect is based on cycloxygenase-1 inhibition and suppression of thromboxane A2 production (50,51). This effect is dose-related; an almost complete suppression of thromboxane A2 is achieved by 100 mg of aspirin (52) relatively fast and which persists for about 10 days (lifespan of platelets). The Antiplatelet Trialists' Collaboration study provided evidence that aspirin therapy reduces by one-half the odds of graft occlusion in patients who have undergone different vascular operations (53).

Aspirin is a weak antiplatelet agent, not being able to inhibit aggregation mediated by thromboxane A2-independent pathways or affect platelet adhesion and secretion. Also, aspirin has no effect on platelet-derived mitogenic factors, and hence cannot prevent restenosis or accelerated atherosclerosis after angioplasty (51).

Ticlopidine and *clopidogrel* are oral antiplatelet agents which inhibit the binding of ADP to its platelet receptor, with the consequent inhibition of fibrinogen binding to the GPIIb/IIIa complex. The effect is dose-dependent: ticlopidine (500 mg/day), and clopidogrel (75 mg/day). Adequate platelet inhibition requires 2–3 days of therapy, with a maximal effect after 4–7 days of treatment (54). Like aspirin, the antiplatelet effect lasts for 8–10 days. The combination with aspirin has a synergistic effect of platelet inhibition (55) and reduces the delay observed with clopidogrel and ticlopidine.

Clopidogrel seems to be more effective than either aspirin or ticlopidine in preventing coronary stent thrombosis (56,57). A loading dose of clopidogrel (with 300 mg, for example) is frequently administered to patients undergoing percutaneous intervention who need more rapid platelet inhibition.

3.3. GPIIb/IIIa Receptor Inhibitors

GPIIb/IIIa receptor inhibitors are receptor-specific antibodies that prevent the binding of fibrinogen to these receptors, thereby inhibiting platelet aggregation initiated by any other metabolic pathway. *Abciximab (ReoPro)* is a fragment of murine monoclonal antibodies that is attached to human immunoglobulin, and directed against GPIIb/IIIa receptors, resulting in a non-competitive receptor blockade (58). It is a short-acting intravenous agent with a half-life of 10 minutes. The antiplatelet effect lasts up to 48 h. Effective reversal can be achieved by transfusion of 10 U of platelets.

Eptifibatide (Integrilin) and *Tirofiban (Aggrastat)* are parenterally administered peptides which competitively inhibit GPIIb/IIIa receptor. When 80% of GPIIb/IIIa receptors are blocked, platelet aggregation is almost completely eliminated with only a mild prolongation of bleeding time; with 90% receptor blockade, prolongation of bleeding time to 15–30 minutes occurs (59,60).

The most significant adverse effect of these agents is bleeding (61) and thrombocytopenia (62). Lower doses of the drug and shorter courses of concomitant heparin may minimize the bleeding complications. Multiple randomized, placebo-controlled trials have demonstrated the efficacy of platelet GPIIb/IIIa inhibitors in preventing thromboembolic complications in patients undergoing coronary balloon angioplasty, stenting, and atherectomy. Abciximab has been demonstrated to reduce significantly (50%) all cardiac events at 30 days (61–66) in patients undergoing coronary interventions. It has been also shown to have a stronger antiplatelet effect than clopidogrel at the time of coronary stent implantation (56). Abciximab therapy reduces the need for stent deployment and improves clinical outcome (assessed at 30 days and 6 months follow-up), without increasing bleeding complications (58). Two other studies have tested the efficacy of eptifibatide (67) and tirofiban (68) in preventing subsequent events after coronary interventions. The relative risk reduction of ischemic complications in IMPACT II was 22% in the eptifibatide group vs. placebo (67), and in RESTORE was 24% in the tirofiban group vs. placebo (68).

The role of GPIIb/IIIa inhibitors in the prevention and treatment of thromboembolic complications of patients undergoing CAS is controversial. Qureshi et al. (69) have reported the result of a small study involving 19 patients undergoing angioplasty in the internal carotid artery ($n = 13$), vertebral artery ($n = 4$), and basilar artery ($n = 2$), followed by stent placement across 13 lesions with abciximab infusion. After a bolus of 0.25 mg/kg, the patients received 12–24 h of intravenous infusion of abciximab at 10 mcg/minute. Intra-procedural heparin was given in all 19 procedures, with partial reversal in 6. Almost all patients received pre-procedural antiplatelet therapy including a combination of aspirin and ticlopidine or clopidogrel. Two patients experienced transient neurological deficit either during ($n = 1$) or immediately after ($n = 1$) the procedure. A third patient developed complete occlusion of the right vertebral artery after the angioplasty followed by complete recanalization with 24 h of abciximab infusion. No major (hemoglobin decrease > 5 g/dL) or minor (hemoglobin decrease 3–5 g/dL) bleeding was observed in any patient. Eight patients developed insignificant bleeding, and thrombocytopenia was observed in only one patient who concomitantly received intravenous heparin (69). A larger study including 37 patients undergoing CAS was designed to assess the safety and efficacy of abciximab as an adjunctive treatment to endovascular interventions (70). All patients received intravenous abciximab 0.25 mg/kg as a single bolus followed by 12 h infusion at the rate of 10 mcg/minute. Another group of 33 patients received intra-procedural intravenous heparin only. All patients received aspirin (325 mg daily) and ticlopidine (250 mg twice daily) or clopidogrel (75 mg daily) 72 h before the procedure. Minor ischemic strokes were observed in one of 37 abciximab-treated patients and in four of 33 heparin-treated patients. No major ischemic stroke was observed in either group. Transient neurological deficits were noted in nine abciximab-treated patients and in one heparin-treated patient. Minor bleeding was observed in three patients from the abciximab group and in four patients treated with heparin. Major bleeding was noted in four patients from each group. Two patients who received abciximab developed intra-cerebral hemorrhage, one of them being fatal. The frequency of ischemic complications in high-risk patients treated with abciximab was lower (3%) than in the low-risk heparin-treated group (12%), but the benefit was lost due to a high rate of intracranial hemorrhage (5%) (70). Qureshi et al. (71) tested the safety of intravenous eptifibatide during CAS in a study that included 10 patients. After access to the artery via femoral artery, a 50 U/kg bolus of heparin was administered to achieve an activated coagulation time (ACT) between 250 and 300 s. Each patient received a single-dose bolus of 135 mcg/kg of eptifibatide, followed by a 20–24 h infusion at 0.5 mcg/kg/m. No post-procedural heparin was given. All patients received combined antiplatelet therapy starting 3 days before the procedure, including aspirin (325 mg daily) and clopidogrel (75 mg daily). One patient developed a minor stroke post-procedurally that improved at 7 days; three patients underwent scheduled coronary artery bypass graft surgery 4–12 days after undergoing carotid stenting, and at 1-month follow-up, no new ischemic events were observed. Major or minor bleeding was not recorded in any patient, and insignificant bleeding was recorded in two patients (71).

3.4. Inhibitors of Thrombin and Fibrinogen

Heparins are glycosaminoglycans composed of a mixture of polysaccharides with weights between 3000 and 40,000 da, with an immediate anticoagulant effect and a half-life of 1.5 h. The most accepted heparin mechanisms of action include the activation and modulation of antithrombin III activity, resulting in thrombin neutralization and inactivation of Factors IXa, Xa, XIa, and XIIa (72). Two major complications are associated with heparin: hemorrhagic complications and immunologically induced thrombocytopenia (73). Thrombocytopenia occurs after 3–15 days of treatment initiation and resolves within 4 days of treatment cessation. It is usually associated with elevated platelet immunoglobulin G levels or heparin-dependent platelet aggregating factor (74). Bleeding complications are dependent on the magnitude of anticoagulation, measured by ACT or activated partial thromboplastin time (PTT). Two studies have demonstrated that thrombosis after coronary stent placement could be related to low ACT levels (75,76). Administration of a 10,000-unit bolus followed by repeated bolus doses to achieve an ACT of more than 300 s is recommended. The use of heparin during the first 24 h after the procedure is controversial. Two randomized trials have failed to demonstrate any benefit in reducing thromboembolic complications within the first 24 h after coronary angioplasty (77,78). In addition, the risk of bleeding from the site of the arterial puncture has been found to be increased with the use of heparin in the post-procedure period (79).

Low molecular weight heparin (LMWH) is formed by the fractionation of heterogenous heparin mixtures to heparin molecules (4000–5500 da). The high-molecular weight heparins bind to endothelial cells and plasma proteins; this non-specific binding limits the amount of heparin available to interact with antithrombin III and decreases the anticoagulant effect of heparin (80). The decreased non-specific binding of LMWH confers to them a higher bioavailability at lower doses and a more predictable anticoagulant effect, obviating the need for laboratory monitoring. Compared to standard unfractionated heparins, LMWH has fewer bleeding complications (81) and a lower risk for heparin-induced thrombocytopenia (82). The preparations approved in the USA are enoxaparin (Lovenox), dalteparin (Fragmin), and tinzaparin (Innohep). Fondaparinux (Arixtra) is also available as a synthetic pentasaccharide which inhibits Factor X. A randomized, double-blind, placebo-controlled multi-center trial designed to assess the safety and efficacy of enoxaparin in patients with a high risk for stent thrombosis (ATLAST) was terminated prematurely after the randomization of 1102 patients (target enrollment was 2000 patients) due to the low incidence of the primary end-point. Stent thrombosis occurred in 1.8% enoxaparin-treated patients vs. 2.7% in the placebo group (all patients received aspirin and ticlopidine). The frequency of stent thrombosis and other ischemic events within 15–30 days after the stent placement was low whether the patients received enoxaparin or not (83).

Warfarin is a derivative of a natural lactone (coumarin) with an anticoagulant effect based on delaying thrombin generation through the inhibition of vitamin K/epoxide reductase-dependent coagulation Factors II, VII, IX, and X. Rapidly absorbed from the gastrointestinal tract, warfarin reaches peak plasma values within 90 minutes; its half-life is approximately 40 h. However, the individual anticoagulant response is highly unpredictable; the anticoagulant effect of warfarin is seen only after the normal coagulation factors are cleared from the plasma, which might last for 72–96 h. Warfarin does not have a role in the prevention of thromboembolic complications following angioplasty/stenting.

3.5. Direct Inhibitors of Thrombin

Hirudin and its analogs are antithrombin III-independent inhibitors of thrombin, which are able to access and inactivate thrombin bound to fibrin (84). These direct thrombin inhibitors increase the rapidity of t-PA-mediated recanalization and have been shown to have a promising role in acute myocardial infarction, unstable angina, and angioplasty (85,86). As an adjunctive therapy in combination with either antiplatelet therapy or GP IIB/IIIA inhibitors in coronary angioplasty, they have revealed efficacy at least comparable to and bleeding rates better than heparin (87–89). Two direct thrombin inhibitors—*bivalirudin* (Angiomax) and *argatroban* have been approved for use in adjunctive therapy for coronary interventions. There is no published experience with the use of these agents in carotid interventions.

3.6. Antiplatelet Therapy Vs. Anticoagulant Therapy in Endovascular Procedures

Patients undergoing angioplasty and stent placement for the treatment of coronary or cerebrovascular diseases who are treated with a variety of anticoagulant agents in attempts to reduce the risk of thromboembolic complications, have consistently demonstrated a considerable risk for bleeding complications without an efficient reduction of thrombotic complications. The standard regimens consisting of aspirin, dipyridamole, dextran, heparin, and warfarin produced bleeding complications especially at the sites of insertion of arterial sheaths at rates of 3–16% (79). The rate of subacute thrombosis remained ~7% and was as high as 28% when stenting was used in conjunction with angioplasty. The length of hospital stay was also increased (90,91). Several groups in France assessed the alternative of replacing the standard anticoagulant treatment with different regimens of antiplatelet agents (heparin as a bolus only, followed by LMWH, low dose of aspirin and ticlopidine, with discontinuation of dipyridamole, dextran, and warfarin). The rate of bleeding complications was reduced by two-thirds and the rate of subacute thrombosis was reduced to one-eighth from the previous rate (to 1.3–1.8% from 10.4%) (92). A study comparing aspirin/warfarin and aspirin/ticlopidine after coronary stent placement, showed a lower incidence of clinical cardiac events and stent occlusion in the aspirin/ticlopidine group than in the aspirin/warfarin group (1.6 vs. 6.2% and 0.8 vs. 5.4% respectively) (93). In conclusion, antiplatelet therapy, as opposed to anticoagulant therapy, has fewer bleeding complications, shorter hospital stay, and lower rates of stent thrombosis and has become the standard of care in the prevention of thromboembolic complications following angioplasty and stenting.

3.7. Combined Antiplatelet Therapy Vs. Antiplatelet Monotherapy

Because of synergistic action, combined antiplatelet therapy has been demonstrated to be superior to monotherapy in stent thrombosis reduction: 1.3–1.8 vs. 10.4% (90). The combination of aspirin plus ticlopidine is associated with a lower rate of stent thrombosis (0.8%) compared with aspirin alone (1.5%) (94,95). In the Stent Antithrombotic Regimen Study, the incidence of myocardial infarction, death, coronary angioplasty, or bypass at 1 month was reduced by 80% in the aspirin/ticlopidine group compared with the aspirin-alone group (91).

The current recommendation for antithrombotic prophylaxis is to administer a combination antiplatelet therapy in the form of aspirin 325 mg PO once daily and clopidogrel 75 mg PO once daily for 3 days prior to the procedure, and heparinization during the procedure to maintain ACT levels beyond 300 s throughout the procedure. Current data do not support the use of GPIIb/IIIa antagonists routinely or long-term anticoagulation (96). The aspirin and clopidogrel regimen described above is also used preferentially in the Carotid Revascularization Endarterectomy vs. Stent Trial (CREST).

4. SHOULD CAROTID ANGIOPLASTY AND STENTING BE PERFORMED WITH CEREBRAL EMBOLIC PROTECTION?

The use of embolic cerebral protection was first introduced by Theron et al. (97), and since then, the use of embolic protection has been considered to be an important advancement in the endovascular treatment of carotid stenosis. The rationale for using such devices is based on the idea that the embolic shower released from the carotid plaque during CAS is responsible for the majority of perioperative neurological deficits after CAS. Up to 29% of patients undergoing CAS without cerebral embolic protection have been reported to have cerebral ischemia detected by diffusion-weighted magnetic resonance (MR) images (98). This number could be substantially reduced (7.1%) with the use of embolic protection devices (99).

Initial studies demonstrating the potential benefit of distal embolic protection have been already published. In a multi-center experiment with 75 patients (100) treated using a balloon device (Percusurge GuardWire, Percusurge Inc., Sunnyvale, CA), no single case of perioperative death or major stroke was noted. Several devices are currently being studied (101–104) and initial reports suggest that they might prove to be a major technical advance in carotid endovascular treatment.

In a recent meta-analysis, Kastrup et al. (105) compared the outcome of 2537 CAS procedures without protection devices in 2357 patients (26 series of patients) with 896 CAS with cerebral protection in 839 patients (11 series of patients), performed between January 1990 and June 2002. Both groups were similar with respect to age, sex, risk factors, and indications for CAS. The combined stroke and death rate within 30 days in both symptomatic and asymptomatic patients was 1.8% in patients treated with protection devices vs. 5.5% in patients treated with CAS without cerebral protection. Since then, Mudra et al. (106) have reported the outcome of 100 CAS procedures, all performed with the use of embolic protection (28 cases with balloon occlusion and 72 cases with filter device). During the procedure, 4% of patients developed a transient ischemic attack (TIA) and 2% had a minor stroke. In 90% of the interventions, debris was collected from the embolic protection device.

Two randomized, controlled trials are evaluating the efficacy of protected carotid angioplasty and stenting: CREST, which is jointly sponsored by the National Institutes of Health and Guidance Corporation (Indianapolis, IN), and the Study of Angioplasty with Protection in Patients at High Risk for Endarterectomy (SAPPHIRE) supported by Cordis Corporation

(Miami Lakes, FL). The SAPPHIRE trial has been discussed earlier in the chapter on stenting for symptomatic carotid stenosis. At the time of this writing, the 1 year outcome results were not published. The 30 day results, however, showed that CAS with emboli protection might be preferable to CEA in patients with significant co-morbid conditions. The current level of evidence on embolic protection devices suggests an important role for these devices during the performance of CAS almost every time the procedure is performed unless the arterial anatomy precludes its safe use.

5. SUMMARY

Carotid angioplasty and stenting particularly when combined with embolic protection devices has emerged as a safe and viable alternative to carotid endarterectomy in patients with certain risk factors including severe coronary artery disease, congestive heart failure, severe chronic obstructive pulmonary disease, contralateral carotid occlusion, post-endarterectomy carotid restenosis, radiation-induced carotid disease, and prior history of radical neck dissection. Whether it has comparable long-term efficacy and durability in high-risk individuals and whether similar results could be extended to all patients with carotid stenosis who require revascularization is controversial at this time, and is being addressed in current clinical trials.

REFERENCES

1. Hanel RA, Xavier AR, Kirmani JF, Yahia AM, Qureshi AI. Management of carotid artery stenosis: comparing endarterectomy and stenting. Curr Cardiol Rep 2003; 5(2):153–159.
2. Phatouros CC, Higashida RT, Malek AM, Meyers PM, Lempert TE, Dowd CF, Halbach VV. Carotid artery stent placement for atherosclerotic disease: rationale, technique, and current status. Radiology 2000; 217(1):26–41.
3. Roubin GS, New G, Iyer SS, Vitek JJ, Al-Mubarak N, Liu MW, Yadav J, Gomez C, Kuntz RE. Immediate and late clinical outcomes of carotid artery stenting in patients with symptomatic and asymptomatic carotid artery stenosis: a 5-year prospective analysis. Circulation 2001; 103(4):532–537.
4. Yadav JS, Roubin GS, Iyer S, Vitek J, King P, Jordan WD, Fisher WS. Elective stenting of the extracranial carotid arteries. Circulation 1997; 95(2): 376–381.
5. Diethrich EB, Ndiaye M, Reid DB. Stenting in the carotid artery: initial experience in 110 patients. J Endovasc Surg 1996; 3(1):42–62.
6. Henry M, Amor M, Masson I, Tzvetanov K, Chati Z, Khanna N. Angioplasty and stenting of the extracranial carotid arteries. J Endovasc Surg 1998; 5(4):293–304.
7. Kerber CW, Cromwell LD, Loehden OL. Catheter dilatation of proximal carotid stenosis during distal bifurcation endarterectomy. Am J Neuroradiol 1980; 1(4):348–349.

8. Mathias K. A new catheter system for percutaneous transluminal angioplasty (PTA) of carotid artery stenoses. Fortschr Med 1977; 95(15):1007–1011.
9. Mullan S, Duda EE, Patronas NJ. Some examples of balloon technology in neurosurgery. J Neurosurg 1980; 52(3):321–329.
10. Vitek JJ, Morawetz RB. Percutaneous transluminal angioplasty of the external carotid artery: preliminary report. Am J Neuroradiol 1982; 3(5):541–546.
11. Freitag G, Freitag J, Koch RD, Wagemann W. Percutaneous angioplasty of carotid artery stenoses. Neuroradiology 1986; 28(2):126–127.
12. Tsai FY, Matovich V, Hieshima G, Shah DC, Mehringer CM, Tiu G, Higashida R, Pribram HF. Percutaneous transluminal angioplasty of the carotid artery. Am J Neuroradiol 1986; 7(2):349–358.
13. Brown MM, Butler P, Gibbs J, Swash M, Waterston J. Feasibility of percutaneous transluminal angioplasty for carotid artery stenosis. J Neurol Neurosurg Psychiatr 1990; 53(3):238–243.
14. Eckert B, Zanella F, Thie A, Steinmetz J, Zeumer H. Angioplasty of the internal carotid artery: results, complications and follow-up in 61 cases. Cerebrovasc Dis 1996; 6:97–105.
15. Gil-Peralta A, Mayol A, Marcos JR, Gonzalez A, Ruano J, Boza F, Duran F. Percutaneous transluminal angioplasty of the symptomatic atherosclerotic carotid arteries. Results, complications, and follow-up. Stroke 1996; 27(12): 2271–2273.
16. Wholey MH, Wholey M, Bergeron P, Diethrich EB, Henry M, Laborde JC, Mathias K, Myla S, Roubin GS, Shawl F, Theron JG, Yadav JS, Dorros G, Guimaraens J, Higashida R, Kumar V, Leon M, Lim M, Londero H, Mesa J, Ramee S, Rodriguez A, Rosenfield K, Teitelbaum G, Vozzi C. Current global status of carotid artery stent placement. Cathet Cardiovasc Diagn 1998; 44(1):1–6.
17. Yadav JS, Wholey MH, Kuntz RE, Fayad P, Katzen BT, Mishkel GJ, Bajwa TK, Whitlow P, Strickman NE, Jaff MR, Popma JJ, Snead DB, Cutlip DE, Firth BG, Ouriel K. Protected carotid-artery stenting versus endarterectomy in high-risk patients. N Engl J Med 2004; 351(15):1493–1501.
18. Harbaugh RE, Stieg PE, Moayeri N, Hsu L. Carotid-coronary artery bypass graft conundrum. Neurosurgery 1998; 43(4):926–931.
19. Ringer A, Lanzino G, Fessler R, Qureshi A, Guterman L, Hopkins L. Carotid angioplasty and stenting. In: Whittemore A, Bandyk D, Cronenwett J, Hertzer N, White R, eds. Advances in Vascular Surgery. Vol. 9. St. Louis, MO: Mosby, 2001.
20. Paciaroni M, Eliasziw M, Kappelle LJ, Finan JW, Ferguson GG, Barnett HJ. Medical complications associated with carotid endarterectomy. North American Symptomatic Carotid Endarterectomy Trial (NASCET). Stroke 1999; 30(9):1759–1763.
21. Goldstein LB, Samsa GP, Matchar DB, Oddone EZ. Multicenter review of preoperative risk factors for endarterectomy for asymptomatic carotid artery stenosis. Stroke 1998; 29(4):750–753.
22. Moore WS, Barnett HJ, Beebe HG, Bernstein EF, Brener BJ, Brott T, Caplan LR, Day A, Goldstone J, Hobson RW, 2nd, et al. Guidelines for carotid

endarterectomy. A multidisciplinary consensus statement from the ad hoc Committee, American Heart Association. Stroke 1995; 26(1):188–201.

23. Goldstein LB, McCrory DC, Landsman PB, Samsa GP, Ancukiewicz M, Oddone EZ, Matchar DB. Multicenter review of preoperative risk factors for carotid endarterectomy in patients with ipsilateral symptoms. Stroke 1994; 25(6):1116–1121.

24. Lopes DK, Mericle RA, Lanzino G, Wakhloo AK, Guterman LR, Hopkins LN. Stent placement for the treatment of occlusive atherosclerotic carotid artery disease in patients with concomitant coronary artery disease. J Neurosurg 2002; 96(3):490–496.

25. Waigand J, Gross CM, Uhlich F, Kramer J, Tamaschke C, Vogel P, Luft FC, Dietz R. Elective stenting of carotid artery stenosis in patients with severe coronary artery disease. Eur Heart J 1998; 19(9):1365–1370.

26. Thomas M, Otis SM, Rush M, Zyroff J, Dilley RB, Bernstein EF. Recurrent carotid artery stenosis following endarterectomy. Ann Surg 1984; 200(1): 74–79.

27. Meyer FB, Piepgras DG, Fode NC. Surgical treatment of recurrent carotid artery stenosis. J Neurosurg 1994; 80(5):781–787.

28. AbuRahma AF, Jennings TG, Wulu JT, Tarakji L, Robinson PA. Redo carotid endarterectomy versus primary carotid endarterectomy. Stroke 2001; 32(12):2787–2792.

29. Yadav JS, Roubin GS, King P, Iyer S, Vitek J. Angioplasty and stenting for restenosis after carotid endarterectomy. Initial experience. Stroke 1996; 27(11):2075–2079.

30. Lanzino G, Mericle RA, Lopes DK, Wakhloo AK, Guterman LR, Hopkins LN. Percutaneous transluminal angioplasty and stent placement for recurrent carotid artery stenosis. J Neurosurg 1999; 90(4):688–694.

31. Gasecki AP, Eliasziw M, Ferguson GG, Hachinski V, Barnett HJ. Long-term prognosis and effect of endarterectomy in patients with symptomatic severe carotid stenosis and contralateral carotid stenosis or occlusion: results from NASCET. North American Symptomatic Carotid Endarterectomy Trial (NASCET) Group. J Neurosurg 1995; 83(5):778–782.

32. Beneficial effect of carotid endarterectomy in symptomatic patients with high-grade carotid stenosis. North American Symptomatic Carotid Endarterectomy Trial Collaborators. N Engl J Med 1991; 325(7):445–453.

33. Mathur A, Roubin GS, Gomez CR, Iyer SS, Wong PM, Piamsomboon C, Yadav SS, Dean LS, Vitek JJ. Elective carotid artery stenting in the presence of contralateral occlusion. Am J Cardiol 1998; 81(11):1315–1317.

34. Kim S, Mericle R, Lanzino G, Qureshi A, Guterman L, Hopkins L. Carotid angioplasty and stent placement in patients with tandem stenosis. Neurosurgery 1998; 43:708A.

35. Loftus CM, Biller J, Hart MN, Cornell SH, Hiratzka LF. Management of radiation-induced accelerated carotid atherosclerosis. Arch Neurol 1987; 44(7): 711–714.

36. Melliere D, Becquemin JP, Berrahal D, Desgranges P, Cavillon A. Management of radiation-induced occlusive arterial disease: a reassessment. J Cardiovasc Surg (Torino) 1997; 38(3):261–269.

37. Al-Mubarak N, Roubin GS, Iyer SS, Gomez CR, Liu MW, Vitek JJ. Carotid stenting for severe radiation-induced extracranial carotid artery occlusive disease. J Endovasc Ther 2000; 7(1):36–40.
38. Parsons TJ, Haycraft DL, Hoak JC, Sage H. Interaction of platelets and purified collagens in a laminar flow model. Thromb Res 1986; 43(4): 435–443.
39. Hynes RO. Integrins: a family of cell surface receptors. Cell 1987; 48(4): 549–554.
40. Lefkovits J, Plow EF, Topol EJ. Platelet glycoprotein IIb/IIIa receptors in cardiovascular medicine. N Engl J Med 1995; 332(23):1553–1559.
41. Fuster V, Jang IK. Role of platelet-inhibitor agents in coronary artery disease. In: Topol EJ, ed. Textbook of Interventional Cardiology. 2nd ed. Philadelphia: WB Saunders Co., 1994:3–22.
42. Barry WL, Sarembock IJ. Antiplatelet and anticoagulant therapy in patients undergoing percutaneous transluminal coronary angioplasty. Cardiol Clin 1994; 12(3):517–535.
43. Lijnen HR, Collen D. Fibrinolytic agents: mechanisms of activity and pharmacology. Thromb Haemost 1995; 74(1):387–390.
44. Granger CB, Califf RM, Topol EJ. Thrombolytic therapy for acute myocardial infarction. A review. Drugs 1992; 44(3):293–325.
45. Booth NA. The natural inhibitors of fibrinolysis. In: Bloom AL, Forbes CD, Thomas DP, Tuddenham EGD, eds. Haemostasis and Thrombosis. 3rd ed. Edinburgh: Churchill Livingstone, 1994:669–717.
46. Ghigliotti G, Waissbluth AR, Speidel C, Abendschein DR, Eisenberg PR. Prolonged activation of prothrombin on the vascular wall after arterial injury. Arterioscler Thromb Vasc Biol 1998; 18(2):250–257.
47. More RS, Rutty G, Underwood MJ, Brack MJ, Gershlick AH. A time sequence of vessel wall changes in an experimental model of angioplasty. J Pathol 1994; 172(3):287–292.
48. Ferns GA, Stewart-Lee AL, Anggard EE. Arterial response to mechanical injury: balloon catheter de-endothelialization. Atherosclerosis 1992; 92(2–3): 89–104.
49. Van Belle E, Tio FO, Chen D, Maillard L, Kearney M, Isner JM. Passivation of metallic stents after arterial gene transfer of phVEGF165 inhibits thrombus formation and intimal thickening. J Am Coll Cardiol 1997; 29(6):1371–1379.
50. Roth GJ, Stanford N, Majerus PW, Acetylation of prostaglandin synthase by aspirin. Proceedings of the National Academy Sciences of the United States of America. 1975; 72(8):3073–3076.
51. Theroux P. Antiplatelet therapy: do the new platelet inhibitors add significantly to the clinical benefits of aspirin? Am Heart J 1997; 134(5 Pt 2):S62–S70.
52. Patrignani P, Filabozzi P, Patrono C. Selective cumulative inhibition of platelet thromboxane production by low-dose aspirin in healthy subjects. J Clin Invest 1982; 69(6):1366–1372.
53. Antiplatelet Trialists' Collaboration. Collaborative overview of randomised trials of antiplatelet therapy—II: maintenance of vascular graft or arterial patency by antiplatelet therapy. Br Med J 1994; 308(6922):159–168.

54. Coukell AJ, Markham A. Clopidogrel. Drugs 1997; 54(5):745–750; discussion 751.
55. Harker LA, Bruno JJ. Ticlopidine's mechanism of action on platelets. In: Hass WK, Easton JD, eds. Ticlopidine, Platelets and Vascular Diseases. New York: Springer-Verlag, 1993:41–59.
56. Claeys MJ, Van Der Planken MG, Michiels JJ, Vertessen F, Dilling D, Bosmans JM, Vrints CJ. Comparison of antiplatelet effect of loading dose of clopidogrel versus abciximab during coronary intervention. Blood Coag Fibrinol 2002; 13(4):283–288.
57. Sharis PJ, Cannon CP, Loscalzo J. The antiplatelet effects of ticlopidine and clopidogrel. Ann Intern Med 1998; 129(5):394–405.
58. Kereiakes DJ, Lincoff AM, Miller DP, Tcheng JE, Cabot CF, Anderson KM, Weisman HF, Califf RM, Topol EJ. Abciximab therapy and unplanned coronary stent deployment: favorable effects on stent use, clinical outcomes, and bleeding complications. EPILOG Trial Investigators. Circulation 1998; 97(9): 857–864.
59. Cox D, Aoki T, Seki J, Motoyama Y, Yoshida K. The pharmacology of the integrins. Med Res Rev 1994; 14(2):195–228.
60. Coller BS, Scudder LE, Beer J, Gold HK, Folts JD, Cavagnaro J, Jordan R, Wagner C, Iuliucci J, Knight D. Monoclonal antibodies to platelet glycoprotein IIb/IIIa as antithrombotic agents. Ann NY Acad Sci 1991; 614:193–213.
61. Use of a monoclonal antibody directed against the platelet glycoprotein IIb/IIIa receptor in high-risk coronary angioplasty. The EPIC Investigation. N Engl J Med 1994; 330(14):956–961.
62. Vorchheimer DA, Badimon JJ, Fuster V. Platelet glycoprotein IIb/IIIa receptor antagonists in cardiovascular disease. JAMA 1999; 281(15):1407–1414.
63. Platelet glycoprotein IIb/IIIa receptor blockade and low-dose heparin during percutaneous coronary revascularization. The EPILOG Investigators. N Engl J Med 1997; 336(24):1689–1696.
64. Randomised placebo-controlled trial of abciximab before and during coronary intervention in refractory unstable angina: the CAPTURE Study. Lancet 1997; 349(9063):1429–1435.
65. Brener SJ, Barr LA, Burchenal JE, Katz S, George BS, Jones AA, Cohen ED, Gainey PC, White HJ, Cheek HB, Moses JW, Moliterno DJ, Effron MB, Topol EJ. Randomised, placebo-controlled trial of platelet glycoprotein IIb/IIIa blockade with primary angioplasty for acute myocardial infarction. ReoPro and Primary PTCA Organization and Randomised Trial (RAPPORT) Investigators. Circulation 1998; 98(8):734–741.
66. Randomised placebo-controlled and balloon-angioplasty-controlled trial to assess safety of coronary stenting with use of platelet glycoprotein-IIb/IIIa blockade. The EPISTENT Investigators. Evaluation of platelet IIb/IIIa inhibitor for stenting. Lancet 1998; 352(9122):87–92.
67. Randomised placebo-controlled trial of effect of eptifibatide on complications of percutaneous coronary intervention: IMPACT-II. Integrilin to minimise platelet aggregation and coronary thrombosis-II. Lancet 1997; 349(9063): 1422–1428.

68. Effects of platelet glycoprotein IIb/IIIa blockade with tirofiban on adverse cardiac events in patients with unstable angina or acute myocardial infarction undergoing coronary angioplasty. The RESTORE Investigators. Randomised Efficacy Study of Tirofiban for Outcomes and REstenosis. Circulation 1997; 96(5):1445–1453.

69. Qureshi AI, Suri MF, Khan J, Fessler RD, Guterman LR, Hopkins LN. Abciximab as an adjunct to high-risk carotid or vertebrobasilar angioplasty: preliminary experience. Neurosurgery 2000; 46(6):1316–1324.

70. Qureshi AI, Suri MF, Ali Z, Kim SH, Lanzino G, Fessler RD, Ringer AJ, Guterman LR, Hopkins LN. Carotid angioplasty and stent placement: a prospective analysis of perioperative complications and impact of intravenously administered abciximab. Neurosurgery 2002; 50(3):466–473.

71. Qureshi AI, Ali Z, Suri MF, Kim SH, Fessler RD, Ringer AJ, Guterman LR, Hopkins LN. Open-label phase I clinical study to assess the safety of intravenous eptifibatide in patients undergoing internal carotid artery angioplasty and stent placement. Neurosurgery 2001; 48(5):998–1004.

72. Hirsh J. Heparin. N Engl J Med 1991; 324(22):1565–1574.

73. Bell WR, Tomasulo PA, Alving BM, Duffy TP. Thrombocytopenia occurring during the administration of heparin. A prospective study in 52 patients. Ann Intern Med 1976; 85(2):155–160.

74. Kelton JG, Sheridan D, Brain H, Powers PJ, Turpie AG, Carter CJ. Clinical usefulness of testing for a heparin-dependent platelet-aggregating factor in patients with suspected heparin-associated thrombocytopenia. J Lab Clin Med 1984; 103(4):606–612.

75. Narins CR, Hillegass WB Jr, Nelson CL, Tcheng JE, Harrington RA, Phillips HR, Stack RS, Califf RM. Relation between activated clotting time during angioplasty and abrupt closure. Circulation 1996; 93(4):667–671.

76. Bittl JA, Ahmed WH. Relation between abrupt vessel closure and the anticoagulant response to heparin or bivalirudin during coronary angioplasty. Am J Cardiol 1998; 82(8B):50P–56P.

77. Ellis SG, Roubin GS, Wilentz J, Douglas JS Jr, King SB 3rd. Effect of 18- to 24-hour heparin administration for prevention of restenosis after uncomplicated coronary angioplasty. Am Heart J 1989; 117(4):777–782.

78. Friedman HZ, Cragg DR, Glazier SM, Gangadharan V, Marsalese DL, Schreiber TL, O'Neill WW. Randomised prospective evaluation of prolonged versus abbreviated intravenous heparin therapy after coronary angioplasty. J Am Coll Cardiol 1994; 24(5):1214–1219.

79. Lincoff AM, Tcheng JE, Califf RM, Bass T, Popma JJ, Teirstein PS, Kleiman NS, Hattel LJ, Anderson HV, Ferguson JJ, Cabot CF, Anderson KM, Berdan LG, Musco MH, Weisman HF, Topol EJ. Standard versus low-dose weight-adjusted heparin in patients treated with the platelet glycoprotein IIb/IIIa receptor antibody fragment abciximab (c7E3 Fab) during percutaneous coronary revascularization. PROLOG Investigators. Am J Cardiol 1997; 79(3):286–291.

80. Weitz JI. Low-molecular-weight heparins. N Engl J Med 1997; 337(10):688–698.

81. Cade JF, Buchanan MR, Boneu B, Ockelford P, Cater CJ, Cerskus AL, Hirsh J. A comparison of the antithrombotic and haemorrhagic effects of low molecular weight heparin fractions: the influence of the method of preparation. Thromb Res 1984; 35(6):613–625.

82. Warkentin TE, Levine MN, Hirsh J, Horsewood P, Roberts RS, Gent M, Kelton JG. Heparin-induced thrombocytopenia in patients treated with low-molecular-weight heparin or unfractionated heparin. N Engl J Med 1995; 332(20):1330–1335.

83. Berger PB, Mahaffey KW, Meier SJ, Buller CE, Batchelor W, Fry ET, Zidar JP, The AI. Safety and efficacy of only 2 weeks of ticlopidine therapy in patients at increased risk of coronary stent thrombosis: results from the Antiplatelet Therapy alone versus Lovenox plus Antiplatelet therapy in patients at increased risk of Stent Thrombosis (ATLAST) trial. Am Heart J 2002; 143(5):841–846.

84. Mirshahi M, Soria J, Soria C, Faivre R, Lu H, Courtney M, Roitsch C, Tripier D, Caen JP. Evaluation of the inhibition by heparin and hirudin of coagulation activation during r-tPA-induced thrombolysis. Blood 1989; 74(3):1025–1030.

85. Cannon CP, Braunwald E. Hirudin: initial results in acute myocardial infarction, unstable angina and angioplasty. J Am Coll Cardiol 1995; 25(Suppl 7): 30S–37S.

86. Lidon RM, Theroux P, Lesperance J, Adelman B, Bonan R, Duval D, Levesque J. A pilot, early angiographic patency study using a direct thrombin inhibitor as adjunctive therapy to streptokinase in acute myocardial infarction. Circulation 1994; 89(4):1567–1572.

87. Topol EJ, Bonan R, Jewitt D, Sigwart U, Kakkar VV, Rothman M, de Bono D, Ferguson J, Willerson JT, Strony J. Use of a direct antithrombin, hirulog, in place of heparin during coronary angioplasty. Circulation 1993; 87(5): 1622–1629.

88. Lincoff AM, Kleiman NS, Kottke-Marchant K, Maierson ES, Maresh K, Wolski KE, Topol EJ. Bivalirudin with planned or provisional abciximab versus low-dose heparin and abciximab during percutaneous coronary revascularization: results of the Comparison of Abciximab Complications with Hirulog for Ischemic Events Trial (CACHET). Am Heart J 2002; 143(5):847–853.

89. Lincoff AM, Bittl JA, Harrington RA, Feit F, Kleiman NS, Jackman JD, Sarembock IJ, Cohen Dj, Spriggs D, Ebrahimi R, Keren G, Carr J, Cohen EA, Betriu A, Desmet W, Kereiakes DJ, Rutsch W, Wilcox RG, de Feyter PJ, Vahanian A, Topol EJ, Investigators R-. Bivalirudin and provisional glycoprotein IIb/IIIa blockade compared with heparin and planned glycoprotein IIb/IIIa blockade during percutaneous coronary intervention: REPLACE-2 randomized trial. JAMA 2003; 289(7):853–863.

90. Karrillon GJ, Morice MC, Benveniste E, Bunouf P, Aubry P, Cattan S, Chevalier B, Commeau P, Criber A, Eifeman C, Grollier G, Guerin Y, Henry M, Lefevre T, Livarek B, Louvard Y, Marco J, Makowski S, Monassier JP, Pernes JM, Rioux P, Spaulding C, Zemour G. Intracoronary stent implantation without ultrasound guidance and with replacement of conventional anticoagulation by antiplatelet therapy. 30-day clinical outcome of the French Multicenter Registry. Circulation 1996; 94(7):1519–1527.

91. Zidar JP. Rationale for low-molecular weight heparin in coronary stenting. Am Heart J 1997; 134(5 Pt 2):S81–S87.

92. Jordan C, Carvalho H, Fajadet J, Cassagneau B, Robert G, Marco J, Pasteur C. Reduction of subacute thrombosis rate after coronary stenting using a new anticoagulant protocol. Circulation 1994; 90(Suppl I):124 (abstract).

93. Schomig A, Neumann FJ, Kastrati A, Schuhlen H, Blasini R, Hadamitzky M, Walter H, Zitzmann-Roth EM, Richardt G, Alt E, Schmitt C, Ulm K. A randomised comparison of antiplatelet and anticoagulant therapy after the placement of coronary-artery stents. N Engl J Med 1996; 334(17):1084–1089.

94. Hall P, Nakamura S, Maiello L, Itoh A, Blengino S, Martini G, Ferraro M, Colombo A. A randomized comparison of combined ticlopidine and aspirin therapy versus aspirin therapy alone after successful intravascular ultrasound-guided stent implantation. Circulation 1996; 93(2):215–222.

95. Goods CM, al-Shaibi KF, Liu MW, Yadav JS, Mathur A, Jain SP, Dean LS, Iyer SS, Parks JM, Roubin GS. Comparison of aspirin alone versus aspirin plus ticlopidine after coronary artery stenting. Am J Cardiol 1996; 78(9): 1042–1044.

96. Qureshi AI. Editorial comment—Thromboembolic events during neuroendovascular procedures. Stroke 2003; 34(7):1728–1729.

97. Theron J, Raymond J, Casasco A, Courtheoux F. Percutaneous angioplasty of atherosclerotic and postsurgical stenosis of carotid arteries. Am J Neuroradiol 1987; 8(3):495–500.

98. Jaeger HJ, Mathias KD, Hauth E, Drescher R, Gissler HM, Hennigs S, Christmann A. Cerebral ischemia detected with diffusion-weighted MR imaging after stent implantation in the carotid artery. Am J Neuroradiol 2002; 23(2):200–207.

99. Mathias K. A vast single center experience from Europe: immediate and late outcome in > 1400 patients. Paper presented at: Trans Catheter Therapeutics, 2002, Washington, DC.

100. Whitlow PL, Lylyk P, Londero H, Mendiz OA, Mathias K, Jaeger H, Parodi J, Schonholz C, Milei J. Carotid artery stenting protected with an emboli containment system. Stroke 2002; 33(5):1308–1314.

101. Parodi JC, La Mura R, Ferreira LM, Mendez MV, Cersosimo H, Schonholz C, Garelli G. Initial evaluation of carotid angioplasty and stenting with three different cerebral protection devices. J Vasc Surg 2000; 32(6):1127–1136.

102. Al-Mubarak N, Roubin GS, Vitek JJ, Iyer SS, New G, Leon MB. Effect of the distal-balloon protection system on microembolization during carotid stenting. Circulation 2001; 104(17):1999–2002.

103. Reimers B, Corvaja N, Moshiri S, Sacca S, Albiero R, Di Mario C, Pascotto P, Colombo A. Cerebral protection with filter devices during carotid artery stenting. Circulation 2001; 104(1):12–15.

104. Ohki T, Veith FJ, Grenell S, Lipsitz EC, Gargiulo N, McKay J, Valladares J, Suggs WD, Kazmi M. Initial experience with cerebral protection devices to prevent embolization during carotid artery stenting. J Vasc Surg 2002; 36(6):1175–1185.

105. Kastrup A, Groschel K, Krapf H, Brehm BR, Dichgans J, Schulz JB. Early outcome of carotid angioplasty and stenting with and without cerebral

protection devices: a systematic review of the literature. Stroke 2003; 34(3): 813–819.

106. Mudra H, Ziegler M, Haufe MC, Hug M, Knape A, Meurer A, Pitzl H, Buchele W, Spes C. Percutaneous carotid angioplasty with stent implantation and protection device against embolism—a prospective study of 100 consecutive cases. Dtsch Med Wochenschr 2003; 128(15):790–796.

Index

[Recurrent carotid stenosis]
  neo-intimal hyperplasia, 269
  serial surveillance, 268
  serial ultrasound imaging, 268
Recurrent cerebral ischemic events, 279
Recurrent ischemic stroke, 277, 278, 279
Recurrent stroke, 155
Red meat, 176
RDA. *See* Recommended daily
  allowance.
Remodeling, possible mechanisms of, 93
Restenosis, surveillance and
  management of, 268–270
Risk factors, 12–14
  associated with stroke, 21
  cholesterol, 13
  population studies, 12
    age, 13
    gene–environment interaction, 13
    male sex, 13
  risk analysis, 13
  systolic hypertension, 13
  cigarette smoking, 13
Risk models, 6
Risk of CEA, 197–203
  age, 201, 202
  degree of ill health, 201
  old patients, 201
  perioperative death, 202
  for asymptomatic stenosis, 199, 200
  in ACAS trial, 200
  depends on type of symptom, 200
  lower operative mortality, 200
  related to sex, 200–201
  case-fatality score, 201
  in ECST, 200–201
  patch graft in women, 201
  in women, 201
  for symptomatic stenosis, 197–199
  in ECST, 197–199
  fatal stroke, 198
  in NASCET, 198, 199
  neck hematoma, 198
  non-fatal myocardial infarctions, 198
  nonfatal strokes, 197
  unstable angina, 198
  time, 202, 203

[Risk of CEA]
  clinical guidelines, 203
  delay in CEA, 202
  from ECST and NASCET data, 202
  for evolving symptoms, 202
  for stable symptoms, 202
  in TIA or non disablingstroke, 202
Role for perioperative monitoring,
  265–268
  blood flow threshold, 266
  completion angioscopy, 267
  intimal flaps, 266
  middle cerebral artery velocities, 267
  neurological deficit, 266
  neuronal electrical activity, 266
  perioperative monitoring, role of, 267
  quality control techniques, 266
  angiography, 266
  angioscopy, 266
  retained luminal thrombus, 266
  transcranial Doppler monitoring, 267
  transcranial Doppler ultrasound, 266
Role of cerebral protection devices,
  297, 298
  anti-embolism system, 297
  cerebral blood flow, 298
  distal protection devices, 297
  embolic debris, 297
  temporary cerebral protection, 297
RTKs. *See* Receptor tyrosine kinases.

S-adenosyl homocysteine, 160
S-adenosyl methionine, 162
SAH. *See* S-adenosyl homocysteine.
SALT. *See* Swedish aspirin
  low dose trial.
SAM. *See* S-adenosylmethionine.
Sample size calculations, 299
SEARCH. *See* Study of the effectiveness
  of additional reductions in
  cholesterol and homocysteine.
Severity/stage of the illness, 249
Shunt and patch usage, 245
Shunt deployment, 257–260
  cerebral perfusion, 257
  Circle of Willis, 257

Milton Keynes UK
Ingram Content Group UK Ltd.
UKHW020016071024
449327UK00031B/2804